D0989996

Pathways to Quality Health Care

MEDICARE'S QUALITY IMPROVEMENT ORGANIZATION PROGRAM

Maximizing Potential

Committee on Redesigning Health Insurance Performance Measures, Payment, and Performance Improvement Programs

Board on Health Care Services

INSTITUTE OF MEDICINE
OF THE NATIONAL ACADEMIES

THE NATIONAL ACADEMIES PRESS
Washington, D.C.
www.nap.edu

THE NATIONAL ACADEMIES PRESS   500 Fifth Street, N.W.   Washington, DC 20001

NOTICE: The project that is the subject of this report was approved by the Governing Board of the National Research Council, whose members are drawn from the councils of the National Academy of Sciences, the National Academy of Engineering, and the Institute of Medicine. The members of the committee responsible for the report were chosen for their special competences and with regard for appropriate balance.

This study was supported by Contract No. HHSM-500-2004-00010C between the National Academy of Sciences and the United States Department of Health and Human Services through the Centers for Medicare and Medicaid Services. Any opinions, findings, conclusions, or recommendations expressed in this publication are those of the author(s) and do not necessarily reflect the view of the organizations or agencies that provided support for this project.

Library of Congress Cataloging-in-Publication Data

Medicare's quality improvement organization program : maximizing potential / Committee on Redesigning Health Insurance Performance Measures, Payment, and Performance Improvement Programs, Board on Health Care Services.
    p. ; cm. — (Pathways to quality health care)
    "This study was supported by Contract No. HHSM-500-2004-00010C between the National Academy of Sciences and the United States Department of Health and Human Services through the Centers for Medicare and Medicaid Services"—T.p. verso.
    Includes bibliographical references and index.
    ISBN 0-309-10108-5 (hardback)
    1. Medicare—Quality control. 2. Medical care—United States—Quality control. 3. Health care reform—United States. I. Institute of Medicine (U.S.). Committee on Redesigning Health Insurance Performance Measures, Payment, and Performance Improvement Programs.
II. Series.
    [DNLM: 1. Medicare—organization & administration. 2. Quality Assurance, Health Care—organization & administration—United States. 3. Health Care Reform—organization & administration—United States. 4. Quality of Health Care—organization & administration—United States. WT 31 M4898 2006]
    RA412.3.M449 2006
    368.4'260068—dc22
                                  2006014099

Additional copies of this report are available from the National Academies Press, 500 Fifth Street, N.W., Lockbox 285, Washington, DC 20055; (800) 624-6242 or (202) 334-3313 (in the Washington metropolitan area); Internet, http://www.nap.edu.

For more information about the Institute of Medicine, visit the IOM home page at: www.iom.edu.

Copyright 2006 by the National Academy of Sciences. All rights reserved.

Printed in the United States of America.

The serpent has been a symbol of long life, healing, and knowledge among almost all cultures and religions since the beginning of recorded history. The serpent adopted as a logotype by the Institute of Medicine is a relief carving from ancient Greece, now held by the Staatliche Museen in Berlin.

FLORIDA GULF COAST
UNIVERSITY LIBRARY

"Knowing is not enough; we must apply.
Willing is not enough; we must do."
—Goethe

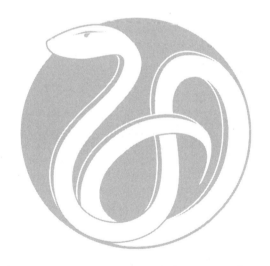

INSTITUTE OF MEDICINE
OF THE NATIONAL ACADEMIES

Advising the Nation. Improving Health.

THE NATIONAL ACADEMIES
Advisers to the Nation on Science, Engineering, and Medicine

The **National Academy of Sciences** is a private, nonprofit, self-perpetuating society of distinguished scholars engaged in scientific and engineering research, dedicated to the furtherance of science and technology and to their use for the general welfare. Upon the authority of the charter granted to it by the Congress in 1863, the Academy has a mandate that requires it to advise the federal government on scientific and technical matters. Dr. Ralph J. Cicerone is president of the National Academy of Sciences.

The **National Academy of Engineering** was established in 1964, under the charter of the National Academy of Sciences, as a parallel organization of outstanding engineers. It is autonomous in its administration and in the selection of its members, sharing with the National Academy of Sciences the responsibility for advising the federal government. The National Academy of Engineering also sponsors engineering programs aimed at meeting national needs, encourages education and research, and recognizes the superior achievements of engineers. Dr. Wm. A. Wulf is president of the National Academy of Engineering.

The **Institute of Medicine** was established in 1970 by the National Academy of Sciences to secure the services of eminent members of appropriate professions in the examination of policy matters pertaining to the health of the public. The Institute acts under the responsibility given to the National Academy of Sciences by its congressional charter to be an adviser to the federal government and, upon its own initiative, to identify issues of medical care, research, and education. Dr. Harvey V. Fineberg is president of the Institute of Medicine.

The **National Research Council** was organized by the National Academy of Sciences in 1916 to associate the broad community of science and technology with the Academy's purposes of furthering knowledge and advising the federal government. Functioning in accordance with general policies determined by the Academy, the Council has become the principal operating agency of both the National Academy of Sciences and the National Academy of Engineering in providing services to the government, the public, and the scientific and engineering communities. The Council is administered jointly by both Academies and the Institute of Medicine. Dr. Ralph J. Cicerone and Dr. Wm. A. Wulf are chair and vice chair, respectively, of the National Research Council.

www.national-academies.org

COMMITTEE ON REDESIGNING HEALTH INSURANCE PERFORMANCE MEASURES, PAYMENT, AND PERFORMANCE IMPROVEMENT PROGRAMS

STEVEN A. SCHROEDER (*Chair*), Distinguished Professor of Health and Health Care, University of California, San Francisco

BOBBIE BERKOWITZ, Alumni Endowed Professor of Nursing, Psychosocial and Community Health, University of Washington, Seattle

DONALD M. BERWICK, President and Chief Executive Officer, Institute for Healthcare Improvement, Cambridge, MA

BRUCE E. BRADLEY, Director, Health Care Strategy and Public Policy, Health Care Initiatives, General Motors Corporation, Pontiac, MI

JANET M. CORRIGAN,[1] President and Chief Executive Officer, National Committee for Quality Health Care, Washington, DC

KAREN DAVIS, President, The Commonwealth Fund, New York

NANCY-ANN MIN DePARLE, Senior Advisor, JPMorgan Partners, LLC, Washington, DC

ELLIOTT S. FISHER, Professor of Medicine and Community Family Medicine, Dartmouth Medical School, Hanover, NH

RICHARD G. FRANK, Margaret T. Morris Professor of Health Economics, Harvard Medical School, Boston, MA

ROBERT S. GALVIN, Director, Global Health Care, General Electric Company, Fairfield, CT

DAVID H. GUSTAFSON, Research Professor of Industrial Engineering, University of Wisconsin, Madison

MARY ANNE KODA-KIMBLE, Professor and Dean, School of Pharmacy, University of California, San Francisco

ALAN R. NELSON, Special Advisor to the Executive Vice President, American College of Physicians, Fairfax, VA

NORMAN C. PAYSON, President, NCP, Inc., Concord, NH

WILLIAM A. PECK, Director, Center for Health Policy, Washington University School of Medicine, St. Louis, MO

NEIL R. POWE, Professor of Medicine, Epidemiology and Health Policy, The Johns Hopkins University School of Medicine and Johns Hopkins Bloomberg School of Public Health, Baltimore, MD

CHRISTOPHER QUERAM, President and Chief Executive Officer, Wisconsin Collaborative for Healthcare Quality, Madison

ROBERT D. REISCHAUER, President, The Urban Institute, Washington, DC

---

[1]Appointed to the committee beginning June 1, 2005.

WILLIAM C. RICHARDSON, President Emeritus, The Johns Hopkins University and W.K. Kellogg Foundation, Hickory Corners, MI
CHERYL M. SCOTT, President Emerita, Group Health Cooperative, Seattle, WA
STEPHEN M. SHORTELL, Blue Cross of California Distinguished Professor of Health Policy and Management and Dean, School of Public Health, University of California, Berkeley
SAMUEL O. THIER, Professor of Medicine and Professor of Health Care Policy, Harvard Medical School, Massachusetts General Hospital, Boston
GAIL R. WILENSKY, Senior Fellow, Project HOPE, Bethesda, MD

Study Staff

JANET CORRIGAN,[2] Project Director
ROSEMARY A. CHALK,[3] Project Director
KAREN ADAMS,[4] Senior Program Officer, Lead Staff for the Subcommittee on Performance Measurement Evaluation
DIANNE MILLER WOLMAN, Senior Program Officer, Lead Staff on Quality Improvement Organization Program Evaluation
CONTESSA FINCHER,[5] Program Officer
TRACY A. HARRIS, Program Officer
SAMANTHA M. CHAO, Senior Health Policy Associate
DANITZA VALDIVIA, Program Associate
MICHELLE BAZEMORE, Senior Program Assistant

---

[2]Served through May 2005.
[3]Served beginning May 2005.
[4]Served through February 2006.
[5]Served through July 2005.

Reviewers

This report has been reviewed in draft form by individuals chosen for their diverse perspectives and technical expertise, in accordance with procedures approved by the National Research Council's Report Review Committee. The purpose of this independent review is to provide candid and critical comments that will assist the institution in making its published report as sound as possible and to ensure that the report meets institutional standards for objectivity, evidence, and responsiveness to the study charge. The review comments and draft manuscript remain confidential to protect the integrity of the deliberative process. We wish to thank the following individuals for their review of this report:

BRUCE BAGLEY, Medical Director for Quality Improvement, American Academy of Family Physicians, Leawood, KS

LAWRENCE P. CASALINO, Assistant Professor, University of Chicago, Department of Health Studies, Chicago, IL

BARBARA B. FLEMING, Chief, Office of Quality and Performance, Veterans Health Administration, Washington, DC

MARY ANNE KEHOE, Chief Operating Officer, Lincoln Lutheran Home, Racine, WI

PETER V. LEE, President and Chief Executive Officer, Pacific Business Group on Health, San Francisco, CA

RICARDO MARTINEZ, Executive Vice President of Medical Affairs, The Schumacher Group, Kennesaw, GA

MYLES MAXFIELD, Associate Director of Health Research, Mathematica Policy Research, Inc., Washington, DC

ELIZABETH A. MCGLYNN, Associate Director, Center for Research on Quality Health Care, RAND Corporation, Santa Monica, CA

DON NIELSEN, Senior Vice President for Quality Leadership, American Hospital Association, Washington, DC

L. GREGORY PAWLSON, Executive Vice President, National Committee for Quality Assurance, Washington, DC

MICHAEL ROBBINS-ROTHMAN, Senior Consultant, Clinical Systems Improvement, University of Mississippi Medical Center, Jackson

TIMOTHY SIZE, Executive Director, Rural Wisconsin Health Cooperative, Sauk City

ANDREW WEBBER, President and Chief Executive Officer, National Business Coalition on Health, Washington, DC

ALAN ZASLAVSKY, Professor of Statistics, Department of Health Care Policy, Harvard Medical School, Boston, MA

Although the reviewers listed above provided many constructive comments and suggestions, they were not asked to endorse the report's conclusions or recommendations, nor did they see the final draft of the report before its release. The review of this report was overseen by coordinator **DONALD M. STEINWACHS,** Professor and Chair, Johns Hopkins Bloomberg School of Public Health, Baltimore, Maryland, and monitor **HAROLD C. SOX,** Editor, *Annals of Internal Medicine*, Philadelphia, Pennsylvania. Appointed by the National Research Council and the Institute of Medicine, they were responsible for making certain that an independent examination of this report was carried out in accordance with institutional procedures and that all review comments were carefully considered. Responsibility for the final content of this report rests entirely with the authoring committee and the institution.

Foreword

Transformation of the U.S. health care system will not come easily. It will require concerted action by many public- and private-sector participants working toward the goals of safety, effectiveness, efficiency, patient-centered care, timeliness, and equity, which the Institute of Medicine (IOM) has previously identified as the critical aims of health care quality.

This report is part of a new IOM series titled *Pathways to Quality Health Care*. The series of reports explores how to transition between the existing health care system and the system we should create if we are to reduce waste and unnecessary procedures while fostering value and performance. The present report aims to help individual and institutional providers improve their clinical performance and achieve higher levels of quality as assessed by purchasers and consumers. The report highlights the important roles that a national program with private organizations in each state can play in supporting higher-quality care, especially for those providers who serve Medicare beneficiaries.

As discussed in the first report in the *Pathways* series, *Performance Measurement: Accelerating Improvement*, more visible and consistent measures of quality must be associated with specific providers and health care settings to support better decisions and investments in health care. In this second report, the committee looks closely at the sources of technical assistance that encourage providers to improve their performance. In the early history of quality improvement, Congress thought it best to review individual case records of beneficiaries in seeking to improve care in the Medicare system. More recent experience in other sectors of the economy suggests that such retrospective record reviews are only one dimension of what is needed to achieve higher levels of performance from a complex enterprise. Broader system-level interventions frequently offer better ways to nurture behavioral and organizational change that can improve performance.

Many health care providers and organizations have made great strides in improving their quality of care. But the pace of progress is uneven. Some providers want and deserve technical assistance in eliminating key barriers that impede their progress. All providers and their patients can benefit from opportunities to learn from one another and to share lessons learned from experience in implementing higher standards of care.

In this report, the IOM Committee on Redesigning Health Insurance Performance Measures, Payment, and Performance Improvement Programs carefully examines the Quality Improvement Organizations that serve every state, as well as the national program that guides and supports them. The committee's recommendations deserve careful consideration as our elected leaders and health care purchasers seek to reward high-performing providers. The committee recommends focusing public resources for technical assistance to achieve better quality on those providers that demonstrate the potential for change, with priority given to those in greatest need. The report suggests public- and private-sector collaborations that can strengthen the foundation for this valuable technical assistance. It is important to note that, consistent with IOM policy and procedures, one member of the study committee who currently serves on the board of a Quality Improvement Organization did not participate in the committee deliberations that led to the development of this report.

This report is a further step from the "what" of quality improvement to the "how." By providing an in-depth assessment of the federal experience with quality improvement, the report helps point the way for those who strive to create higher quality and better value in health care.

Harvey V. Fineberg, M.D., Ph.D.
President, Institute of Medicine
February 2006

Preface

This report, *Medicare's Quality Improvement Organization Program: Maximizing Potential*, is the second in the Institute of Medicine's (IOM) *Pathways to Quality Health Care* series and was authored by the IOM's Committee on Redesigning Health Insurance Performance Measures, Payment, and Performance Improvement Programs. The committee concludes that the changing environment of health care, with the increased public reporting of performance measures and payment incentives for providers who meet certain quality standards, will create a growing demand from providers for technical assistance with the reporting of performance measures and analysis, as well as with process and systems improvements.

The *Pathways to Quality Health Care* series builds on earlier IOM studies, known collectively as the *Quality Chasm* series, which highlight the importance of strengthening key elements of the health care infrastructure to dramatically improve the quality of care delivered to patients across all health care settings. The *Pathways to Quality Health Care* series addresses the critical role of performance measurement and reporting, quality improvement, and payment incentives in reducing the fragmentation of the health care delivery system and improving care. In 2005, the IOM released the first report in the *Pathways to Quality Health Care* series, *Performance Measurement: Accelerating Improvement*, which recommends adoption of leading performance measures, identifies gaps in performance measures and areas for further development, and calls for a coherent national system to support robust performance measurement and public reporting. The congressional request for a comprehensive evaluation of the Medicare Quality Improvement Organization (QIO) program provided a timely opportunity to examine how the QIO program fits within the evolving performance improvement efforts in the nation's health care system. The third report of the series, to be released in 2006, will examine payment strategies that the Centers for Medicare and Medicaid Services (CMS) could use to stimulate higher levels of performance within the health care system and improve the quality of services offered to Medicare beneficiaries.

The committee's study of the QIO program shows that the program has the potential to play an important role in this new environment, but that a major restructuring is essential to enhance the program's ability to promote quality improvement. Recognizing the critical need for quality improvements in health care, the committee presents recommendations to strengthen the QIO program for the future.

The committee concludes that the quality of health care for Medicare beneficiaries has been improving slowly but that gaps in quality persist. The QIO program could become an important national resource to accelerate the improvement of quality on the basis of its presence in each state, programwide support centers, and national support services for performance measurement. The current program, however, needs updating and a major restructuring. The U.S. Congress, the U.S. Department of Health and Human Services, and CMS should create an improved structure for the QIOs and a program environment that promotes QIO assistance to more providers more effectively.

A strong, focused QIO network is essential to the effective implementation of performance measurement and reporting. The QIO program should help the national board proposed in the first report in the *Pathways to Quality* series implement the system for performance measurement and reporting, and assist providers with the development of their own capacity to measure and improve their performance. CMS should encourage and expect continuous performance improvement among all Medicare providers, and the QIOs should aid those providers requesting assistance.

To realize their potential in the emerging health care environment, QIOs should focus on technical assistance for performance measurement and improvement; their effectiveness is currently diluted by competing interests and activities. Therefore, CMS should develop separate contracts with other capable organizations to conduct reviews of beneficiary complaints, appeals, and other cases. This devolution of functions will ensure that beneficiaries and the Medicare Trust Funds receive primary attention and that case reviews are conducted more efficiently.

The committee trusts that its recommendations will provide guidance to both the U.S. Congress and the U.S. Department of Health and Human Services on how to restructure the QIO program so that it will be better positioned to serve as Medicare's main program for quality improvement. The report includes as well both a broad and detailed overview of the current QIO program that should be useful to members of Congress and the federal executive branch, as well as the QIO community, seeking to understand this complex program. The report should also serve as a useful foundation upon which future studies can build.

All Americans deserve what CMS has set as its vision: the right care for every person every time. We do not yet benefit from that level of quality, and it is clear that science-based guidelines are not followed consistently. To the extent that the QIO program can assist health care facilities and practitioners with measurement and improvement of the quality of the health care they provide, we will all benefit.

As chairman of the committee, I thank all committee members, IOM staff, and the Subcommittee for Quality Improvement Organization Program Evaluation for their contributions of expertise and insight. They all voluntarily spent considerable time and effort on the study and on shaping the report. I particularly would like to recognize the contributions of the chair of the subcommittee, Steve Shortell, and IOM senior program officer Dianne Miller Wolman, who directed this study.

Steven A. Schroeder, M.D.
Chairman
February 2006

Acknowledgments

Medicare's Quality Improvement Organization Program: Maximizing Potential benefited from the contributions of many people. The committee takes this opportunity to recognize those who helped develop the data and analyses on which the report is based.

The committee acknowledges the members of the Subcommittee on Quality Improvement Organization Program Evaluation, who contributed so much to this report: Stephen M. Shortell, Chair, University of California, Berkeley; Anne-Marie J. Audet, The Commonwealth Fund; Jack L. Cox, consultant; David H. Gustafson, University of Wisconsin; Jeff Kang, CIGNA HealthCare; Alan R. Nelson, American College of Physicians; Gregg Pane, District of Columbia Department of Health; Barbara R. Paul, BEI; William A. Peck, Washington University School of Medicine; Eric D. Peterson, Duke University School of Medicine; and Shoshanna Sofaer, Baruch College. All members of the subcommittee gave much time and advice in designing the original data collection tools and procedures, in performing the critical literature review that supports this report's findings and conclusions, and in reviewing and critiquing primary research articles. John Ring and Clyde Behney also contributed as directors of the Board on Health Care Services of the Institute of Medicine.

The committee benefited from presentations made by a number of experts. The following individuals shared their research, experience, and perspectives with the committee: Marc M. Boutin, National Health Council; Elizabeth Bradley, Yale School of Public Health; David Brailer, U.S. Department of Health and Human Services; Donald W. Fisher, American Medical Group Association, Inc.; Nancy Foster, American Hospital Association; Larry A. Green, American Academy of Family Physicians; Maulik Joshi, Delmarva Foundation; Barbara B. Manard, American Association of Homes and Services for the Aging; Mark McClellan, Centers for Medicare and Medicaid Services; Gordon Mosser, Institute for Clinical Systems Improvement; Peter Pronovost, The Johns Hopkins University School of Medicine; and Andrew Webber, National Business Coalition on Health.

The American Health Quality Association was an important source of information and support. Many staff and members, especially the following individuals, generously gave their time and knowledge and made presentations to further the committee's aims: David Adler, Dale Bratzler, Todd Ketch, David Schulke, and Jonathan Sugarman.

The committee acknowledges the particular contributions of Allyson Ross Davies, consultant, in the development and implementation of a web-based data collection tool, and Cheryl Ulmer, consultant, in the conduct and analysis of 20 telephone interviews. Timothy Jost, professor, Washington and Lee University School of Law, provided valuable legal advice. Eric Lawrence, Assistant Professor of Political Science, The George Washington University, offered guidance on research methodologies and statistics. Rona Briere, Alisa Decatur, and Michael K. Hayes provided editorial assistance and assistance with the preparation of the manuscript for publication.

The committee extends special thanks to all 53 Quality Improvement Organizations for their willing and active participation in multiple interviews, site visits, and data collection efforts.

Funding for the project came from the Centers for Medicare and Medicaid Services (CMS). The committee appreciates the assistance and information received from CMS staff around the country and particularly recognizes Gary Christopherson, Steve Jencks, Joyce Kelly, and Bill Rollow for their extra support throughout the project.

Contents

APPENDIXES

MEDICARE'S QUALITY IMPROVEMENT ORGANIZATION PROGRAM

Summary

In the Medicare Prescription Drug, Improvement, and Modernization Act of 2003 (P.L. 108-173, section 109), the U.S. Congress requested that the Institute of Medicine (IOM) conduct an evaluation of the Quality Improvement Organization (QIO) program administered by the Centers for Medicare and Medicaid Services (CMS). The QIO program consists of a set of federally administered contracts that support QIO services in each state, as well as special studies and program support services at the national level. This report responds to the congressional request by providing an overview of the QIO program and an assessment of its impact on the quality of health care for Medicare beneficiaries, funding levels and sources for QIO activities, CMS oversight of those activities, and the extent to which other organizations could perform similar functions. (The congressional request to the IOM did not include a fiscal integrity review.) This report builds on the IOM's *Quality Chasm* series, which outlines a vision for a better health care system meeting six key aims: health care should be safe, effective, patient-centered, timely, efficient, and equitable.

The IOM Committee on Redesigning Health Insurance Performance Measures, Payment, and Performance Improvement Programs conducted this assessment during a time of significant change in the health care environment in the United States, characterized by increased attention to safety, beneficiary protection, quality improvement, efficiency, and performance measurement. In preparing this report, the committee considered how the QIO program can best participate in this new health care environment and contribute to the achievement of higher quality in provider performance and in the health care received by Medicare beneficiaries.

BACKGROUND

The Medicare Context

Medicare is the single largest purchaser of health care in the United States; in 2004 the program paid more than $295 billion in benefits to care for 41.7 million beneficiaries. CMS has an obligation to ensure that the care received by all Medicare beneficiaries meets the standards all Americans deserve. As the original *Quality Chasm* report makes abundantly clear, however, Medicare beneficiaries, like Americans generally, too often do not receive quality care that meets scientifically established guidelines and suffer worse health outcomes as a result. At the same time, per capita spending on health care in the United States is higher than that in any other developed country. Americans deserve greater value from their expensive investments in health care. To this end, it will be necessary to close the large gap remaining between the quality of care that is provided and the quality of care that all Americans should receive.

Among those over age 65, the primary Medicare population, 87 percent have at least one chronic condition, and more than 36 percent have three or more such conditions. Transitions in care from one provider setting to another, particularly important for individuals with chronic conditions, are not efficient and well coordinated in the current health care system. Adverse drug events in hospitals and ambulatory care settings are a serious problem and may be more likely to occur among chronically ill individuals and during transitions in care.

As administrator of Medicare, CMS has an opportunity to lead other federal and private insurers and purchasers in stimulating improvements in health care practices. In addition to the QIO program, CMS has certain mechanisms at its disposal that can promote the diffusion of best-care practices, including Conditions of Participation, Survey and Certification requirements, and other regulatory and research authorities. All these mechanisms should be focused on improving the quality of U.S. health care in the 21st century and implementing a national performance measurement and reporting system that can support quality improvement efforts.

The QIO program encompasses 41 organizations that hold 53 contracts with CMS to provide services in all 50 states, Puerto Rico, the Virgin Islands, and the District of Columbia. The contracts require each QIO to offer technical assistance to nursing homes, home health agencies, hospitals, prescription drug plans, pharmacies, and physician practices to help them improve the quality of care they provide to Medicare beneficiaries. The QIOs also have the responsibility to protect beneficiaries and the Medicare Trust Funds by reviewing individual cases. In addition to the 53 QIOs, the QIO program funds several QIO Support Centers (QIOSCs), which serve as national resources and provide assistance to the QIOs in carrying out these responsibilities. The QIO program also funds numerous special studies and contracts to support existing program functions and to conduct research and develop materials for quality-related activities.

Over time, the QIO program has evolved to address new requirements and expectations. It now constitutes a multifaceted enterprise that deserves a thorough analysis to:

- Highlight significant assets that can be used to shape the future of health care.
- Identify functions that might be discarded or reassigned to other appropriate agencies.
- Recommend actions to strengthen the program and CMS management practices.

The recommendations offered in this report for restructuring the QIO program are intended to spur more rapid improvement in health care quality. This restructuring of the QIO program, in coordination with the use of performance measurement, reporting, and payment incentives (addressed in the other reports in the IOM's *Pathways to Quality Health Care* series), should enable great strides in closing the quality gap.

History and Current Status of the QIO Program

Over the course of more than 35 years, federal priorities for the QIO program have changed from quality assurance and retrospective utilization review of individual case records to systemic collaboration with providers for the improvement of overall patterns and processes of care. Observations drawn from the history of the program offer several key insights:

- Many QIO staff, boards, and executives have a long history with the program and established relationships with health care providers on which they can draw for valuable resources and perspectives.
- Although the views of many providers have changed along with the program's evolution, some hospital executives and physicians still perceive the QIOs primarily as regulators.
- Frequent changes in the required activities of the QIOs demand that contractors demonstrate flexibility and adaptability. They also create significant challenges to any assessment of the program.

In this report, the IOM committee focused on activities performed during the 7th and 8th contract periods (2002–2005 and 2005–2008, respectively), also referred to as scopes of work (SOWs).[1] Most of the data collected to assess the program relates to the 7th SOW.

KEY FINDINGS AND CONCLUSIONS

Extensive variations in the organizational structures and the specific services of the QIOs make generalizations difficult. Nonetheless, the committee's assessment led to the following conclusions:

- The quality of the health care received by Medicare beneficiaries has improved over time.
- The existing evidence is inadequate to determine the extent to which the QIO program has contributed directly to those improvements.
- The QIO program provides a potentially valuable nationwide infrastructure dedicated to promoting quality health care.
- The value of the program could be enhanced through the use of strategies designed to focus the QIOs' attention on the provision of technical assistance in support of quality improvement, to broaden their governance base and structure, and to improve CMS's management of related data systems and program evaluations.

Following is a discussion of the key findings that led to these conclusions. First, though, it is important to note that in the process of examining the QIO program, the committee considered a number of options for and alternatives to the program, including restructuring or reorganizing the federal program and contracting with other private organizations. The committee's recommendations concerning the future of the QIO program are based on an assessment of these options and alternatives.

Quality Improvement in Medicare

Published evidence indicates improvements in the quality of care received by Medicare beneficiaries between 1998 and 2004, although the numbers of quality measures studied are limited, and those examined focus

---

[1]CMS contracts with private organizations for QIO services in each state for 3-year periods. CMS uses the acronym SOW for both "scope of work" and "statement of work." In this report, the committee uses SOW only for "scope of work" and adopts the general usage of SOW by the QIO community, in which the term denotes either tasks required in general or the time period of a contract. When discussing specific details of QIO work, the committee refers to the contract itself. For example, the 7th SOW was from 2002 to 2005. It required all QIOs to provide technical assistance to nursing homes, and the contract for this SOW stipulated that QIOs must recruit 30 percent of nursing homes to develop a plan of action.

primarily on the quality of care provided in hospitals. Improvements have occurred in areas targeted as national priorities (and for QIO attention), such as rates of mammography, care provided after a heart attack, and rates of screening and treatment for diabetes. Managed care organizations have also demonstrated improvements in the care provided to Medicare beneficiaries. As noted above, however, there is substantial room for further improvement. In addition to the deficiencies in care transitions and unacceptable rates of adverse events mentioned earlier, many people do not receive appropriate preventive care, and the quality of other services varies greatly among providers and by the geographic location, race, and income of the beneficiary.

Studies conducted to date cannot be used to determine the cause of the improvements that have occurred because of limitations in the study designs, the complexity of the programs being evaluated, and conflicting results. Yet the difficulty of attributing quality improvement to any specific intervention or program is not limited to the QIO program; rather, it is characteristic of quality improvement interventions in general and applies to improvement efforts of other organizations as well. The lack of evidence does not mean the interventions undertaken by the QIOs and other organizations have had no impact. The committee was unable to document conclusively whether individual QIOs or the program as a whole has had a positive impact, a negative impact, or no impact on the quality of care during the period of the 7th SOW. However, CMS's preliminary reports of performance on quality measures during the 7th SOW suggest that providers that worked intensely with a QIO on an intervention showed greater improvement than those that did not.

Are some QIOs more effective than others? There appears to be a common perception that some QIOs are outstanding, while others are mediocre. According to performance measures, some QIOs are better than others at improving quality on a particular care dimension or a specific task. Objective global measures of QIOs, however, do not exist, and CMS's contract performance scores for QIOs neither indicate which fall into each level of performance nor highlight significant differences in overall performance.

Despite these uncertainties, the committee concluded that the QIO program has the potential to help meet the crucial need of improving the quality of health care. As implementation of a broad national performance measurement system proceeds and payments increasingly reward quality improvement, the need for technical assistance for quality improvement efforts will increase. The QIO program's nationwide coverage, support resources, and partnering relationships with providers are distinct assets. A major restructuring of the program should enhance its ability both to meet this need for assistance and to document the resulting impact on quality of care. A sharper focus on technical assistance and more systematic and rigorous evaluations of the program's current and future efforts would provide a stronger evidence base that could be used to guide future decisions about the program. At the same time, the other organizations performing QIO-like functions in the private sector deserve further scrutiny, as CMS's implementation of the recommended structural reforms to increase open competition might allow such organizations to complement, augment, or in some cases replace current organizations holding QIO contracts.

Structural Issues

The presence of organizations with trained experts dedicated to providing quality improvement services in every state is a significant asset at both the local and national levels. The committee notes that the QIOs and CMS have established important relationships with providers, their professional associations, and various other stakeholder groups, thus promoting concerted, coordinated quality improvement efforts. Some providers, such as small physician practices, will have a particular need for assistance with reporting of performance measures and quality improvement in the future. In sum, the potential exists for a reconfigured QIO program to have a measurable positive impact on the quality of care for Medicare beneficiaries. To realize this potential, however, it will be necessary to address a number of structural issues.

QIO Board Composition, Functions, and Structure

The boards of organizations holding QIO contracts are heavily dominated by physicians. Most QIO boards have only one (mandated) consumer representative, which is insufficient to influence the attainment of more patient-centered care. The committee concluded that QIO governance generally lacks (1) sufficient representation of individuals with the required expertise other than physicians, and of individuals from outside the health care field; (2) tools for assessment of the performance of individual board members and the board as a whole; (3) important committees for finance, auditing, and strategic planning; and (4) adequate transparency.

Physician-Access or Physician-Sponsored Organizations

The legislative requirement that eligible organizations attain specific levels of local physician involvement is outmoded, and reflects the historical use of case review to identify local outliers instead of the goal of raising all care to the level of evidence-based national guidelines and standards. Elimination of this requirement could increase competition for QIO contracts.

Conflicts of Interest

A QIO is restricted from contracting with health care providers in its state for technical assistance or review services similar to those covered by its core Medicare contract. QIOs would be able to serve more providers and beneficiaries if they could contract for additional services and supplement their CMS funds with those from providers and other sources.

Confidentiality Restrictions

Confidentiality restrictions on the QIOs' treatment of clinical data reflect the protective attitudes of the predecessor programs and provider interests. Given the current interest in transparency, public reporting, and consumer access to information, those restrictions are largely inappropriate and constrain use of the data for intervention programs.

Functions and Impacts of the QIOs

The QIOs had three main functions under the 7th SOW:

- Offer providers technical assistance in improving the quality of care through collaboratives or other interventions by supporting process redesign, data collection and interpretation for internal quality improvement, and dissemination activities related to the use of publicly available comparative quality data.
- Provide education and communications for beneficiaries.
- Protect beneficiaries and the Medicare Trust Funds by reviewing complaints and appeals and performing other case reviews to estimate payment error rates and address other billing concerns.

The 8th SOW (2005–2008) retains the technical assistance and protection functions of the 7th SOW, but the education and communications function has been subsumed under the other two. Indeed, the QIOs contribute indirectly to beneficiary education—an integral part of quality health care—through the technical assistance they offer to providers. Moreover, many stakeholder groups in the community, as well as other CMS programs, work directly with beneficiaries, and QIOs often partner with them to reach beneficiaries through public information campaigns. The contract for the 8th SOW was designed to encourage quality improvement through organizational "transformations" intended to produce more rapid, measurable improvements in care. The QIOs must work intensively with subsets of individual providers to help them redesign care processes and make internal systemic changes, such as the adoption and implementation of health information and communications technologies, so as to narrow the gap between current and ideal standards of care. The contract also includes new activities related to the Medicare Part D prescription drug benefit.

Strengthening beneficiary protection is critical, and some case review is needed, but CMS could manage those functions more appropriately through contracts with other organizations. The evidence indicates that QIOs have not publicized beneficiary rights effectively and have issued fewer provider sanctions in recent years. This may be the result of inherent conflicts of interest: QIOs consider providers, not beneficiaries, to be their primary clients, and a QIO may not want to antagonize the providers it needs to participate in its interventions and satisfaction surveys.

Beneficiaries have multiple avenues at the state level for pursuing complaints, such as state survey and certification agencies, ombudsman programs, state insurance oversight bodies, and state medical boards. Medicare needs to do a better job of educating beneficiaries about their rights under federal law and directing them to an agency that will handle their complaints expeditiously and fairly, with an emphasis on improving the quality of health care in the future and with a focus on the beneficiary as the primary client. For example, CMS could consolidate complaints, appeals, and case reviews into four regional centers, each having a larger staff with more expertise than would be possible for any single QIO currently. The competitors for these regional contracts might include some of the QIOs most capable of performing such reviews, as well as other organizations. The committee could not determine the cost-effectiveness of the various categories and types of case reviews from the available program data.

The current concentration in the QIOs of all three functions—technical assistance, beneficiary education and communications, and protection of beneficiaries and the trust funds—contributes to several shortcomings:

- Hostile attitudes among some providers and a reluctance to participate in QIO quality improvement activities.
- Possible conflicts of interest that could limit the QIOs' aggressive pursuit of complaints, appeals, and problematic cases.
- Inefficient operations concerning staffing, particularly with regard to on-call physicians who are needed 24 hours a day, 7 days a week to review urgent appeals for the coverage of services.

Given the growing demand for external reporting of quality and efficiency measures and the increasing number of programs offering financial rewards for quality improvements, providers are likely to increase their requests for technical assistance. QIOs would have greater value if they concentrated their limited resources on the provision of technical assistance to support performance measurement and quality improvement. Providers' needs for such assistance are substantial, and internal and commercial resources to meet these needs are frequently unavailable or unaffordable. The committee therefore concluded that the regulatory functions of the various case reviews should not remain in the core SOW for every QIO and should devolve to other appropriate organizations.

Management of the QIO Program

CMS has the challenge of managing the QIO program in the field, as well as integrating it into the operational responsibilities of the Medicare program. The committee identified several areas in which management changes could improve the effectiveness of the QIOs.

Lack of Program Priorities

The contract for the 8th SOW does not set overall program or QIO priorities, although it specifies the individual tasks in great detail. The complex evaluation formulas provided are of little use to the QIOs for prioritizing their work and reflect the absence of overall strategic priorities, a comprehensive evaluation plan, and program guidance.

Strategic Planning

The QIO program has begun a promising long-range strategic planning process that includes stakeholders and staff and involves meeting separately with representatives of each provider setting. This separate engagement with specific provider settings, however, is inconsistent with the IOM vision of integrated care. As noted earlier, Medicare patients, particularly those with chronic conditions, need care that is coordinated across provider settings. Thus quality and efficiency measure sets should include measures for multiple provider settings and reward all providers accordingly. The QIO program's strategic planning process should contribute to the alignment of the QIOs' technical assistance efforts with performance measurement, payment, and pay for performance. The new Part D prescription drug benefit represents another opportunity for QIOs to focus on the coordination of care across provider settings, because maintaining appropriate drug therapies is critical as a patient receives health care in multiple settings.

Lack of an Overall Program Evaluation

Previous IOM reports on the CMS programs that preceded today's QIO program called for overall program evaluations, as well as formative studies to guide tasks in progress. To date, CMS has not conducted a comprehensive program evaluation, and only a few published evaluations of specific QIO quality interventions exist, although some evaluations are being planned for the 8th SOW. This lack of evaluations limited the information available for the present study and constrains the program's internal planning.

Overly Complex Contract Performance Evaluations

Assessments of a QIO's contract performance are based on complex formulas and separate calculations for each task. The increased complexity of tasks in the 8th SOW is reflected in a set of formulas and incentive awards more complicated than those used for the 7th SOW. These formulas indicate an excessive level of process management of the QIOs on the part of CMS and the need for greater strategic guidance.

Lack of Evaluation of QIOSC and Other Contracts

Nearly one-third of the total QIO program funding is allocated to contracts for QIOSCs, special studies, and support services. In contrast to the detailed formulas used to evaluate the QIOs' performance on the core contract, there are no clear criteria for the evaluation of contractor performance under these other contracts, and little formal evaluation of these contractors has taken place. At present, coordination among these contracts is lacking, and no management system for dissemination of the results of special studies and other research contracts is available.

Slow Data Processing

The Standard Data Processing System supports a range of communications tools, as well as the flow, processing, and storage of data from medical records. This system is essential to the QIO program and could become a critical component of a national system for performance measurement and reporting. A major concern of the QIOs and providers is that the data used to monitor provider progress often are not reported in a timely manner. As CMS increases the number of measures required for public reporting, the volume of data will grow, generating an increased need for timely and useful reports.

Late Issuance of the 8th SOW

The 8th SOW was released without sufficient time for the QIOs or other potential applicants to prepare properly for the new contract. Changes in the contract and uncertainties about future changes have persisted, with a major revision being issued more than 3 months after the contract's start date.

Three-Year Contract Length

The current 3-year contract length is problematic given the startup efforts required in response to the changes in each new contract; time lags in the availability of provider performance data; the time needed by CMS, the Department of Health and Human Services, and the Office of Management and Budget to develop the next contract; and the time required to conduct more rigorous evaluations of program interventions. Longer contract periods with increased interim monitoring would be more suitable for the management of the QIO program. In addition, extending the contract period beyond 3 years would allow the QIOs to focus on a consistent set of priorities for achieving basic transformation of the systems within provider settings.

RECOMMENDATIONS

Focus on Quality Improvement and Performance Measurement

Recommendation 1: The Quality Improvement Organization (QIO) program must become an integral part of strategies for future performance measurement and improvement in the health care system. The U.S. Congress, the secretary of the U.S. Department of Health and Human Services (DHHS), and the Centers for Medicare and Medicaid Services (CMS) should strengthen and reform key dimensions of the QIO program, emphasizing the provision of technical assistance for performance measurement and quality improvement. These changes will enable the program to contribute to improved quality of care for Medicare beneficiaries as they move through multiple health care settings over time.

- Quality improvement should embrace all six aims for health care established by the Institute of Medicine (IOM) (safety, effectiveness, patient-centeredness, timeliness, efficiency, and equity).
- QIO services should be available to all providers, Medicare Advantage organizations, and prescription drug plans.
- QIO services should emphasize hands-on and other technical assistance aimed at building provider capacity as needed by each provider setting, such as:
  - Instruction in how to collect, aggregate, and interpret data on the measures to be used for internal quality improvement, public reporting, and payment.
  - Instruction in how to conduct root-cause analyses and deep case studies of sentinel events or other problems.

- Advice and guidance on how to bring about, sustain, and diffuse internal system redesign and process changes, particularly those related to the use of information technology for quality improvement and those that promote care coordination and efficiency through an episode of care.
- Enhancement of and technical support for the direct role of providers in beneficiary education as an integral component of improved care, better patient experiences, and patient self-management.
- Assistance with convening and brokering cooperation among various stakeholders.

......

Recommendation 2: QIOs should actively encourage all providers to pursue quality improvement and should assist those providers requesting technical assistance; if demand exceeds resources, priority should be given to those providers who demonstrate the most need for improvement or who face significant challenges in their efforts to improve quality. CMS should encourage and expect all providers to continuously improve the quality of care for Medicare beneficiaries.

......

Recommendation 3: Congress and CMS should strengthen the organizational structure and governance of QIOs to reflect the new, narrower focus on technical assistance for performance measurement and quality improvement. Congress should eliminate the requirement that QIO governing boards be physician-access or physician-sponsored, while also enhancing the boards' ability to provide oversight and direction.

- Congress and CMS should improve QIO governance by requiring (1) broader representation of all stakeholders on QIO boards, including more beneficiaries and consumers with the requisite training and executive-level representatives of providers; (2) expansion of the areas of expertise represented on QIO boards through the inclusion of individuals from various health professional disciplines, group purchasers, and professionals in information management; and (3) greater diversity of quality improvement professionals on QIO boards through the inclusion of experts from outside the health care field and beyond the local community.

- QIO boards should strengthen their committee structures and consider development plans for individual members, implementation of annual performance evaluations, and annual assessments of the board as a whole as well as plans for its improvement.
- Organizations holding QIO contracts should include on their websites a listing of members of their boards of directors, along with information on the compensation provided to those members and the chief executive officer.

......

Recommendation 4: Congress and CMS should develop mechanisms other than those already in place to better manage complaints and appeals of Medicare beneficiaries, as well as other case reviews. The QIO in each state should no longer have responsibility for handling beneficiary complaints, appeals, and other case reviews for payment or other purposes.

- Reviews of beneficiary complaints regarding the quality of care received are critical and should be a top priority for contractors that treat the beneficiary as their primary client. CMS should consolidate the review functions into a few regional or national competitive contracts or determine the most appropriate agencies with which to contract for the purpose in each state.
- To handle beneficiaries' appeals and other case reviews more efficiently, CMS could contract at the national or regional level with a limited number of appropriate organizations, such as fiscal intermediaries or individual QIOs. This devolution of responsibilities would allow QIOs to concentrate their resources on quality improvement efforts with providers.

......

Data Processing

Recommendation 5: The secretary of DHHS and CMS should revise the QIO program's data-handling practices so that data will be available to providers and the QIOs in a timely manner for use in improving services and measuring performance.

- CMS should initiate a comprehensive review of its data-sharing systems, processes, and regulations to identify and correct practices and procedures, including abstraction of medical chart data, that restrict the sharing of data by the QIOs for quality improvement purposes or that inhibit prompt feedback to the QIOs and providers on provider performance.

- The QIO program should support the processes of national reporting of performance measures, data aggregation, data analysis, and feedback.
- The secretary of DHHS should allow and encourage the sharing of medical claims data when the sharing of such data is not precluded by the privacy protections of the Health Insurance Portability and Accountability Act, as well as the sharing of more detailed complaint-resolution data with complainants.
- CMS should work toward the ultimate goal of integrating more care data from all providers and public and private payers to create both records of patient care over time and population-level data.
- Independently of the core QIO contract, CMS should be responsible for ensuring and auditing the accuracy of the data submitted by providers that participate in the Medicare program. Providers should be accountable for the validity and accuracy of the quality measurement data they submit. The QIOs should supply providers with technical assistance to improve the validity and accuracy of the data collected.

......

QIO Program Management

Recommendation 6: CMS should establish clear goals and strategic priorities for the QIO program. Congress, the secretary of DHHS, and CMS should improve their management of the QIO program as necessary to support those goals, especially by enhancing contracting processes for the QIO core contract and QIO Support Center (QIOSC) contracts; integrating the program's core, support, and special study contracts; and improving coordination and communication within the program.

- CMS should provide the QIOs with a coherent and feasible scope of work that sets forth clear priorities for quality improvement and performance measurement.
  - CMS's priorities and planning efforts should focus on integrating QIO collaboration with various types of providers to improve the coordination of patient care across multiple settings.

- To prepare for the 9th scope of work, CMS should consider conducting a national survey of the main provider settings (nursing homes, home health agencies, hospitals, outpatient physician practices, end-stage renal disease facilities, prescription drug plans, and pharmacies) to determine specific unmet needs for technical assistance. Such information might be complemented by information from focus groups conducted with a mix of representatives from the various settings.
- The QIO core contracts and the QIOSC contracts should include incentives aimed at promoting a broader transfer of knowledge concerning successful quality improvement interventions and more rapid improvement.
- The QIOs should have the resources they need to conduct at least one locally initiated quality improvement project on the basis of demonstrated need and the design and evaluation criteria established by CMS.

- Congress and CMS should change the contract structure for core QIO services for the 9th scope of work:
  - Strong incentives and penalties that reward high performance and penalize poor performance should be included. CMS should encourage sufficient competition for the core contracts to permit the selection of a QIO contractor on the basis of contractor-proposed interim and final performance measures and goals. During the contract period, there should be less process management of internal QIO operations by CMS.
  - Congress should permit extension of the core contract from 3 to 5 years to allow for the measurement, refinement, and evaluation of technical assistance efforts and the achievement of transformational goals.
  - There should be greater competition for each new contract. CMS should consider previous experience and performance as a QIO among the selection criteria; demonstrated capacity to support quality improvement on the part of any eligible organization should predominate.
  - Performance periods should be consistent. All QIOs should begin and end the contract cycle on the same date so the planning, implementation, and evaluation of each scope of work can be applied nationally.
  - A timetable should be established for goal setting, program planning, and funding processes for the core QIO contracts. The schedule should ensure that new scopes of work are issued in a timely fashion, and that contracts and funding levels are developed and finalized so as to allow sufficient time

for QIOs and competing organizations to prepare in advance for the new contract without major program and staff disruptions.

- CMS should award QIOSC contracts several months in advance of a new QIO contract cycle to allow for the preparation of tools and materials for QIO use, definition of the required tasks and deliverables that will serve the QIOs and the Government Task Leaders, and inclusion of explicit methods for assessment of the contractor's performance. Congress and CMS should allow entities other than QIOs with expertise in quality improvement to bid on QIOSC contracts; familiarity with QIO work, the capability to carry out the work, and experience in performing the required functions should be appropriately weighted when the bids are assessed.

- The QIO core contract and contracts for special studies, support services, and QIOSCs should all reflect the explicit goals and priorities of the program.

- CMS and the Agency for Healthcare Research and Quality should establish ongoing mechanisms for sharing quality improvement knowledge and research results, especially through QIOSCs.

- CMS should take steps to improve coordination and communications within the QIO program and with QIOs. In particular, the roles and responsibilities of and communications among Project Officers, Contract Officers, Government Task Leaders, Scientific Officers, and QIO executives and their staff should be clarified.

  - CMS should build self-assessment, transparency, clearer communications, and continuous quality improvement into the daily workings of the team overseeing the QIO program, just as the QIOs expect providers to do.

  - The contracting function should be subordinate to and support the program management and business functions.

  - Ongoing program evaluations (see Recommendation 7) should provide guidance for the continuous improvement of program management, coordination, and communications.

......

QIO Program Evaluations

Recommendation 7: CMS should develop four types of evaluation to assess the QIO program. CMS should conduct three of these four types of evaluation internally to assess QIO performance against predetermined goals and priorities at the following levels: (1) the program as a whole, (2) individual QIOs with respect to the core contract, and (3) selected quality improvement interventions implemented by QIOs. DHHS should periodically commission the fourth type of evaluation—independent, external evaluations of the QIO program's overall contributions.

- The QIOs should be learning organizations, continually improving the assistance they offer to health care providers. CMS should develop explicit benchmarks for use in ongoing measurement of progress on the effectiveness and costs of the program.
- CMS should form a technical expert panel to offer ongoing guidance on the design of the three types of internal CMS evaluations, including options for identifying optimally performing QIOs, as well as methodologies for attributing quality improvements to the QIO program's interventions.
- CMS should ensure that evaluations of the effectiveness of quality improvement interventions are conducted. The committee suggests that CMS should use the most rigorous evaluation designs practicable, including randomized controlled trials. This approach should also contribute to CMS's overall program evaluation.
  - Evaluations should include concurrent, qualitative descriptions and assessments of the nuanced nature of the QIOs' role in quality improvement interventions and the roles of other players.
  - As appropriate, evaluations should be stratified among provider settings and across states and regions.
  - CMS should assess the cost-effectiveness of each type of intervention to assist with the allocation of resources.
- The secretary of DHHS should allocate adequate funds from the QIO apportionment to carry out, on an ongoing basis, both internal and external evaluations.

......

QIO Program Funding

Recommendation 8: Congress and the secretary of DHHS should focus all QIO resources on supporting health care providers' performance measurement and quality improvement efforts. The secretary should remove from QIO core contracts funds sufficient to support case reviews, appeals, and beneficiary complaints when those functions are devolved to other organizations. The secretary should increase the remaining funds to allow for inflation, the incorporation of evaluations into all QIO work, the increased numbers of providers and beneficiaries being served, and the labor-intensive nature of technical assistance and quality improvement activities.

- The multiple evaluations undertaken during the 8th and 9th SOWs should guide future funding decisions, with budget increases or decreases being provided according to the evaluation findings. If the evaluations demonstrate that no positive impact is attributable to the QIO program's efforts, CMS will need to rethink its quality improvement approach and the possible benefit of transitioning funds to an alternative structure and strategy for Medicare.
- Once a national performance measurement and reporting system has been established, its priorities should help guide the funding levels and policy direction of the QIO program, recognizing that adequate funding is necessary to reach the goals set for the QIO program.
- The secretary of DHHS should ease the conflict-of-interest restriction with regard to supplementing the QIO quality improvement budgets with external funds. Given the limits of federal funding, the QIOs should be allowed to seek funds for quality improvement activities from providers and other organizations as appropriate.

Introduction

This introduction provides background on the Institute of Medicine (IOM) study that produced this report on the Quality Improvement Organization (QIO) program, the congressional mandate for the study, and the overall study context. It includes a brief review of a predecessor report and its implications for the QIO program, as well as a summary of the methodology used for the present study and an overview of this report's organization.

Section 109 of the Medicare Prescription Drug, Improvement, and Modernization Act of 2003 (P.L. 108-173) requested an evaluation of the QIO program by the IOM and added new responsibilities for the QIOs related to the Part D prescription drug benefit included in that legislation. This study was undertaken in response to that request. It was sponsored by the Department of Health and Human Services and funded through the Quality Improvement Group of the Centers for Medicare and Medicaid Services (CMS), which manages the QIO program. The IOM integrated ·this study into its Redesigning Health Insurance project, which was initiated in 2004 to perform in-depth analyses of the structural and finance mechanisms that can be used to promote health care quality and performance improvement. The Committee on Redesigning Health Insurance Performance Measures, Payment, and Performance Improvement Programs (referred to as the Committee on Redesigning Health Insurance) is the most recent IOM committee to study health care quality and to build on the findings and conclusions of two earlier IOM reports—*To Err Is Human: Building a Safer Health System* (IOM, 2000) and *Crossing the Quality Chasm: A New Health System for the 21st Century* (IOM, 2001). Those and the subsequent series of 10 reports, known as the *Quality Chasm* series, concluded that the fragmentation of the health care system inhibited the delivery of high-quality care and that care was not being delivered in a patient-centered, effective manner. This new series of reports being produced under the Redesigning Health Insurance project—the *Pathways to Quality Health Care* series—builds on the vision of those previous reports by laying out the steps needed to drive fundamental change in the environmental factors affecting health care delivery to enhance quality and performance.

The first report of the Committee on Redesigning Health Insurance, *Performance Measurement: Accelerating Improvement,* was published in 2005 in response to P.L. 108-173, section 238 (IOM, 2006). That report offers a set of performance measures that can be used to track improvements in health care quality. It also recommends the creation of a national system for measurement of and reporting on the quality of health care that would establish national health care goals, develop standardized measures, and formulate data collection and public reporting procedures designed to foster health care quality.

This is the second report produced by the Committee on Redesigning Health Insurance. Focusing on performance improvement, it considers the history, role, and effectiveness of the QIO program and its potential to promote quality improvement within a changing environment that includes standardized performance measures and new data collection and reporting requirements.

A third report, like the *Performance Measurement* report based on section 238 of P.L. 108-173, is planned as part of the Redesigning Health Insurance project. That report will focus on payment strategies that can be used to incentivize performance and quality improvement and will be published in 2006.

BACKGROUND

Health care spending in the United States is higher than that in any other industrialized country (Reinhardt et al., 2004). Yet the quality of health care in America is not what it should be, a gap well documented by the IOM and health policy researchers (IOM, 2000, 2001, 2006). For example:

- Adults, on average, receive just more than half of the clinical services known to be beneficial for their conditions and tend to receive many unnecessary services (McGlynn et al., 2003).
- Wide disparities exist in the use of health care services and patterns of health care based on geographic location, the supply of health care ser-

vices, and race and ethnicity (Fisher et al., 2003a,b). Ethnic disparities in the treatment of Medicare beneficiaries are evident, with minorities receiving lower-quality mental health and preventive care services, on average, than whites and Asians (Leatherman and McCarthy, 2005).

• Adverse drug events for patients in hospitals and ambulatory care settings are a serious problem, and many such events are preventable (Leatherman and McCarthy, 2005).

• Reporting of serious quality problems in nursing homes varies widely, ranging from 6 percent of nursing homes cited in one state to 54 percent in another; serious deficiencies are generally understated (GAO, 2006).

• Sicker adults in the United States are more likely to report medical, medication, and laboratory errors than their counterparts in Australia, Canada, New Zealand, Germany, and the United Kingdom (Schoen et al., 2005).

• The United States is among the few industrialized countries that does not ensure access to health care services for its population; in 2004, 45.8 million people in the United States lacked health insurance (U.S. Census Bureau, 2005).

• Health information and communications technologies which could contribute to improved quality are available, but their adoption by providers has been slow. Among physician practices generally, only 18 percent of physicians use electronic health records; for those in solo or small-group practices, the figure is just 13 percent (Miller and Sim, 2004).

These examples illustrate the magnitude of the need to improve the quality of care offered by all types of providers and practitioners. Medicare can and should play an important role in meeting this need.

The Medicare program provides coverage for health care services for an estimated 41.7 million people who are disabled, have end-stage renal disease, or are aged 65 and older; the program spent more than $295 billion on benefits in 2004 (CMS, 2004; KFF, 2005). Chronic conditions are common among the noninstitutionalized Medicare population: 87 percent have at least one such condition, 36 percent have three or more, and 32 percent have limitations in activities of daily living (KFF, 2005). Care for patients with chronic conditions often should, but often does not, include coordination among practitioners in different care settings and smooth transitions as patients move from one setting to another.

Medicare, through CMS, currently manages 53 QIO contracts (one for each state, Puerto Rico, the District of Columbia, and the Virgin Islands; for simplicity, this report refers to "53 states"). The QIO program is aimed at improving the quality of Medicare through national oversight and monitoring of Medicare services and billing, as well as through state-based efforts in which the QIOs work directly with health care providers (SSA,

1935a). The national and state levels of the program are charged with a variety of functions:

- Improving the quality of care provided to Medicare beneficiaries by ensuring that providers meet professionally recognized, evidence-based standards and guidelines.
- Protecting beneficiaries' rights, responding to their complaints, and investigating evidence of poor-quality care.
- Protecting the Medicare Trust Funds by reviewing claims patterns and suspicious cases for the inappropriate use of services or incorrect billing codes.
- More recently, improving prescription drug therapy under the Medicare Part D prescription drug benefit (SSA, 1935b; CMS, 2002).

QIOs offer technical assistance to health care providers—including home health care agencies, hospitals, nursing homes, and physician practices—to improve the quality of care they offer. QIOs also serve as conveners of and collaborators with the relevant organizations in their local communities to promote better-quality care.

The Medicare program includes other quality-related functions, such as the Survey and Certification of providers to ensure that they meet CMS's Conditions of Participation. Separate End-Stage Renal Disease Networks, similar to the QIOs, have quality improvement responsibilities for the care of beneficiaries who qualify for Medicare because they have end-stage renal disease. CMS also supports the development, implementation, and reporting of quality measures and the development of consumer satisfaction surveys. This report recognizes these other quality activities within CMS but focuses mainly on the QIO program.

Congressional Mandate for This Study

The legislative request for an IOM evaluation of the QIO program (see Box I.1) came at a time when the U.S. Congress was examining various strategies for the promotion of quality improvement within CMS. Congress mandated that the IOM provide an overview of the QIO program and assess and report on the following:

- The duties of the QIOs
- The extent to which other organizations could perform these duties at least as well as the QIOs
- The extent to which QIOs improve the quality of care under Medicare
- The effectiveness of QIO case reviews and other actions

- Funding amounts and sources for the QIOs
- Oversight of the QIOs

The congressional request to IOM did not include a fiscal integrity review.

As noted above, the IOM charged the Committee on Redesigning Health Insurance with conducting the QIO study. The committee members

---

BOX I.1   Mandate to the IOM Under the Medicare Prescription Drug, Improvement, and Modernization Act of 2003 (P.L. 108-173)

SEC. 109. EXPANDING THE WORK OF MEDICARE QUALITY IMPROVEMENT ORGANIZATIONS TO INCLUDE PARTS C AND D.

(d) IOM STUDY OF QIOs—

    (1) IN GENERAL—The Secretary shall request the Institute of Medicine of the National Academy of Sciences to conduct an evaluation of the program under Part B of Title XI of the Social Security Act. The study shall include a review of the following:

        (A) An overview of the program under such part.

        (B) The duties of organizations with contracts with the Secretary under such part.

        (C) The extent to which quality improvement organizations improve the quality of care for medicare beneficiaries.

        (D) The extent to which other entities could perform such quality improvement functions as well as, or better than, quality improvement organizations.

        (E) The effectiveness of reviews and other actions conducted by such organizations in carrying out those duties.

        (F) The source and amount of funding for such organizations.

        (G) The conduct of oversight of such organizations.

    (2) REPORT TO CONGRESS—Not later than June 1, 2006, the Secretary shall submit to Congress a report on the results of the study described in paragraph (1), including any recommendations for legislation.

    (3) INCREASED COMPETITION—If the Secretary finds based on the study conducted under paragraph (1) that other entities could improve quality in the Medicare program as well as, or better than, the current quality improvement organizations, then the Secretary shall provide for such increased competition through the addition of new types of entities which may perform quality improvement functions.

have a broad range of expertise in and experience with many aspects of the health care system and the Medicare program (see the biographical sketches of the committee members in Appendix E). A subcommittee comprising individuals with particular expertise in quality improvement issues conducted the data collection and analysis for this study.

In addition to the mandated evaluation of the accomplishments and limitations of the QIO program, the committee assessed the future of the program to determine how it can strengthen its role in the new environment of quality improvement, performance measurement, and payment incentives. The report therefore considers how the QIO program can best contribute to and support growing interest among health plans, purchasers, providers, and consumers in achieving higher levels of performance and health care quality as envisioned by the *Quality Chasm* reports.

The IOM Redesigning Health Insurance Project

Recognizing the deficiencies of the health care system discussed above, earlier IOM studies proposed six quality aims for U.S. health care: it should be safe, effective, patient-centered, timely, efficient, and equitable (IOM, 2001). These aims were subsequently incorporated into the CMS *Quality Improvement Roadmap* (CMS, 2005).

Inconsistencies in the quality of health care services occur at all levels in the health care system and among the various types of providers and clinicians; the problem is not due simply to a few outliers or the bottom quartile of providers. Achievement of the six quality aims will require fundamental reforms within the health care environment that transform relationships at many levels, including those between patients and clinicians, within health care organizations, and within the settings in which practitioners function.

The goal of the IOM Redesigning Health Insurance project is to develop structural and financial reforms for public and private health insurance and other health care systems that will result in a greater emphasis on performance and quality. The committee's reports focus on operational and finance mechanisms that will speed the elimination of current inconsistencies in health care quality, accomplish the six quality aims cited above, and promote and reward performance improvement. The changes needed to achieve these goals encompass performance measurement, the QIO program, and payment incentives.

An earlier IOM report on health care quality highlighted the need for government agencies to pave the way in introducing quality improvements in the public and private sectors of the health care system (IOM, 2002). Medicare, as the largest single purchaser of health care and a national leader in health quality assessment, now has an opportunity to align incentives within CMS to improve the quality of care throughout the health care system by establishing a comprehensive performance measurement and reporting system and rewarding selected providers of high-quality care. Not only could Medicare align these programs now, but it could also promote the spread of best-care practices through Conditions of Participation, Survey and Certification requirements, and other regulatory and research authorities, as well as through the QIO program. In addition, Medicare would greatly magnify its impact by coordinating its policies with those of other major government programs, such as Medicaid, the State Children's Health Insurance Program, and the program of the Veterans Health Administration, as recommended in earlier IOM studies (IOM, 2002, 2006).

Significant opportunities therefore exist for Medicare to create and lead a coordinated approach to quality improvement that encourages private-sector participation. Medicare's policies and practices can influence some private insurers (CMS, 2004). To the extent that private insurers share Medicare's interest in improving quality and adopt Medicare policies, reporting burdens on providers will be reduced, and the potential impact on quality should be amplified. Private insurers could create comparable and consistent programs requiring providers to report their performance measures and could reward quality providers who met certain standards, based on scientific evidence and the recommendations of this committee. A consistent approach to quality among insurers and purchasers of health care could hasten the adoption of improvements by providers.

Performance Measurement Report and Its Implications for the QIO Program

The future of the QIO program is closely intertwined with performance measurement and reporting and with payment incentives for providers. It is therefore useful to review the key conclusions and recommendations of the committee's first report, on performance measurement, as background for an assessment of the history and the future of the QIO program.

Performance Measurement: Accelerating Improvement was produced under a separate congressional mandate (section 238) in P.L. 108-173. That report examined performance measures that could ultimately be used for a Medicare payment system that would reward providers for quality care. The study demonstrated that a multitude of measurement sets currently in use measure the same clinical conditions. However, the specific details of the measures are frequently inconsistent, creating variations that present barriers to effective data collection and reporting and unnecessary burdens on providers. In addition, important areas of care are not yet being measured, nor do accepted measures yet exist for these areas. The *Performance Measurement* report therefore offers a comprehensive strategy that can be used to overcome these barriers to the use of quality measures in health care. This strategy includes the creation of a National Quality Coordination Board (NQCB) to facilitate the coordination of functions currently carried out by various separate organizations, and to take on certain activities necessary at the national level to enhance performance measurement and reporting (IOM, 2006). For further detail, see Chapter 3 of the present report.

The development of a national system for performance measurement and reporting will require strong national- and community-level infrastructures to support the efforts of health care institutions and individual providers to participate in new performance measurement, data collection, and reporting processes. The committee expects that many providers, particularly physicians in small and solo practices, will need assistance both with the collection and use of the new measures and with the adoption and implementation of electronic systems to facilitate record keeping and processes for the improvement of health care. Translation of the recommendations offered in the *Performance Measurement* report into operational procedures represents a unique opportunity for the QIO program as a whole and its core contractors to contribute to the development and implementation of the necessary infrastructure and to help improve the quality of the health care delivery system. If an infrastructure such as that provided by the QIO program were not in place nationally, it would be necessary to create one, because the private market has not met providers' widespread need for assistance in improving quality. This perspective served as a foundation for the committee's review of the assets and capabilities of the QIO program and assessment of the program's potential role in contributing to the future of health care quality improvement.

The committee concluded that the new requirements for health care performance measurement and reporting may help stimulate the adoption of electronic health records by many providers; likewise, realignment of the financial incentives in the health insurance system to reward higher levels of quality and performance improvement will likely stimulate behavioral and institutional reforms that will improve the quality of health care delivery. Yet these strategies are insufficient to create the fundamental transformation necessary to achieve the six aims of the IOM quality initiative. Many providers will need technical assistance to help achieve the aims.

As envisioned in the *Performance Measurement* report, the NQCB will have seven key functions, most of which could benefit from both the support of the QIO program and the involvement of QIOs:

- Specify the purposes and aims of the U.S. health care system.
- Establish short- and long-term national goals for improving the nation's health care system.

• Designate or, if necessary, develop standardized performance measures for evaluating the performance of current providers and monitoring the nation's progress toward these goals.

• Ensure the creation of data collection, validation, and aggregation processes.

• Establish public reporting methods responsive to the needs of all stakeholders.

• Identify and fund an agenda for research on new measures that can be used to address existing gaps.

• Evaluate the impact of performance measurement on pay-for-performance, quality improvement, public reporting, and other policies.

CMS will need to redeploy its resources in the QIO program and beyond to support the implementation of a national system for measurement and reporting and to sustain other performance improvement programs that are rapidly moving forward for Medicare. In the face of these transformational changes, the role and the capacity of the QIO program deserve a critical examination.

AUDIENCES FOR THIS REPORT

This report is intended for multiple audiences, including members of Congress, the federal executive branch, the QIOs, health care providers and clinicians, Medicare beneficiaries, and stakeholder groups. Some audiences will be interested in extensive detail on the QIO program, while others will want only a brief overview of the program and the committee's findings, conclusions, and recommendations. Part II of this report was prepared for those in the former category; in addition, the appendixes to the report include some of the program details reviewed by the committee, including previously unpublished data collected specifically for this study. Part I is intended for those desiring an overview prior to or in lieu of reading the more detailed treatment in Part II.

STUDY APPROACH

The Committee on Redesigning Health Insurance and the Subcommittee on Quality Improvement Organization Program Evaluation gathered data on the highly complex QIO program from a wide variety of sources and compared the conclusions drawn in those sources. The following data collection methods were used:

• A focused review of the literature on the impact of quality improvement and the QIO program's improvement efforts

- The collection of data from all 53 QIOs through the SurveyMonkey website
- Quantitative analyses of QIOs' relative performance on various tasks of the 7th scope of work (SOW),[1] based on CMS contract performance evaluation scores
- Site visits by 18 committee members and IOM staff to 11 different QIOs and one Department of Health and Human Services regional office
- Telephone interviews with the chief executive officers of 20 randomly selected QIOs
- An in-person focus group discussion with the chief executive officers of 11 QIOs
- A 3-day briefing by CMS staff, supplemented by specific data requested from CMS
- A half-day public workshop involving members of the committee and subcommittee, academic researchers, experts on quality improvement who are working in the field, and other stakeholders
- Access to QIOnet, a CMS internal website for the QIO program that includes performance data by state
- Face-to-face interviews with representatives of four selected QIOs, four randomly selected QIO Support Center staff, and the respective chief executive officers
- Formal and informal discussions with staff and members of the American Health Quality Association, the national organization that represents all QIOs
- Informal discussions with representatives of consumer and beneficiary organizations and various providers
- The collection of data at national conferences and meetings related to QIOs
- Soliciting of suggestions from businesses and other entities providing QIO-like services

Each of these methods is described in detail in Chapter 6.

Various constraints, such as the timing of the 7th and 8th SOWs and the budget for this study, made it impossible to build data collection into

---

[1]CMS uses the acronym SOW for both "scope of work" and "statement of work." In this report, the committee uses SOW only for "scope of work" and adopts the general usage of SOW accepted within the QIO community, in which the term denotes either tasks required in general or the time period of a contract. When discussing specific details of QIO work, the committee is referring to the contract itself. For example, the 7th SOW covered the period from 2002 to 2005. It required all QIOs to provide technical assistance to nursing homes, and the contract for this SOW stipulated that QIOs must recruit 30 percent of nursing homes to develop a plan of action.

the QIO contracts: the 7th SOW was under way before the start of the IOM contract, and the 8th would not be able to produce data in time for the present study. Timing and budget also precluded travel to all the QIOs. For the same reasons, the committee was unable to meet federal requirements to conduct formal surveys of consumers and providers, although it recognized the importance of collecting such data. Furthermore, recent changes in the operations of the QIO program that occurred after the preparation of the present report cannot be reflected here. Another constraint was the need for the IOM to agree to maintain confidentiality to gain access to certain data from CMS and individual QIO sources; hence, most of the data are reported in aggregate form and contain no identifiers that could be linked to a particular QIO or state.

Despite the above limitations, the committee's various data collection methods as a whole provided a substantial amount of data and information. The committee was able to use triangulation to check the consistency of the findings derived from various sources and methods, and more than one committee member or IOM staff member was involved with most of the data collection and analysis. The committee gave greatest weight to the data collected uniformly from all the QIOs through the web-based tool, to the telephone interviews used to collect data from a random sample of QIOs, and to the data for each QIO from the Dashboard section of CMS's internal website.

ORGANIZATION OF THIS REPORT

As alluded to above, this report consists of two major sections. Part I consists of five policy-oriented chapters that describe the evolution of the QIO program (Chapter 1), the main findings and conclusions emerging from the committee's evaluation of the program (Chapter 2), a summary of *Performance Measurement: Accelerating Improvement* and its relation to the QIO program and other entities (Chapter 3), and recommendations concerning QIO program activities and oversight of the QIO program by CMS (Chapters 4 and 5, respectively).

Part II of this report, Chapters 6 through 13, provides more detail on the committee's analysis of the QIO program that fulfills the congressional mandate for this study. It begins by further describing the methods used for this study (Chapter 6). Focusing on the 7th and 8th SOWs, from 2002 to the present, Part II then provides an in-depth discussion of the QIO program and its funding, as well as the structure of the state-level organizations (Chapter 7); current program activities and their impacts (Chapters 8 to 12); and CMS oversight of the program (Chapter 13). Collectively, Part II serves as part of the basis for the conclusions and recommendations presented in Part I. The specific tasks of QIOs in the 7th and the 8th SOWs, described in Chapters 8 to 12, encompass technical assistance for quality improvement, beneficiary education and communications, and the protection of beneficiaries and program integrity. In Part II, the committee's evaluation of the program (summarized in Chapter 2) is woven into the detailed descriptions of the program, which reflect a literature review, as well as analyses conducted specifically for this study. The report concludes with several appendixes that present tables with supporting data (Appendix A), describe private-sector organizations offering services related to quality improvement (Appendix B), review various approaches to program evaluation (Appendix C), provide a glossary and listing of acronyms used in the report (Appendix D), and present biographical sketches of committee members (Appendix E).

REFERENCES

CMS (Centers for Medicare and Medicaid Services). 2002. *7th Statement of Work (SOW)*. [Online]. Available: http://www.cms.hhs.gov/qio [accessed April, 9, 2005].

CMS. 2004. *2004 CMS Statistics*. Washington, DC: U.S. Department of Health and Human Services.

CMS. July 2005. *Quality Improvement Roadmap*. [Online]. Available: http://www.medicaldevices.org/public/issues/documents/CMSMedicareroadmap.pdf [accessed December 26, 2005].

Fisher ES, Wennberg DE, Stukel TA, Gottlieb DJ, Lucas FL, Pinder EL. 2003a. The implications of regional variations in Medicare spending. Part 1. The content, quality, and accessibility of care. *Annals of Internal Medicine* 138(4):273–287.

Fisher ES, Wennberg DE, Stukel TA, Gottlieb DJ, Lucas FL, Pinder EL. 2003b. The implications of regional variations in Medicare spending. Part 2. Health outcomes and satisfaction with care. *Annals of Internal Medicine* 138(4):288–298.

GAO (U.S. Government Accountability Office). 2006. *Despite Increased Oversight, Challenges Remain in Ensuring High-Quality Care and Resident Safety*. Washington, DC: U.S. Government Printing Office.

IOM (Institute of Medicine). 2000. *To Err Is Human: Building a Safer Health System*. Kohn LT, Corrigan JM, Donaldson MS, eds. Washington, DC: National Academy Press.

IOM. 2001. *Crossing the Quality Chasm: A New Health System for the 21st Century*. Washington, DC: National Academy Press.

IOM. 2002. *Leadership by Example: Coordinating Government Roles in Improving Health Care Quality*. Corrigan JM, Eden J, Smith BM, eds. Washington, DC: National Academy Press.

IOM. 2006. *Performance Measurement: Accelerating Improvement*. Washington, DC: The National Academies Press.

KFF (The Henry J. Kaiser Family Foundation). 2005. *Medicare Chart Book 2005*. Washington, DC: The Henry J. Kaiser Family Foundation.

Leatherman S, McCarthy D. May 2005. *Quality of Health Care for Medicare Beneficiaries: A Chartbook*. New York: The Commonwealth Fund.

McGlynn EA, Asch SM, Adams J, Keesey J, Hicks J, DeCristofaro A, Kerr EA. 2003. The quality of health care delivered to adults in the United States. *New England Journal of Medicine* 348(26):2635–2645.

Medicare Prescription Drug, Improvement, and Modernization Act. 2003. *Medicare Prescription Drug, Improvement, and Modernization Act of 2003* (Enrolled as Agreed to or Passed by Both House and Senate). Section 109: Expanding the Work of Medicare Quality Improvement Organizations to Include Parts C and D. Washington, DC: U.S. Congress.

Miller RH, Sim I. 2004. Physicians' use of electronic medical records: Barriers and solutions. *Health Affairs* 23(2):116–126.

Reinhardt UE, Hussey PS, Anderson GF. 2004. U.S. health care spending in an international context. *Health Affairs* 23(3):10–25.

Schoen C, Osborn R, Huynh PT, Doty M, Zapert K, Peugh J, Davis K. 2005. Taking the pulse of health care systems: Experiences of patients with health problems in six countries. *Health Affairs.* Web Exclusive: w5.509.

SSA (Social Security Act). 1935a. U.S. Code 42. H.R. 7260, Section 1862g.

SSA. 1935b. U.S. Code 42. H.R. 7260, Sections 1151–1165.

U.S. Census Bureau. 2005. *Health Insurance Coverage: 2004.* [Online]. Available: http://www.census.gov/hhes/www/hlthins/hlthin04/hlth04asc.html [accessed August 30, 2005].

Part I

INTRODUCTION

The committee's recommendations for the Quality Improvement Organization (QIO) program, presented in Chapters 4 and 5, are built on a dual foundation. First is an extensive study of the QIO program conducted for this project. It included a review of the history and various aspects of the program, based on data gathered from the Centers for Medicare and Medicaid Services (CMS), data gathered directly from the QIOs, information from representatives of the QIO community and stakeholders, a literature review, and original data analyses. The second foundation for the recommendations in this report is the recommendations presented in the committee's first report in the *Pathways to Quality Health Care* series, *Performance Measurement: Accelerating Improvement* (IOM, 2006). That report presents a view of the future of health care delivery that includes a national system for coordinating the measurement and reporting of a broad set of quality measures, some of which will be used to implement provider payment systems designed to reward quality and performance improvement. Provider payment systems are the focus of the committee's next report, which will be published in 2006.

As noted in the introduction to the present report, Part I is policy oriented and includes the committee's judgments, while Part II provides the detailed evidence base on the QIO program, including data collected specifically for this study, that helped inform those judgments. Part I consists of five chapters:

- Chapter 1 presents a historical overview of the QIO program and its predecessor organizations. Because this is the third time the Institute of Medicine has been asked to examine Medicare's quality assurance program, this chapter also includes some details from the previous two reviews.
- Chapter 2 provides a summary of the key findings discussed in detail in Part II and the conclusions the committee drew from those findings.
- Chapter 3 gives a summary of *Performance Measurement: Accelerating Improvement* (IOM, 2006). The first part of the chapter presents that report's key recommendations concerning measure sets and the system needed to promote their use. The second part provides a discussion of what is required to implement a national system for performance measurement and of how QIOs and other entities might carry out some of those tasks.
- Chapter 4 provides recommendations regarding future directions for the QIO program. Included is the rationale for those recommendations, which is based on the findings and conclusions presented in Chapter 2 and the committee's prior recommendations as summarized in Chapter 3, as well as additional information.
- Chapter 5 presents the committee's recommendations on the oversight of the QIO program by CMS. This is a critical topic given that CMS will play a significant role in implementing a national system for performance measurement and payment incentives and has responsibility for the QIO program.

The committee encourages those readers who would like a more in-depth description of the QIO program and its management to turn to Part II for the data used to support the findings, conclusions, and recommendations presented in Part I.

REFERENCE

IOM (Institute of Medicine). 2006. *Performance Measurement: Accelerating Improvement.* Washington, DC: The National Academies Press.

1

A Historical Perspective and the Current QIO Program

CHAPTER SUMMARY

This chapter presents an overview of the health care quality assessment activities of Medicare from the early days of quality assurance through the evolution to quality improvement and the current Quality Improvement Organization (QIO) program. It focuses particularly on the QIO program from 2002 to 2005, the period evaluated in this report, and the next contract period, which is intended to achieve quality improvements through activities that will transform systems, processes, and outcomes of care.

The federal government's interest in ensuring the quality of health care for Medicare beneficiaries in the United States originated with an emphasis on detecting the overuse and inappropriate use of Medicare benefits (primarily for cost-containment purposes). Over time, this interest expanded to include the measurement of improvements in the quality of care because such measurements are more reliable for monitoring the performance of health care providers. The Centers for Medicare and Medicaid Services (CMS) is now in the early stages of promoting transformational changes in the way providers deliver care.[1] Over the course of more than 35 years and these shifts in emphasis, the priorities of the federal quality assurance program changed from utilization reviews of individual case records to collaboration with providers for the improvement of overall patterns and processes of care. Such collaboration allows the federal quality assurance

---

[1]CMS views this transformation as taking place through the adoption of certain strategies (measurement and reporting, implementation of health information technology, process redesign, and changes in organizational culture). CMS believes the QIO program, along with other efforts, can lead to measurable changes in the health care delivery system to align with the six aims set forth by the Institute of Medicine (IOM, 2001) and CMS's vision of "the right care for every patient every time" (Pugh, 2005:2).

program to play a more systemic role in improving the quality of health care and ultimately in yielding better health outcomes for beneficiaries.

The history of the Medicare program for quality improvement offers several key insights that reflect this evolutionary process and are relevant to consideration of how the Quality Improvement Organization (QIO) program might be used most effectively in the future:

- Many QIOs emerged from the antecedent organizations and retain staff, boards, and executive leaders with long histories of involvement in the Medicare quality improvement program (see Chapter 7 for a discussion of the current structure and staffing of QIOs). This continuity represents a strength for most organizations, although in some cases it could lead to a lack of creativity that can accompany low turnover among leaders.
- Although the views of many providers have changed, some hospital executives still perceive QIOs as "regulatory agencies." This perception reflects the previous activities of the organizations (Bradley et al., 2005; NORC, 2004; data from site visits).
- Frequently changing priorities required the QIO program and its contractors to demonstrate a flexibility and an ability to adapt to new priorities, expand activities, shift functions, and acquire new skills in response to tasks and priorities specified in CMS's statements of work. The flexibility and adaptability of the program bode well for its ability to carry out new functions in the future, but its constant changes have also created program discontinuities, stress for staff, and challenges to evaluation of the program (see Chapter 13).

This chapter first provides a brief overview of the history of the QIO program and then describes the evolution of the program from the early days of Medicare. The discussion is most detailed for the two most recent contract periods (the 7th and 8th scopes of work [SOWs]).[2]

HISTORY OF THE QIO PROGRAM

Certain challenges must be addressed when one is evaluating a complex public program with a lengthy history that has evolved in response to shift-

---

[2]CMS contracts with private organizations for QIO services in each state for 3-year periods. CMS uses the acronym SOW for both "scope of work" and "statement of work." In this report, the committee uses SOW only for "scope of work" and adopts the general usage of SOW by the QIO community, in which the term denotes either tasks required in general or the time period of a contract. When discussing specific details of QIO work, the committee refers to the contract itself. For example, the 7th SOW was from 2002 to 2005. It required all QIOs to provide technical assistance to nursing homes, and the contract for this SOW stipulated that QIOs must recruit 30 percent of nursing homes to develop a plan of action.

ing health care priorities. One must choose certain time periods and program features on which to focus and develop criteria for assessment of the program's performance and impact. The evaluation must also be useful to various audiences: policy makers, those managing the program, those working in the program both at the federal level and in contractor organizations, and those providers and practitioners who do and do not participate in the program.

The QIO program has existed in various forms for more than 35 years. As noted earlier, beginning a few years after the creation of Medicare in 1965 and continuing through its first 20 years of existence, the Medicare quality assurance program placed a strong emphasis on utilization control and focused attention on hospital and physician outliers that provided substandard or unnecessary care. In 1990, in response to a congressional mandate, the Institute of Medicine (IOM) completed a major review of quality assurance activities and the Medicare program's contractors for local quality services, called Peer Review Organizations (IOM, 1990). The IOM report recommended a shift away from utilization review and the traditional regulatory approach used to control aberrant providers and toward a focus on health care decision making, health outcomes, and the development of a professional capacity to improve care (IOM, 1990). The adoption of many of that report's recommendations contributed to further changes in the QIO program. One recommendation that was not adopted, however, called for the creation of a technical advisory panel that would assist with the evaluation of the recommended quality assurance program and with program management and operations.

The program also evolved in response to changing definitions of "quality." In a literature review conducted for its 1990 study, the IOM found over 100 definitions of quality of care. In 1974, the IOM had defined quality only in the context of specifying the purpose of a quality assurance system ("to make health care more effective in bettering the health status and satisfaction of a population, within the resources which society and individuals have chosen to spend for that care" [IOM, 1974:1–2]). Definitions of quality were numerous and incongruent. In its 1990 report, the IOM expanded previous definitions to include both individuals and populations, adopted outcome measures that linked processes to outcomes, and recognized the importance of patient and provider satisfaction. The IOM defined quality of care as "the degree to which health services for individuals and populations increase the likelihood of desired health outcomes and are consistent with current professional knowledge" (IOM, 1990:21). Later, in its *Quality Chasm* series, the IOM developed a vision for the future of health care, which was based on six aims for the delivery of quality care: health care should be safe, effective, patient-centered, timely, efficient, and equitable. In addition to these six aims, the *Quality Chasm* report suggested ten rules for how care should be delivered, focusing on the point that health care should be viewed as a relationship between patients and providers aimed at yielding the best health outcomes, and specified various properties of the health care system itself that would help foster that relationship (IOM, 2001).

The Committee on Redesigning Health Insurance considered looking back to 1990 to assess the QIO program's impact, to consider how the program evolved in response to the 1990 IOM report, and to examine the impacts of those changes on the health care system with respect to the vision of high-quality health care set forth in the *Quality Chasm* series. Even if the QIO program had implemented all of the prior IOM report's recommendations, however, it would still be necessary to assess whether the program is now well positioned to foster quality improvement in the present and future health care environments. Fundamental changes in the Medicare program and the practice of medicine, as well as in the broader health care system, have occurred since 1990; these changes have contributed to new expectations and new needs for guidance and assistance in the adaptation of earlier practices and processes to new standards of care.

For example, when the earlier IOM committee began its study nearly 20 years ago, it did not anticipate that Medicare would now be reporting national performance measures publicly by provider name for nearly all hospitals, nursing homes, and home health care agencies. It could not have known that some private purchasers would be implementing pay-for-performance systems or that the Medicare Payment Advisory Commission (MedPAC), created to support Congress with data and advice related to the operation of the Medicare program, would recommend that Medicare consider paying for performance as well. Also, the fact that the QIO program or an individual organization in a particular state did or did not do well during the 4th SOW might have little bearing on its performance during the 7th SOW because the nature of the work and the methods used to measure it have changed substantially.

Rather than comparing the present performance of the QIO program against earlier recommendations and current expectations, the committee decided to supplement its evaluation with an assessment of how the program might contribute to future quality improvement efforts. A key factor in this assessment was the above-noted adaptable nature of the Medicare quality assurance and improvement program and the ability of QIOs to respond to new demands and changes in each CMS contract.

Other, practical reasons influenced the committee's decision to limit its detailed review to a fairly recent period. The QIO program's management shifted direction during previous SOWs from requiring evaluations of local, specific projects to requiring statewide evaluations, which allowed the aggregation of data to show national effects. National measures, however, were not broadly used until the 7th SOW contract period (2002 to 2005). Thus, comparable national data aggregated from each state were limited or nonexistent before the 7th SOW. Also, older data on program operations would have been more difficult to obtain.

The committee determined that it would be most useful to focus attention on describing the history of the QIO program as it existed during the 7th SOW, and, as noted above, the descriptive data and analyses of the program in Part II of this report relate primarily to the 7th and 8th SOWs. Nonetheless, the next section of this chapter describes selected elements of Medicare's quality programs from their beginning to the present contract period. An understanding of the QIO program's evolution can provide guidance for assessing the program's potential value in strengthening the quality improvement efforts of CMS and the role CMS could play in implementing the recommendations formulated in the recent IOM report *Performance Measurement: Accelerating Improvement* (IOM, 2006). Such an understanding can also illuminate reasons for the need to restructure and strengthen the program.

EVOLUTION OF MEDICARE'S QUALITY IMPROVEMENT PROGRAM

Early Quality Review Programs

Experimental Medical Care Review Organizations

Soon after the enactment of the Medicare program in 1965, concerns developed about the quality and cost of health care services provided to beneficiaries (Bhatia et al., 2000). In addition to creating health benefits, the initial Medicare law (P.L. 89-97) focused on patient safety and access to care from competent health care providers. It required hospital-based utilization review, state licensure of physicians, and voluntary hospital accreditation by the Joint Commission on Accreditation of Hospitals (now called the Joint Commission on Accreditation of Healthcare Organizations) or state certification (Jost, 1989). In 1971, the U.S. Congress authorized Experimental Medical Care Review Organizations (EMCROs) to evaluate the use of services provided to Medicare beneficiaries. EMCROs examined individual Medicare cases and sought to reduce the unnecessary utilization of services in inpatient and ambulatory care settings through the education of physicians and research (IOM, 1990). EMCROs were voluntary groups of physicians who received grants from the National Center for Health Services Research (the predecessor agency to the current Agency for Healthcare Research and Quality) to review the services provided through the Medicare and Medicaid programs (Sprague, 2002). The EMCRO program itself existed from 1970 to 1975.

Professional Standards Review Organizations

In 1972, amendments to Title XI of the Social Security Act (P.L. 92-603) authorized the establishment of Professional Standards Review Organizations (PSROs), new locally based organizations, to replace the EMCROs. PSROs were sponsored by physicians, and only local physicians could evaluate cases. Like the EMCROs, they used implicit review (decision making based on individual professional judgment) to determine the medical necessity of the services provided (Sprague, 2002). They targeted egregious cases by comparing the care given by the provider with local standards of care and practice patterns. Physicians regarded the PSROs primarily as adversaries and as enforcers of cost containment that punished individual providers by recommending sanctions (Bhatia et al., 2000; Sprague, 2002).

Although the focus of the PSROs was still on retrospective utilization review of hospital admissions and lengths of stay, PSROs also participated in Medical Care Evaluation Studies (later called Quality Review Studies) to address concerns regarding quality of care (Jost, 1989). PSROs were not viewed as motivators for systemwide quality improvement, however (Sprague, 2002). Moreover, studies conducted in the late 1970s and early 1980s demonstrated that PSROs had little if any impact on the quality of care or the containment of expenditures (IOM, 1990).

Utilization and Quality Control Peer Review Organizations

In 1982, the Peer Review Improvement Act (P.L. 97-248) replaced PSROs with Utilization and Quality Control Peer Review Organizations (PROs). There was a total of 54 PROs, one for each state and territory.[3] The PROs continued the focus on medical necessity and standards of care in the provision of Medicare services. Congress retained elements of local peer review by requiring the PROs to be physician-sponsored (which required at least 10 percent of locally practicing physicians to participate as reviewers) or to be physician-access (which required at least one physician of each specialty in the area to be available to conduct reviews of medical records) (CMS, 2004b). New requirements were that physicians could not review their own close colleagues and that the PROs had to include at least one consumer representative on their governing board. Unlike PSROs, PROs could have for-profit status (Jost, 1989). Funding of the overall program shifted to an apportionment drawn directly from the Medicare Trust Funds instead of annual appropriations (IOM, 1990; Sprague, 2002).

---

[3]PROs were managed for each of the 50 states; the District of Columbia; Puerto Rico; the U.S. Virgin Islands; and the combined area of Guam, American Samoa, and the Northern Marianas.

Although PROs continued to target inappropriate or unnecessary services and cost containment during the 1980s, implementation of the hospital prospective payment system in 1983 drew attention to premature discharges (Rogers et al., 1990) and the potential underuse of necessary services. By the late 1990s, the development of Medicare managed care (Medicare+Choice, now Medicare Advantage) had added a further population of patients whose providers were subject to financial incentives to underuse services and who thus required the attention of the PROs (IOM, 1990; Sprague, 2002).

Early Quality Improvement Contract Cycles

In 1984, the Medicare program established contract cycles for the PROs and eventually lengthened those cycles to 3 years—the period often referred to as the SOW. Once the contracts had been awarded, they could be renewed after 3 years for the next SOW or opened to competitive bidding on the basis of the performance of the PRO. The discussion in this and the next section highlights key features of each SOW.

Each QIO contract is numbered. The 1st SOW, which began in 1984, lasted for 2 years (see Table 1.1). Subsequent SOWs lasted for 3 years each (except for the 3rd SOW, which had a 1-year extension).

1st Scope of Work

The 1st SOW (1984 to 1986) for PROs emphasized reducing inappropriate hospital admissions. PROs compared data from individual retrospective case reviews with implicit, professionally accepted standards and made recommendations for financial sanctions on individual providers (Bhatia et al., 2000). In addition, an offending physician or hospital could be required to create and follow a corrective action plan for improving the quality of care in the future. Providers perceived this as a form of punitive oversight, and it contributed to a hostile relationship between the PROs and providers (Bhatia et al., 2000). Also, some providers perceived this type of quality work as "cookbook" medicine and an affront to their profession (Sprague, 2002).

2nd and 3rd Scopes of Work

The 2nd SOW (1986 to 1989) added more quality-monitoring and review responsibilities. Although most case review activities remained focused on hospital inpatient care, the Omnibus Budget Reconciliation Act (OBRA) of 1986 (P.L. 99-509) extended some review activities to cover other settings, including skilled nursing facilities, home health care agencies, hospi-

TABLE 1.1   QIO Contract Cycles

Cycle or SOW	Dates	Name of Quality Improvement Entities	Name of Responsible Federal Agency
1st SOW	1984–1986	Peer Review Organizations (1983)	Health Care Financing Administration
2nd SOW	1986–1989	Peer Review Organizations	Health Care Financing Administration
3rd SOW	1989–1993	Peer Review Organizations	Health Care Financing Administration
4th SOW	1993–1996	Peer Review Organizations	Health Care Financing Administration
5th SOW	1996–1999	Peer Review Organizations	Health Care Financing Administration
6th SOW	1999–2002	Quality Improvement Organizations	Health Care Financing Administration/Centers for Medicare and Medicaid Services[a]
7th SOW	2002–2005	Quality Improvement Organizations	Centers for Medicare and Medicaid Services
8th SOW	2005–2008	Quality Improvement Organizations	Centers for Medicare and Medicaid Services

[a]The Health Care Financing Administration changed its name in 2001 to become the Centers for Medicare and Medicaid Services.

tal outpatient care settings, and eventually the physician's office setting (Jost, 1989).

OBRA also mandated an IOM study of the current state of quality in Medicare (IOM, 1990). Among other things, the IOM report recommended that the PROs become more proactive in their data collection activities to examine patterns of care and offer feedback to providers. The study concluded that PROs "constitute a potentially valuable infrastructure for quality assurance" that should "be improved and built on, not dismantled" (IOM, 1990:3). The report noted in particular that the PROs had established valuable organizational relationships and provided professional staff expertise. However, the report concluded that certain priorities needed to be revised: quality review and assurance should be emphasized over utilization and cost control; PROs should pay more attention to average practice patterns than to outliers; and PROs should be more involved in health care settings beyond inpatient hospital care. Additionally, the IOM report noted the burdens on providers imposed by the PRO program, its lack of positive incentives and punitive attitude toward providers, the hostile perceptions of the program among many physicians, and its redundancy with other quality assurance programs.

The IOM recognized that the PRO program had a vast and varied list of responsibilities and a budget amounting to less than 0.5 percent of annual Medicare expenditures on services, roughly the same proportion allotted to the PSRO program 10 years earlier. The IOM report concluded that this investment was unlikely to be sufficient to accomplish the tasks assigned to the PROs. The report recommended a reassessment of certain functions, such as some case reviews, appeals, and beneficiary outreach, to determine whether they might be performed nationally or regionally and by other agents (e.g., intermediaries and carriers).

The 1990 IOM report also noted that neither the PSRO nor the PRO program had conducted a comprehensive self-examination or been able to demonstrate its impact on the quality of care for Medicare beneficiaries. The report called for the creation of a technical advisory panel that would, among other things, advise the secretary of the U.S. Department of Health and Human Services on program evaluation. It stressed that the emphasis of the evaluation should be on documenting the impacts of the state organizations on the quality of care and their successes in working with providers on internal quality assurance efforts. Also emphasized was the importance of both the availability of objective evaluation criteria that could be used to assess each state's performance and the use of various methods, such as site visits by a panel of peer experts; however, no specific methods were recommended. Although the intent of the IOM recommendations to increase attention to quality assurance in more care settings was met, and objective criteria for the evaluation of each state's performance were eventually implemented, the impact of the PRO program was not evaluated. In addition, some of the new organizational structures recommended in the IOM report, including a technical advisory panel, were not created.

The 2nd and 3rd SOWs (1986 to 1993) continued to focus on retrospective case reviews and the detection of inappropriate use of services. During that period, however, PROs also shifted toward collaboration with providers to improve the overall delivery of care instead of focusing solely on punishing outliers (IOM, 1990; Bhatia et al., 2000). Prior methods relying on retrospective case data and peer review appeared to be increasingly inadequate for achieving the goal of quality improvement (Rubin et al., 1992). Finally, it became apparent that the standards of care themselves needed attention. In 1992, the Health Care Financing Administration (HCFA), the predecessor of CMS, implemented the Health Care Quality Improvement Initiative to move from targeting individual provider errors toward focusing on practice patterns and care outcomes at the institutional and national levels (Bhatia et al., 2000).

4th and 5th Scopes of Work

PROs continued to evolve by undertaking nationwide quality improvement projects on heart failure, diabetes, and other clinical conditions; improving data collection methods; emphasizing collaboration among governments, providers, and consumers; and dropping some case review activities. PROs did not explicitly promote collaboration with private plans and vendors. The first project under the Health Care Quality Initiative was the Cooperative Cardiovascular Project, which was pilot tested in four states. This project focused on care for acute myocardial infarction in the hospital setting (Sprague, 2002). Pilot efforts were designed to improve care processes through the PROs' development of epidemiological and computer capabilities and the use of new data analysis methods. The PROs worked cooperatively with hospital staff on the development and use of practice guidelines to create quality indicators for patient care (Jencks and Wilensky, 1992). Data abstracted from hospital medical records were used to measure the impact of the quality improvement pilots. The guidelines and the risk-adjusted patterns of care that were obtained were compared, and it was found that the results of the Cooperative Cardiovascular Project had generally been positive. The project became a national effort at the beginning of the 5th SOW (Ellerbeck et al., 1995; Marciniak et al., 1998).

The Health Care Quality Improvement Initiative expanded to include other diseases and incorporated continuous quality improvement and total quality management concepts. Beginning in 1994, HCFA introduced these concepts to its staff and those of the QIOs through special training sessions. The staffs learned how to use the PDSA (Plan, Do, Study, Act) Cycle method to produce more rapid results during interventions with providers. The activities in the 5th SOW were based on accountability through consistent performance measurement. HCFA promoted the development of measures, data collection tools, and reporting systems for uniform tracking of the progress of each state on a few selected clinical conditions (personal communication, J. Kelly, June 29, 2005). HCFA had previously developed two Clinical Data Abstraction Centers to improve the efficiency of data collection efforts and the quality of the data collected (Bhatia et al., 2000).

Recognizing that the PRO program had not been thoroughly evaluated, HCFA planned to conduct such an evaluation internally. To enhance outside acceptance of the evaluation and its credibility, in 1994 HCFA commissioned the IOM to assess HCFA's evaluation strategy. HCFA asked the IOM to review and critique within a very brief time period its preliminary evaluation strategy and then its final, revised evaluation plan. Given the time constraints on this study, the IOM Committee on the Medicare Peer Review Organization Evaluation Plan issued two letter reports, in January and June 1994 (IOM, 1994). The reports welcomed HCFA's plan to measure the quality of care instead of merely obtaining cost savings from the reduced use of services. The committee did note, however, that the "lack of a strong, clear vision of where the agency would like to go with the PRO program over the coming decade or so is a major drawback to the proposed evaluation strategy" (IOM, 1994:5). The committee questioned the programmatic purpose of the evaluation, its criteria for judging the success of PRO projects, and how and to whom the results would be disseminated. The committee encouraged attention to failures as well as successes, because failures could also serve as useful learning experiences. In addition, the committee raised the question of how HCFA would implement the recommendations resulting from the agency's own evaluation. The committee concluded that the effectiveness of the PRO program could not be fully reflected in a simple aggregation of the impacts of the various cooperative improvement projects.

The IOM letter reports advocated the use of a phased approach with a "formative evaluation" as the initial focus. The formative evaluation would include pilot or demonstration projects to provide an iterative learning experience whereby HCFA would use information to modify and improve ongoing projects. The use of a "summative evaluation" of long-term goals was also recommended to evaluate the effectiveness of the completed program in achieving its objectives. The committee observed that the program would benefit from more involvement of informed consumers. It also recommended that HCFA involve people with experience and skills in formal program evaluation and continuous quality improvement as soon as possible.

HCFA used these letter reports as the basis for focusing on formative evaluations, and each PRO conducted evaluations of its individual projects. Because the quality improvement projects varied from state to state and neither uniform data nor consistent methods were used, however, the evaluations were of limited use in assessing the national program or in guiding policy. No summative evaluation was ever conducted.

During the 5th SOW, in addition to case reviews and beneficiary education, PROs worked on both nationally defined and locally selected quality improvement projects in the areas of acute myocardial infarction, diabetes, and preventive care for breast cancer (see Table 1.2). Standardized measures were used to demonstrate statewide improvement in each clinical area (Sprague, 2002). HCFA chose these clinical priority areas because they accounted for a significant amount of morbidity and mortality in the Medicare population, there was strong scientific evidence that specific interventions in these areas would likely lead to improved outcomes, and providers agreed on the recommended care processes (Bhatia et al., 2000).

TABLE 1.2 Evolution of QIO Core Contract

Task	Fifth SOW (1996–1999)	Sixth SOW (1999–2002)

Task 1	National HCQIP
	
	HCFA-directed projects
	• Statewide impact expected
	• Proportional involvement of M+C beneficiaries
	• Projects for:
	  – AMI
	  – Diabetes
	  – Preventive care
	
	PRO-initiated cooperative projects
		National HCQIP
		Projects in specific topic areas with standardized indicators for each setting:
		• AMI
		• Heart failure
		• Pneumonia
		• Stroke
		• Diabetes
		• Breast cancer

Task 2	• PRO designs projects based on local needs • Statewide impact expected • Proportional involvement of M+C beneficiaries	Three required local QI projects: • Choose one indicator from Task 1 and show reduction in a disparity in a disadvantaged group • Develop project in a setting other than acute care hospital or M+C • Develop a project for local needs

Task 3	• Project must include measurable indicators
	
	Beneficiary protection and information activities
	• Education and outreach
	• Hotline
		QI projects with M+C plans
		• Each plan must annually implement two performance improvement projects:
		  – One on a topic of national interest, as selected by HCFA
		  – One selected by the plan on the basis of the needs of its enrollees
		• Projects started each year continue as new projects are added

Task 4	Mandatory case review Multiple categories including: • Beneficiary complaints • HINNs	Payment Error Prevention Program Two projects required: • Unnecessary admissions • Miscoded DRG assignments
Task 5	• EMTALA review • Cataract surgery assistants • Gross violations	Other mandated activities • All mandatory case reviews • Beneficiary outreach and education
Task 6	• Hospital-requested higher-weighted DRG adjustments	Special studies

NOTE: AMI = acute myocardial infarction; DRG = diagnosis-related group; EMTALA = Emergency Medical Treatment and Labor Act; HCQIP = Health Care Quality Improvement

Seventh SOW (2002–2005)	Eighth SOW (2005–2008)
National HCQIP Projects in specific topic areas with standardized indicators for each setting: • Nursing home • Home health • Hospital (AMI, heart failure, pneumonia, surgical infection) • Physician office (diabetes, cancer, immunization) • Underserved or rural populations • M+C (also included in all settings)	Assisting providers with developing capacity for and achieving excellence Projects in specific topic areas with standardized indicators for each setting: • Nursing home • Home health • Hospital (heart failure, pneumonia, AMI, surgical infection) • Rural and critical access hospitals • Physician office (immunization, diabetes, cancer, underserved, Part D, information technology) • Medicare Advantage may be included in all tasks
Information and communication • Promote use of performance data • Transition to hospital-generated data • Other mandated communications activities	Reserved for possible future use

Medicare beneficiary protection activities
• Beneficiary complaint resolution program (includes mediation)
• Hospital Payment Monitoring Program
• Other beneficiary protection activities
  – HINN and NODMAR review
  – M+C appeals and grievances
  – EMTALA review
  – Other mandatory review as needed
	Protect beneficiaries and the Medicare program
	• Beneficiary complaint resolution program (including mediation)
	• Hospital Payment Monitoring Program
	• Other beneficiary protection activities
	  – HINN and NODMAR review
	  – M+C appeals and grievances
	  – EMTALA review
	  – Other mandatory review as needed

Developmental activities (special studies)	Developmental activities (special studies)

Project; HINN = Hospital-Issued Notice of Non-Coverage; M+C = Medicare+Choice; NODMAR = Notice of Discharge and Medicare Appeal Rights; QI = quality improvement.

6th Scope of Work

In the 6th SOW (1999 to 2002), PROs were renamed QIOs, and they continued their individual statewide projects as well as the implementation of national programs. Standardized measures were increasingly introduced to determine the frequencies of either the services provided or the outcomes achieved. QIOs formed national partnerships with the Joint Commission on Accreditation of Healthcare Organizations, the American Hospital Association, and other groups to align quality improvement efforts (CMS, 1999; Bhatia et al., 2000; personal communication, J. Kelly, June 29, 2005). These efforts focused on six national priority areas: acute myocardial infarction, breast cancer, stroke, diabetes, heart failure, and pneumonia. HCFA also promoted a shift from the previous PRO methods of beneficiary and provider education to interventions focused on systemic changes. In addition, the 6th SOW required QIOs to perform certain projects at the local level, including projects in settings other than acute care hospitals. QIOs initiated some quality improvement projects for nursing homes, home health agencies, and organizations participating in Medicare+Choice (Table 1.2).

In addition, a new task, the Payment Error Prevention Program, was aimed at protecting the Medicare Part A Trust Fund from unnecessary admissions and miscoded diagnosis-related group assignments. On the basis of retrospective reviews of medical records, QIOs examined inpatient coding to ascertain both the overpayment and underpayment of claims. The 6th SOW also allowed selected QIOs to conduct special studies (CMS, 1999). During this period, QIOs claimed improvements resulting from two-thirds of more than 2,000 separate projects. However, HCFA failed to demonstrate any overall quantifiable impact of the projects on the quality of care (HCFA, 1998).

QIOs Today[4]

7th Scope of Work

The 7th SOW (2002 to 2005) continued to focus on quality improvement based on the measurement of changes in national performance indicators and the production of incremental changes. At the beginning of the 7th SOW, CMS released the results of performance on a limited set of national measures for the 50 states, Puerto Rico, and the District of

---

[4]This section is a summary of the detailed description of the technical assistance for quality improvement tasks of the 7th and 8th SOWs in Chapter 8, the beneficiary education and communications tasks in Chapter 11, and the protection of beneficiaries and program integrity tasks in Chapter 12.

Columbia.[5] The aggregate national performance results showed improved quality between 1998–1999 and 2000–2001 on 20 of 22 indicators for Medicare fee-for-service inpatient and outpatient care, and all states showed improvement on a majority of the indicators (Jencks et al., 2003). However, the study identified considerable room for improvement and noted that cross-sectional data could not show conclusively that the improvements had resulted specifically from QIO quality improvement efforts.

The 7th SOW was a performance-based contract that used evaluation criteria more detailed and specific than those used in the 6th SOW. In addition, evaluation of the performance of each QIO was based on its achievement of specific targets and was unrelated to the performance of the other QIOs (see Chapter 10 and Table A.3 in Appendix A).

Throughout the 7th SOW, the QIOs continued to provide technical assistance for quality improvement through collaborations with providers (see Chapter 8 for definitions and discussion of technical assistance). The SOW expanded to include required projects in different health care settings: home health agencies and nursing homes, as well as managed care plans and physician offices, in addition to hospitals (CMS, 2002). QIOs continued to improve their data collection and dissemination activities related to the use of performance data. The QIO program set national goals for each indicator, and each state's QIO had to comply with every task of the SOW, using a nationally consistent set of indicators and measures. Each QIO had discretion in determining how to carry out the required projects, but all had to meet the formal national targets, regardless of local demographics and provider differences. The QIOs were no longer required to perform projects to serve local needs, and they did not receive funds in their core budget for projects initiated locally. Home health care–related tasks addressed measures of health status improvement. Hospital-related tasks focused on acute myocardial infarction, heart failure, pneumonia, and the prevention of post-surgical infections. Nursing home–related tasks addressed chronic care and post–acute care concerns, such as pain management and improvement in mobility. Physician office–related tasks encompassed diabetes care, mammography screening, and adult immunizations (CMS, 2002). Many of the quality improvement tasks from the 6th SOW were sustained. The QIOs were also expected to pay special attention to rural and underserved populations as well as Medicare+Choice beneficiaries (CMS, 2002). Participation in QIO quality improvement projects by providers and practitioners continued to be voluntary (Sprague, 2002).

---

[5]The total number of QIOs is 53; data for this study were not available for the U.S. Virgin Islands.

Public reporting was a major driver of the activities performed under the 7th SOW (see Chapter 11). In November 2002, CMS launched the Nursing Home Quality Initiative, which included making nursing home performance measures available to the public. This effort sought to help beneficiaries and their families make informed choices, as well as to encourage nursing homes to improve upon the quality of care they delivered. CMS also initiated public reporting in home health care and hospital settings (CMS, 2004a). The public's increased awareness of and access to information about a provider's performance motivated providers to pay attention to performance measurement. Particularly for hospitals, CMS worked with the National Quality Forum, the Joint Commission on Accreditation of Healthcare Organizations, the National Committee for Quality Assurance, and other organizations to ensure that the performance indicators used by CMS and the QIOs were consistent with other commonly used measures. This collaborative effort was first attempted in the hospital setting and was then expanded to other settings so providers could collect and report the same data to Medicare and the QIOs in addition to other agencies (CMS, 2004a) (see the discussion of the Hospital Quality Alliance in Chapter 11).

Another important QIO function under the 7th SOW was the education of beneficiaries on the publicly reported performance measures. As part of this function, beneficiaries had greater involvement as QIO advisors. Consumer representatives were added to advisory panels, and QIO hotlines were made available for beneficiaries. Other tasks aimed at improving the information provision and communications activities of QIOs continued, as did specific beneficiary protection functions, such as the mediation of complaints.

All QIOs participated in Medicare beneficiary protection activities (CMS, 2002, 2004a). A new beneficiary complaint resolution program was aimed at resolving quality concerns raised by Medicare beneficiaries through alternative means (see Chapter 12). The complainant could choose mediation instead of the normal administrative case review process if the case involved no serious safety concerns. With mediation, beneficiary and provider were brought together voluntarily to resolve the issues, which often involved communication problems.

The Hospital Payment Monitoring Program (HPMP) was designed to protect the Medicare Part A Trust Fund as well as Medicare beneficiaries (CMS, 2004a) (see Chapter 12). Under this program, QIOs reviewed a random sampling of cases to estimate statewide payment error rates. The review focused on coding validity, the medical necessity of the services provided, and the appropriateness of the setting used for the provision of those services. Finally, all QIOs were still bound to traditional case review functions for a growing range of case categories (CMS, 2002) (see Chapter 12).

During the 7th SOW, CMS formally designated a separate QIO to serve as a national resource on each specific task and for each provider setting. Often, the QIO had conducted a special study or other work related to the task during the previous SOW. The QIO was funded as a QIO Support Center (QIOSC), in addition to its core contract, to provide background educational materials, tools, and scientific evidence; facilitate communications among practice communities; and train all QIOs to help them perform the given task (see Chapter 8).

8th Scope of Work

When the 8th SOW was developed, the prior rates of improvement were viewed as neither fast enough nor deep enough to achieve the program's goal of "the right care for every person every time" before the year 2024 (Jencks and Rollow, 2004). Under the 8th SOW (2005 to 2008), therefore, the QIOs are required to create an environment in which quality improvement will occur more quickly and with a greater impact (see Part II for a more detailed discussion of the tasks in the 8th SOW). This approach is aimed at creating "transformational change" (Rollow, 2004), and CMS considers it to be the next program phase necessary to achieve "results, processes, and care outcomes that are both person centered and reliable" (Pugh, 2005:3). The QIO apportionment of $1.265 billion for the 3-year contract includes approximately 68 percent for the 53 core QIO contracts. The remaining 32 percent of the total apportionment funds the QIOSCs; special studies conducted by selected QIOs; and support contracts to other entities for program operations, such as the data system for the whole QIO program. Many of the support contracts relate to broad issues of quality improvement in the Medicare program, such as the development of a series of consumer surveys of patient experiences.

The QIOs are directed to work intensively with a subset of individual providers. Statewide quality improvement measures are given less emphasis. During the 8th SOW, the program aims to initiate changes with the identified participants that will close the recognized gap between current and ideal standards of care. The main change for the QIOs is working with providers and practitioners to help them redesign care delivery systems and care processes and to implement organizational changes that will promote more rapid quality improvement. Provider assistance is focused on areas that represent both a discrepancy between known best and actual practices and a great potential for improved performance. Some of the clinical areas of focus include adult immunization, breast cancer screening, prevention of pressure ulcers, elimination of restraints and surgical complications, promotion of vascular access for hemodialysis, and workforce retention (CMS, 2005). Additional clinical areas receive attention in each provider setting. The physician office setting is the focal point for major changes, with a particular emphasis on small practices and on those caring for underserved populations. Also, QIOs are initiating the Doctor's Office Quality–Information Technology program nationally to promote the use of health information technology. Finally, with physician office projects, QIOs are also to pay special attention to Medicare Advantage beneficiaries and the new Medicare Part D prescription drug benefit (CMS, 2005).

The 8th SOW, like the 7th SOW, uses performance-based contracting, includes tasks in a variety of inpatient and outpatient provider settings, and addresses issues related to protecting beneficiaries and the Medicare Trust Funds. CMS recognizes the increased complexity of the 8th SOW, and therefore includes options for subcontracting those tasks for which the QIOs have been unable to demonstrate competency (competency is demonstrated through successful evaluation of performance under a previous SOW or other CMS-approved means). In the 8th SOW, the distribution of the federal apportionment among the QIO core contracts, QIOSCs, special studies, and the support contract is roughly similar to that in the 7th SOW. Overall, the 8th SOW is aimed at achieving transformational change rather than sustaining the current rate of incremental change (CMS, 2005).

SUMMARY

The evolution of the quality assurance program into a quality improvement program and the functions of the QIO in each state reflect the shifting priorities and changing approaches to quality care among health care managers and policy makers. Over the last 35 years, the overall philosophy of the QIO program has shifted from quality assurance (which focuses on individual cases) to quality improvement (which aims to improve overall patterns of care). A 2002 MedPAC report describes the difference as follows: "Quality assurance standards are designed to ensure a minimum level of quality and to identify and potentially punish individuals within the system who may be providing sub-standard care. In contrast, quality improvement standards are designed to ensure that the entities have an effective process for continually measuring and improving the care delivered by all providers" (MedPAC, 2002:5).

In the 8th SOW, the QIO program's philosophy has changed, as the term "quality of care" has evolved to include the transformation of systems and processes, as well as the development of tools for improving care (Rollow, 2004). These changes are propelled by the increasing interest in public reports of quality and related performance measures and programs that reward providers financially for offering better-quality care. More public reporting requirements and rewards for performance will likely encourage greater provider participation in quality improvement projects. They will also create an increased need for beneficiaries to understand how the use of publicly reported quality information can improve their health. In this new phase, CMS and its QIO program aim to achieve transformational change, focusing on the overarching processes and systems of health care delivery instead of individual episodes of care to create a new culture and environment in which the ideals of quality of care can thrive.

REFERENCES

Bhatia AJ, Blackstock S, Nelson R, Ng TS. 2000. Evolution of quality review programs for Medicare: Quality assurance to quality improvement. *Health Care Financing Review* 22(1):69–74.

Bradley EH, Carlson MDA, Gallo WT, Scinto J, Campbell MK, Krumholz HM. 2005. From adversary to partner: Have quality improvement organizations made the transition? *Health Services Research* 40(2):459–476.

CMS (Centers for Medicare and Medicaid Services). 1999. *6th Statement of Work (SOW)*. [Online]. Available: http://www.cms.hhs.gov/qio [accessed April 9, 2005].

CMS. 2002. *7th Statement of Work (SOW)*. [Online]. Available: http://www.cms.hhs.gov/qio [accessed April 9, 2005].

CMS. 2004a. *CMS Briefing on QIO Programs*. Unpublished. June 22. Baltimore, MD: Centers for Medicare and Medicaid Services.

CMS. 2004b. *Quality Improvement Organization Manual*. [Online]. Available: http://www.cms.hhs.gov/manuals/110_qio/qio110index.asp [accessed May 11, 2005].

CMS. 2005. *8th Statement of Work (SOW), Version 080105-1*. [Online]. Available: http://www.cms.hhs.gov/qio [accessed November 4, 2005].

Ellerbeck EF, Jencks SF, Radford MJ, Kresowik TF, Craig AS, Gold JA, Krumholz HM, Vogel RA. 1995. Quality of care for Medicare patients with acute myocardial infarction: A four-state pilot study from the Cooperative Cardiovascular Project. *Journal of the American Medical Association* 273(19):1509–1514.

HCFA (Health Care Financing Administration, Office of Clinical Standards and Quality). 1998. *PRO Results: Bridging the Past with the Future*. Washington, DC: Health Care Financing Administration.

IOM (Institute of Medicine). 1974. *Advancing the Quality of Health Care*. A Policy Statement by a Committee of the Institute of Medicine. Washington, DC: National Academy Press.

IOM. 1990. *Medicare: A Strategy for Quality Assurance*, Vol. 1. Washington, DC: National Academy Press.

IOM. 1994. *An Assessment of the HCFA Evaluation Plan for the Medicare Peer Review Organization*. Washington, DC: National Academy Press.

IOM. 2001. *Crossing the Quality Chasm: A New Health System for the 21st Century*. Washington, DC: National Academy Press.

IOM. 2006. *Performance Measurement: Accelerating Improvement*. Washington, DC: The National Academies Press.

Jencks SF, Rollow WC. 2004. *What CMS Hopes to Learn from the IOM Study of the QIO Program*. PowerPoint Presentation to the Committee on Redesigning Health Insurance, August 3, Washington, DC.

Jencks SF, Wilensky GR. 1992. The health care quality improvement initiative. A new approach to quality assurance in Medicare. *Journal of the American Medical Association* 268(7):900–903.

Jencks SF, Huff ED, Cuerdon T. 2003. Change in the quality of care delivered to Medicare beneficiaries, 1998–1999 to 2000–2001. *Journal of the American Medical Association* 289(3):305–312.

Jost TS. 1989. Administrative law issues involving the Medicare utilization and quality control peer review organization (PRO) program: Analysis and recommendations. *Ohio State Law Journal* 50:1–71

Marciniak TA, Ellerbeck EF, Radford MJ, Kresowik TF, Gold JA, Krumholz HM, Kiefe CI, Allman RM, Vogel RA, Jencks SF. 1998. Improving the quality of care for Medicare patients with acute myocardial infarction: Results from the Cooperative Cardiovascular Project. *Journal of the American Medical Association* 279(17):1351–1357.

MedPAC (Medicare Payment Advisory Commission). 2002. *Report to the Congress: Applying Quality Improvement Standards in Medicare*. Washington, DC: Medicare Payment Advisory Commission.

NORC (National Organization for Research at the University of Chicago). 2004. *Final Report: Physician Meetings on Take-Up of Electronic Health Records*. Unpublished. Washington, DC: National Organization for Research at the University of Chicago.

Pugh MD. 2005. *Final Report: CMS Quality Group Planning Project QIOSC Contract 500-02-WA02 Final Report*, Revised. Unpublished. Pueblo, CO: Pugh Ettinger McCarthy Associates, LLC.

Rogers WH, Draper D, Kahn KL, Keeler EB, Rubenstein LV. 1990. Quality of care before and after implementation of the DRG-based prospective payment system. A summary of effects. *Journal of the American Medical Association* 264(15):1989–1994.

Rollow WC. 2004. *Evaluating the HCQIP Program*. PowerPoint Presentation to Quality Improvement Organization Subcommittee, October 4, Baltimore, MD.

Rubin HR, Rogers WH, Kahn KL, Rubenstein LV, Brook RH. 1992. Watching the doctor-watchers. How well do peer review organization methods detect hospital care quality problems? *Journal of the American Medical Association* 267(17):2349–2354.

Sprague L. 2002. Contracting for Quality: Medicare's Quality Improvement Organizations. *National Health Policy Forum Issue Brief 774*. Washington, DC: National Health Policy Forum.

2

Assessment of the QIO Program: Findings and Conclusions

CHAPTER SUMMARY

This chapter describes the study's evaluation approach, summarizes the key findings discussed in detail in Part II, and presents the committee's conclusions about the impact of the Quality Improvement Organization program. The committee concludes that although the evidence regarding the program's effects on quality of care is limited and inconclusive, the program has the potential to be a valuable asset as providers become more involved with public reporting and incentive payments from Medicare and other insurers.

The historical overview of the Quality Improvement Organization (QIO) program in Chapter 1 describes a public program that has changed direction, functions, and methods frequently over its 35-year history. Given the absence of earlier evaluations of the program, uncertainties exist with regard to its potential roles in the future. As a base for the recommendations for the future of the program presented in Chapters 4 and 5, this chapter details the committee's findings and conclusions concerning the program's impacts. Specifically, the chapter addresses whether:

• There has been improvement in the quality of health care services provided to Medicare beneficiaries.
• The QIO program has contributed to that improvement.
• Certain components of the QIO program should be eliminated or strengthened.
• There should be a continuing federal role in technical assistance for quality improvement and, if so, whether that role should be stronger.

It becomes clear from the descriptive details presented in Part II that the

QIO program is richly varied. The organizations holding the QIO contracts for each state often differ dramatically in structure, in the services they provide, and in their quality intervention programs, perhaps reflecting differences in the health care services in their communities. This variation makes it difficult to generalize about all QIOs and the program at the national level, as well as to determine what changes in structure might be of most benefit to the program and yield the greatest improvements in the quality of care.

The historical overview presented in the previous chapter shows how the program has changed over time. Nonetheless, many of the organizations holding state contracts and some of their key leadership have persisted with the program through much of its evolution and have demonstrated remarkable flexibility in adapting to each new statement of work. Through that evolution, the QIOs have built partnerships with the providers and other key stakeholders in their states, such as state departments of health and local chapters of the American Association for Retired Persons. The committee gathered anecdotal evidence of many favorable and some less favorable relationships between QIOs and providers, brought to the committee's attention at national conferences, site visits, and informal discussions with providers and consumers. In addition, results of large national surveys of physicians, hospitals, nursing homes, and home health agencies reveal generally favorable attitudes toward their local QIO. (The provider surveys are discussed in detail in Chapter 10.) The committee finds these relationships and the QIOs' capacity for adaptability to be valuable assets.

The remainder of this chapter begins with a discussion of the first two questions raised above: (1) whether care for Medicare beneficiaries has improved, and (2) whether the improvements, if any, can be attributed to the QIO program. Alternatives to the current QIO program, along with their advantages and disadvantages, are considered next. The chapter then addresses program infrastructure at both the national and state levels. Next is a discussion of the main functions of the QIOs, followed by a review of structural issues, such as funding and board composition. Finally, the chapter addresses the oversight responsibilities of the Centers for Medicare and Medicaid Services (CMS). Detailed data and analyses supporting the committee's findings and conclusions are presented mainly in Part II and the appendixes, relevant portions of which are referenced throughout the discussion here.

EVIDENCE OF QUALITY IMPROVEMENT IN MEDICARE

The Medicare program has carefully tracked the growth in the numbers of beneficiaries, the expenditures made on their behalf, and the increasing variety and use of covered services over the history of the program; however, it has produced much less information on the quality of those services. The former director of the QIO program in CMS examined Medicare services by comparing data for 22 clinical inpatient and outpatient measures against state baseline performance reported through the QIO program from 1998–1999 to 2000–2001. It was found that the weighted national average, as well as the state with the median performance, had improved on 20 of the 22 indicators (Jencks et al., 2003). A recent national study employing 9 of the same hospital quality indicators used by Jencks and colleagues (2003), along with publicly reported data on Medicare and all other patients, found that the level of hospital performance had improved on all but 1 measure (Jha et al., 2005). Although these studies were less than ideal—in particular, the number of measures used in each study was limited, and the measures focused primarily on care provided within hospitals—their results indicate that health care for Medicare beneficiaries has improved. There are signs of improvement as well in clinical activities targeted as national priorities on which QIOs and other organizations have focused, such as mammograms and care for heart attacks and diabetes (Leatherman and McCarthy, 2005). Improvements in care for beneficiaries in managed care were also noted from 2000 to 2004 (NCQA, 2005). On the other hand, much evidence, cited in Chapter 1 of this report and in *Performance Measurement: Accelerating Improvement* (IOM, 2006), indicates that the quality of care varies greatly from provider to provider by geographic location, race or ethnicity, and income of the beneficiary and that many people do not receive all the services they need, particularly appropriate preventive care. There is substantial room for further improvement.

Can the gradual improvements in care that have been accomplished be attributed to the QIO program? Because of the nature of their evaluation designs, the studies mentioned above cannot be used to determine the cause of the improvements documented or attribute them to the QIO program. During site visits and focus group discussions conducted for this study, the committee heard frequent anecdotal evidence from providers and the QIOs regarding positive impacts on quality resulting from the multiple forms of technical assistance provided by the QIOs (see Chapter 8). Some studies of specific, limited QIO interventions or collaboratives have also documented improvements over time, but likewise cannot be used to conclude that the improvements were due to the QIOs' efforts (Marciniak et al., 1998; Kiefe et al., 2001; Gould et al., 2002; Chu et al., 2003; Daniel et al., 2004; Dellinger et al., 2005). In addition, preliminary data on several measures of the quality of care under the 7th scope of work (SOW) suggest that the QIOs may have had a positive impact on the care received from nursing home, home health agency, and hospital providers that participated intensively with their QIOs ("identified participants") in comparison with that received from all such providers statewide. The data also suggest that those identified participants achieved greater improvements on measures related to the clinical area of their particular intervention relative to improvements achieved by participants who collaborated with QIOs on interventions unrelated to those measures (personal communication, W. C. Rollow, July 8, 2005; personal communication, J. Kelly, September 8, 2005). The analyses were incomplete as of this writing, however, and it is unclear whether these apparent differences will be significant.

Given the lack of consistent and conclusive evidence in scientific journals and the lack of strong findings from the committee's analyses, it is not possible to determine definitively the extent of the impact of the QIOs and the national QIO infrastructure on the quality of health care received by beneficiaries. Many confounding factors make it difficult to attribute the results obtained thus far. Also, the literature does not address the QIO program as a whole; rather, it merely addresses the impacts of specific quality improvement activities of individual QIOs or quality measures aggregated at the state or national level. Other aspects of the program, such as the impact of QIO case reviews on quality and the value of QIO Support Centers (QIOSCs), have received little or no scrutiny from evaluators. (See Chapter 8 for a discussion of QIOSCs.)

One challenge to evaluating the QIO program is that QIOs recruit voluntary participants and generally partner with multiple stakeholder organizations to conduct quality improvement interventions (see Chapter 8). It would be difficult to identify true control groups; random assignment has not been tried because of practical and political implications; studies often rely only on changes that have been observed compared with performance at the baseline; it is difficult to measure impacts within the time frame of the study; and it is nearly impossible to distinguish the impacts of a QIO from those of its partners and other environmental factors. Also, the nature of the interventions varies depending on the provider type and the QIO, as well as from one provider to another, because the intervention methods used are determined largely by each QIO. The voluntary nature of provider participation with QIOs introduces the possibility of bias in the self-selection of participants, which in turn limits the value of comparisons of the rates of change for identified participant groups with the rates for the entire state. Also, because the QIO has the responsibility to raise the level of quality statewide as well as for identified participants, a large difference between the two rates of quality improvement may indicate a particularly successful program for identified participants but a very weak statewide program. These research limitations and inconclusive findings in the literature are not limited to studies of the QIO program, but also hamper other studies of improvements in health care quality.

In addition to studies related to the QIOs, the literature review performed for this study focused on more generic quality improvement studies in health care. In addition to 23 studies focused specifically on the QIO program and various QIO-led quality improvement interventions, the committee examined 9 articles, including 2 Cochrane reviews (the latter systematically assessed a wide range of studies according to explicit, high standards). (This literature review is discussed further in Chapter 9, and selected articles are summarized in Tables A.1 and A.2 in Appendix A.) The studies paint an inconclusive picture of the effectiveness of quality improvement programs, whether the interventions are conducted by QIOs or other organizations, for both Medicare and non-Medicare services. In part, this lack of conclusive data results from the research challenges mentioned above. Few of the studies used randomized controlled trials or control groups.

An examination of additional literature on the transfer of knowledge about various quality improvement methods also provided inconclusive findings on the effectiveness of these methods; no specific method has been identified as best. Studies do show the importance of commitment on the part of an organization's leadership, staff empowerment, and the development of a plan to promote quality improvement (Bradley et al., 2005; CMS, 2005a). Analysis of the management literature on effecting change to improve patient safety in health care organizations reveals that several human resource management practices are helpful in that process. In particular, to promote successful change and the adoption of new practices, it is important for management to promote "ongoing communication; training; use of mechanisms for measurement, feedback, and redesign; sustained attention; and worker involvement" (IOM, 2004:118).

Knowledge transfer is considered an important part of the QIO program, although evidence that it occurs is meager. A significant portion of the functions of the QIOSCs relates to knowledge transfer among the QIOs: training the trainer, the establishment and maintenance of communities of practice, and the identification and promotion of best practices.

During the site visits, telephone interviews, and focus group discussions conducted by the committee, the chief executive officers (CEOs) of the QIOs emphasized the need to include early adopters, leaders, and champions, in addition to middle and late adopters, in quality interventions to promote their uptake by practitioners and institutions beyond those involved in the interventions. On the other hand, focusing solely on providers that are leaders and champions and may be relatively easy to recruit to a QIO technical assistance program could limit the participation of providers that may need the QIO's assistance the most.

The QIO program considers sharing among QIOs to be important and has established mechanisms for this purpose. For example, the shift in the 7th SOW from a relative failure rate definition for QIOs that must recompete to an absolute target for automatic renewal meant that QIOs were more willing to share and help each other. They were no longer competing to avoid the penalty associated with being in the bottom quartile; they were all trying to meet absolute targets and could cooperate without jeopardy. The 8th SOW maintains similar incentives.

While the QIO contracts and QIO collaboratives are based on sharing and knowledge transfer, other forces in health care are pushing providers in the opposite direction, toward more competition. Under the pressures of public reporting, no providers will want to see their name on the bottom half of the quality-of-care list, which would indicate that the care they provide is of below-average quality. Pay-for-performance schemes are likely to reinforce that competition, depending on the reward structure. Unintended consequences of public reporting and pay for performance should be examined, but no evidence yet exists on what impacts, if any, these programs will have on competition, and it is unclear how QIO collaboratives will work as the environment becomes more competitive for providers. In some communities, providers may welcome the use of public reporting and use it to benchmark and identify other providers from which they could learn. In any case, the program should be considering new options for QIO interventions and mechanisms, such as web-based training and self-guided study tools, to extend the QIOs' reach to more providers.

Because of the limitations of the scientific literature, the committee attempted to use program-generated data, including the performance scores used by CMS to evaluate each QIO's contract performance, to identify high- and low-performing QIOs (see Chapter 10). CMS conducts separate performance assessments for each SOW task and subtask. The scores related to Task 1 (technical assistance for quality improvement) define "quality" for the program. The scores used by the committee are based on specified clinical measures for hospitals, nursing homes, home health care agencies, and physician offices during the 7th SOW through December 2004. To retain its QIO contract during the next SOW without competing, a QIO must attain a passing score for each task; no total or average score based on all tasks is assigned to each QIO. The committee's analyses revealed the following:

• A QIO's score in one provider setting did not correlate with that in any other setting.
• No correlation existed between spending per beneficiary in a state on the QIO's technical assistance in a particular setting and the QIO's performance measure for that setting.
• No correlation existed between the state performance score in a particular setting and measures of the provider's satisfaction with the QIO.
• Some regional variations in the performance scores were noted, as were variations in contract rounds for the home health care provider scores (see Chapter 13 for a discussion of contract rounds).

The committee was unable to ascertain why one QIO might have a higher performance score than another in a particular setting. One might expect that many skills needed to carry out a quality improvement intervention would be transferable from one provider setting to another. They may in fact be transferable, but perhaps some QIO staffs are not well organized to effect that transfer of knowledge, or the provider communities and their stakeholder organizations may differ in ways that affect the success of the QIOs' interventions. Also, the role played by providers' voluntary participation in the impacts of the QIO program is unclear. One study of hospital and ambulatory care measures showed that absolute improvement on 21 of the 22 measures tracked was greater for those states starting at a lower-quality baseline than for those starting at a higher-quality baseline (Jencks et al., 2003). While many inferences can be drawn about why a trend cannot be identified to link improvement and setting of care, it must be noted that some skills and expertise required to provide assistance in each setting are not necessarily the same. Given limited resources and the need to complete other tasks, such as communications and beneficiary protection, QIOs must choose how best to allocate their resources.

The committee heard consistent reports of extensive variations among the QIOs: some are outstanding, while others are mediocre. These judgments appear to reflect an overall perspective on the organizations rather than the QIOs' performance on specific tasks. Yet there are no objective global measures, based on contract performance scores for quality improvement, that could indicate which QIOs belong in which category or even whether there are in fact significant differences in overall performance. For example, some QIOs score high on improving care in one setting but not in others. The complex and detailed formulas used by CMS to assess each state's performance on the core tasks of the SOW can be used to determine the QIOs' performance only on each task separately. For example, 6 of the 36 QIOs in the first two contract rounds failed on at least one assessment standard (task or subtask) and had to recompete for an 8th SOW contract. Those 6 QIOs included some that would not generally be viewed as belonging in the bottom tier on overall performance, some that had received substantial contracts from CMS to conduct special studies or to serve as a QIOSC, and some that were named "best" at particular tasks by other CEOs according to the committee's web-based data collection tool.

ALTERNATIVES TO THE CURRENT QIO PROGRAM

In considering alternatives to the current QIO program, the committee decided it was necessary to step back and ask some fundamental questions.

First, should the federal government exercise a stronger role in the provision of technical assistance to health care providers to promote more rapid improvements in health care quality? The evidence base for the committee's *Performance Measurement* report (IOM, 2006) and for the present study (see the introduction to this report) indicates that the health care received by Americans is seriously inadequate, and that the health care system needs to produce better-quality care that meets standards supported by the best scientific evidence. While these shortcomings have been in the headlines and discussed extensively in the provider community for many years, progress toward improved quality continues to be painfully slow. The committee concludes that the public sector needs to play a substantial role in improving the quality of care for all Americans. This is especially so for those who depend upon federal programs, such as Medicare, Medicaid, the State Children's Health Insurance Program, the Department of Defense's TRICARE, and the programs of the Veterans Health Administration and the Indian Health Service, which provide coverage and care to roughly 100 million people (IOM, 2002). The creation of a performance measurement and reporting system and the implementation of payment systems that reward quality care are important steps in accelerating improvement, but they are insufficient to achieve the six quality aims outlined by the IOM (IOM, 2000, 2001). The committee believes the federal government is well suited to promote better-quality care for all Americans because it spends more than $513 billion annually on their care. The magnitude of this investment can generate positive changes in quality throughout the health care system (IOM, 2002). As the IOM concluded previously, "the federal government *must* assume a stronger leadership role to address quality concerns" (IOM, 2002:x).

Second, given a role for the federal government in providing technical assistance for quality improvement, should that assistance be offered at no cost to providers, as is now the case through the QIOs, or should providers be expected to pay for the assistance? The following findings can help answer this question:

• Many providers have resources that allow them to purchase technical assistance from private organizations, such as those discussed in Chapter 3 and listed in Table B.1 in Appendix B. Also, many providers spend considerable sums to hire quality improvement experts and to conduct improvement programs internally. While the extent and distribution of such expenditures are unknown, they are generally considered to be more common among hospitals, large physician groups, and managed care organizations than among medium and small physician practices and other provider settings. The committee does not wish to discourage such behavior.

• At the same time, particular attention needs to be paid to disparities in access to and use of technical assistance resources within the provider community. Some providers are ready and willing to undertake the internal changes needed to improve quality but lack the resources to purchase the technical assistance they need to achieve these reforms.

• Continuing to achieve improvement at the current rate would be costly in lives and dollars and is therefore unacceptable.

• Regardless of the current level of expenditures by providers for technical assistance to improve quality, the end result is clear—improvements in quality nationally are progressing too slowly. While many providers may be willing to expend their own resources to improve quality when payment becomes based on such improvements, others are likely to be left behind. Some providers simply do not have sufficient resources to purchase the necessary services readily. The expansion of pay-for-performance systems to cover a greater portion of a provider's revenues is likely to worsen this situation. Providers with low levels of quality according to the given metrics may receive no increase or perhaps even a decrease in reimbursements.

• In some areas, poor-quality providers may be the only ones available to a portion of the population, and their failure would further exacerbate disparities in health care access and quality.

The committee concludes that it is important to improve the level of care offered by all providers, even if they cannot afford to purchase technical assistance privately, and that some level of technical assistance should be available through the federal government as a public good. As providers improve their care processes for Medicare beneficiaries, it is likely that other patients will benefit as well.

PROGRAM INFRASTRUCTURE

Given the committee's limited ability to attribute quality improvements in Medicare directly to the efforts of the QIO program, it is necessary to consider whether the current program should continue. Although it may appear obvious, the committee believes the existence of 41 separate organizations holding QIO contracts dedicated to providing quality improvement services in every state, the District of Columbia, Puerto Rico, and the Virgin Islands is a significant asset. The cadre of trained experts in QIOs (see Chapter 7) is a potentially valuable resource for offering technical assistance in quality improvement and for helping hospitals, nursing homes, home health agencies, and outpatient physician practices collect data on their performance and aggregate and analyze those data to improve the care they deliver.

The QIO program has created an infrastructure across the United States with staff trained and experienced in various quality improvement techniques. The QIO program serves as a focal point within CMS for assisting health care service providers in improving the care they offer to Medicare beneficiaries and others. It is also the only program within CMS that actively addresses health disparities (Jost, 2005). The following are examples of the QIOs' expertise and experience drawn from the committee's QIO and Regional Office site visits, telephone interviews, and web-based data collection tool:

- All but seven QIO contracts are staffed with at least one employee who is a Certified Professional in Healthcare Quality (through the Healthcare Certification Board, the National Association for Healthcare Quality, or a similarly recognized professional accreditation in quality improvement). Eleven QIOs have from 10 to 34 such certified staff.
- Eighty-eight percent of QIO CEOs believe their leadership staff have substantial competencies for such functions as collaboration, relationship building, team development, and performance measurement. Many CEOs stated that their QIOs have individuals with other leadership skills available to carry out the tasks of the 8th SOW.
- A national survey of the QIOs by the Best Practices QIOSC (Qualis Health, 2004) showed that the quality improvement management staff of many QIOs were familiar at a minimum with various quality improvement techniques and programs, such as the Baldrige criteria, a collaborative methodology, human factors, International Standards Organization (ISO) 9000 criteria, Lean principles, and the Six Sigma program (see Chapter 7 for a discussion of QIO staff training and Chapter 9 for a description of each method). Some QIOs indicated having used some of those tools; only a small number of QIOs reported having staff certification for specific programs, such as Six Sigma. Collaboratives were a major method used in the 6th and 7th SOWs, and many QIO staff were trained in its use. This is reflected in the fact that 98 percent of the QIOs reported being familiar with the method, and 95 percent of the QIOs reported having used it (personal communication, J. Kelly, June 29, 2005). Almost half of the respondents were familiar with even the least common methods—those based on ISO 9000 criteria and Lean principles (Qualis Health, 2004).
- The QIOs had a separate task in the 7th SOW to reduce disparities between an identified group, such as a particular underserved or rural population, and a reference group. In the 8th SOW, the disparities task was folded into all the quality improvement technical assistance tasks rather than remaining separate (see Chapter 8).
- All QIOs gained experience in assisting hospitals with reporting measures during the 7th SOW, when nearly all hospitals decided to participate voluntarily in public reporting to avoid a payment reduction. QIOs were also involved with the public rollout of comparative nursing home measures (see Chapter 11).

Not only does each QIO have technical expertise in quality improvement, data management, and data analysis, but significant expertise in these areas also exists within CMS at the national and regional levels (see Chapter 13). The Central and Regional Office program staff may appear to be small (132 full-time equivalents) relative to the size of the program they oversee, the variety of tasks they perform, and their responsibilities for improving the quality of care for Medicare beneficiaries. Among the staff, however, are people with advanced training and experience in medicine, nursing, quality improvement, epidemiology, scientific research, and data systems (CMS, 2004; personal communication, J. Kelly, September 8, 2005).

Although frustration and complaints with regard to the staff at CMS were voiced frequently during the committee's site visits to QIOs, telephone interviews, and other informal meetings, 85 percent of the QIOs rated their Project Officer "good" or "excellent" on expertise; the Scientific Officers received similarly high ratings on their performance (see Chapter 13). The QIO program's administrator reported that the program has sufficient staff and expertise to conduct the work required under the 8th SOW (personal communication, W. C. Rollow, July 8, 2005). In addition, the program has established potentially useful national communications networks and a data repository that currently serve both the QIOs and the public reporting of hospital data (CMS, 2004) (see Chapter 13 for further discussion of the data systems).

The committee notes that at both the state and the national levels, the QIOs and CMS have established important working relationships with providers, their professional associations, and various other stakeholder groups and convened parties around specific issues (CMS, 2004; Westat, 2005; National Health Policy Forum, 2004). The QIOs and CMS have also been major participants in such collaborative efforts as the Hospital Quality Alliance and the Ambulatory Care Quality Alliance. Both the convening ability of the QIOs and the clout of CMS to bring national organizations to the table are key ingredients for promoting widespread, coordinated quality improvement.

The committee recognizes the expertise available within the QIO program and the enthusiasm, commitment, and dedication to quality improvement exhibited by staff and leadership from the Central Office at CMS, the Regional Offices, and all the organizations holding QIO contracts. The committee concludes that the potential exists for the QIO program to have a measurable positive impact on improving the quality of care for Medicare beneficiaries, serving useful and important functions in the rapidly changing world of Medicare.

FUNCTIONS OF THE QIOs

QIOs have three main functions: (1) offering technical assistance to providers to help them improve the quality of care they deliver; (2) providing education for beneficiaries and communications; and (3) protecting beneficiaries and the Medicare Trust Funds through the review of complaints, appeals, and other cases.

Technical Assistance for Quality Improvement

As discussed above and in detail in Chapters 9 and 10, the existing evidence concerning the impact of QIO quality improvement interventions is insufficiently robust to permit the attribution of improvements to QIO activities. This lack of evidence neither supports nor refutes the effectiveness of the QIO program, nor does the evidence make clear which QIOs are doing a better job of providing technical assistance for quality improvement. Over time, a QIO may show major improvements on statewide measures in one provider setting but not in others. Even if a state excels on all the measures, the improvements cannot be attributed to the QIO with confidence with current data. Research concerning the various quality improvement methods used by QIOs and other organizations is also meager, is unclear about what methods work the best, and does not support the use or avoidance of any particular methods.

Offering technical assistance to a broad variety of providers is a significant challenge for QIOs. In the 7th SOW, technical assistance was provided to nursing homes, home health agencies, physician practices, hospitals, and Medicare Advantage plans. The Medicare Prescription Drug, Improvement, and Modernization Act (P.L. 108-173) added more provider settings related to the new drug benefit, beginning in the 8th SOW with specific projects related to physicians' medication therapy management and to pharmacies working with prescription drug plans. The committee concludes that the current variety of provider settings is sufficiently demanding of QIO staff, and indeed includes more providers than the QIOs are likely to be able to reach. Thus it would be imprudent to expand this task to encompass additional types of Medicare providers, such as clinical laboratories or therapists, at this time. The biggest challenge faced by the QIOs may be delivering technical assistance to the existing range of providers that helps improve quality across all settings, enhances patient transitions from one provider setting to the next, and promotes public health. Expanding the scope of technical assistance and including additional provider settings might be considered in the future should the QIOs achieve sufficient success with their current responsibilities and should there be a compelling need for technical assistance to improve quality in other areas.

During the committee's site visits and telephone interviews, most CEOs of QIOs stated a preference for working with providers considered early adopters, champions, or opinion leaders—or at least providers at a mix of readiness levels—since they believe early adopters are key to the increased diffusion of ideas (see Chapter 8). Concerning the recruitment of providers to QIO improvement projects, CEOs generally agreed that working mainly with the worst-performing providers would be more difficult, slower, and more costly and would result in less diffusion of improvements to other providers. They recommended against focusing QIO resources solely on poor performers because the stigma of being labeled the "worst" would create problems with attracting willing participants.

The committee recognizes that focusing QIO technical assistance on a mix of providers—early adopters and leaders, as well as slower adopters—may have certain benefits. Indeed, ideally there should be sufficient resources for QIOs to assist all providers requesting help. The committee considers it important for the QIO program to focus on assisting providers at a low quality level or those that would be unable to obtain assistance through the private market, particularly with the expansion of public reporting and pay-for-performance programs; however, those providers would not necessarily be unwilling, unready for change, or the slowest adopters of change. Some CEOs also noted that those providers starting a collaborative with the lowest quality measures often make the greatest improvement.

Beneficiary Education and Communications

The 7th SOW reduced funding for education functions, activities targeting beneficiaries and communications, and the 8th SOW shifts a greater proportion of funding to communications than to education. Nonetheless, under the 7th SOW the QIOs conducted communications campaigns to inform the media, hospital discharge planners, and beneficiaries about the rollout of Nursing Home Compare, Home Health Compare, and Hospital Compare,[1] as well as to promote the use of quality information on providers (see Chapter 11). Although some QIOs used communications to beneficiaries to promote the use of preventive services, most reported to the committee that they are oriented more toward providers, and most do not perceive beneficiaries as their primary customers even though improved health outcomes for beneficiaries is the ultimate goal (CMS, 2004).

---

[1]CMS created websites, designed for beneficiary use, that include comparative data on each provider by name.

Protection of Beneficiaries and Trust Funds

The fact that QIOs conduct case reviews of local providers for Medicare payment and coding purposes causes some providers to view them in a regulatory light; this perception can hinder QIOs' attempts to gain the cooperation of providers for quality improvement (NORC, 2004; Bradley et al., 2005). Although some anecdotal evidence suggests that QIO relations with providers have improved substantially since the early days of the program, when the role of the Utilization and Quality Control Peer Review Organizations (PROs) was predominantly regulatory and led to the imposition of significant sanctions, there appears to be lingering resistance among some providers to working with their QIO (National Health Policy Forum, 2004). CMS's surveys of quality improvement officers among providers who both did and did not work intensively with QIOs showed a generally high level of satisfaction (80 percent or better according to QIONet, CMS's internal Dashboard website) in most states and nationally among all provider types except nonidentified nursing home participants (personal communication, M. G. Wang, July 7, 2005). However, the views of the CEOs may differ from those of their quality improvement officers. Indeed, the committee is concerned about the inherent conflict between the QIOs' regulatory and quality improvement roles (see recommendation 4 in Chapter 4).

Nearly all QIO CEOs consider case reviews to be a useful adjunct to the provision of technical assistance for quality improvement. The committee finds that reviews of appeals requiring consideration of a patient's record should not require local physicians to review the record. Local physicians and their representatives may choose to be involved in the development of national measures, guidelines, and quality standards, but once those standards have been set, a local interpretation would be superfluous. Since national guidelines and quality standards should be used, the reviews could be conducted at a central point, although some beneficiary complaints involving mediation would require a local presence. Various agencies and organizations in each state, such as the state medical board and the state department of insurance or health, carry out similar functions. If the bulk of case reviews were conducted at the regional or national level, aberrations at the state level could be perceived more clearly. Also, case reviews at the regional or national level would be more efficient because at present, each QIO must support a full range of on-call specialists 24 hours a day, 7 days a week for appeals requiring a rapid turnaround.

It is not possible to determine the cost-effectiveness of the various categories and types of case reviews given the available data. The abstracting of case records for payment reviews, the staffing of on-call specialists 24 hours a day, 7 days a week for urgent appeals, and the intensity of the labor required for all reviews are costly elements of the QIO review process, whose value is not clear. CMS has not measured the impact of case reviews on the quality of care received by beneficiaries, nor has the program tracked the costs and savings associated with the QIO reviews through to the end of the process to determine the costs and benefits of the various categories of reviews throughout the Medicare program.

Recent data show that QIOs receive relatively few complaints—about 1 for every 14,000 beneficiaries (Gaul, 2005). Additionally, only about one-fourth of these complaints are found to be justified as quality problems, and even fewer sanctions are imposed; today, an average of only 1 sanction per year is imposed (compared with an average of 31 sanctions per year two decades ago). CMS data on the effectiveness of complaint reviews are insufficient for determining trends (see Chapter 12). Additionally, few analyses have been done to determine the effectiveness of payment reviews in terms of cost savings overall.

STRUCTURAL ISSUES

Program Funding

The QIO program is funded through an apportionment from the Medicare Trust Funds rather than an annual appropriation.[2] (Structural issues are discussed in detail in Chapter 7.) The apportionment mechanism allows the U.S. Department of Health and Human Services (DHHS) and the federal Office of Management and Budget to determine the program's needs and to draw on existing resources for that support. Yet the funding level for the QIO program has been very small relative to the Medicare program's level of spending on benefits, shrinking to approximately 0.1 percent in the 8th SOW. The committee was unable to find comparable data for Medicare Advantage plans or other private health plans.

Under the 7th SOW, funding for the 53 QIO core contracts was approximately two-thirds of the estimated total funding for the QIO program of $1.154 billion (see Chapter 7 for detailed discussion of funding). Tasks focused directly on technical assistance for quality improvement consumed more than half of the core contract amount—approximately $449 million from 2002 to 2005. The remaining one-third of the total apportionment went to contracts for the QIOSCs, special studies conducted by selected QIOs, and support for data systems as well as other CMS quality-related activities (personal communication, C. Lazarus, March 17, 2005). The stud-

---

[2]Much of the data on these issues is drawn from the committee's web-based data collection tool and telephone interviews.

ies conducted with these funds have not been systematically disseminated among the QIO community, and their value has not been assessed.

Under the 8th SOW, technical assistance tasks are expected to receive a slightly smaller proportion of the total budget, although the number of such tasks has increased, because responsibilities and funding for case reviews have expanded. The 3-year budget for the overall QIO program increased to $1.265 billion in the 8th SOW, a 9.6 percent increase over the budget under the 7th SOW—roughly a flat budget plus inflation (personal communication, D. Adler, May 23, 2005).

QIO Board Composition, Function, and Structure

Consumer Representation on QIO Boards

The boards of the 41 organizations holding QIO core contracts surveyed for this study vary considerably in size and are heavily dominated by physicians and other clinicians and providers (see Chapter 7 for further discussion of QIO boards and their membership). As noted above, most QIO CEOs consider health care providers, not consumers, to be their main audience. Although consumer representation was mandated more than 20 years ago in the Peer Review Improvement Act (P.L. 97-248), QIO boards rarely have more than the one mandated consumer representative, who is identified primarily as a consumer or beneficiary. The Consumer Advisory Council in each QIO, established under the 7th SOW, is not a substitute for a stronger consumer–beneficiary presence on the board, since the council is only advisory to the board and has a limited focus on policy direction for consumer-related issues (CMS, 2002:35). The committee concludes that, given the growing role for patients in the management of their own care, the need for patients to choose caregivers on the basis of publicly reported quality measures, and an accepted definition of quality health care that includes patient-centeredness, a single consumer on a QIO board is unlikely to have sufficient influence on QIO activities. Also, cultural sensitivity to the diversity of the population is important if QIOs are going to create successful technical assistance programs for providers. Although the QIOs' focus on providers is appropriate and reflects their historical and current functions, greater consumer input on the boards is needed to help shift providers toward the provision of more patient-centered care.

Other Board Issues

Several other elements of the operations of QIO boards may affect their capacity to offer the QIO leadership and guidance. Four areas involving board oversight and direction would benefit from closer attention:

- *Broader representation of various disciplines and expertise*—The QIOs have diverse constituents, including hospitals, physician practices, nursing homes, and home health care agencies. However, the QIO boards appear to have relatively few members from health professions other than physicians. The committee found that physicians dominated nearly all the QIO boards, that two-thirds of all board members listed in the IOM's web-based data collection tool were physicians, and that all responding QIO CEOs (39 of 41) listed representatives of office-based practices on their boards. In particular, nurses (especially those in home health care), physician assistants, pharmacists, and physical and occupational therapists appear to be in short supply on QIO boards and are nonexistent on most boards, even though these types of health care professionals could play critical roles in improving the quality of care. Boards need to become more inclusive, encouraging participation from a variety of stakeholders and relevant experts. The growing responsibilities of QIOs during the 7th SOW included assisting stakeholders with data measurement, collection, aggregation, analysis, and reporting as part of their provision of technical assistance for quality improvement. The committee expects those functions to increase in importance, and the minimal representation of QIO board members with expertise and experience in information technology management and oversight is a concern. Board members from outside the health care sector with experience in quality improvement, process measurement, and performance accountability could also contribute to the governance of QIOs. At the same time, when considering the addition of consumers, health professionals, and others to its board, a QIO must balance the need to keep the board's membership to a workable number. The creation of alternative mechanisms, such as advisory committees, may be necessary to obtain the varied input needed while keeping the board to a manageable size.

- *Board member development and assessment*—Studies have shown that organizational leadership can benefit from the implementation of a systematic plan for individual board member development, an annual assessment of each board member's performance, and an evaluation of the board as a whole (Orlikoff and Totten, 2005). Such assessments are particularly important in light of recent scandals involving both for-profit and not-for-profit health care entities; passage of the Sarbanes-Oxley Act of 2002 (P.L. 107-204), which brings greater accountability and transparency to the for-profit corporate world; and efforts in the not-for-profit sector by Board Source, Independent Sector, the Aspen Institute, and the Center for Healthcare Governance, which have recommended new requirements for board accountability. Just under a quarter of the 41 organizations holding contracts under the 7th SOW reported that they had formal mechanisms in place for evaluating the performance of individual board members; the same proportion of QIOs evaluate the overall performance of their boards.

- *Financial oversight and strategic guidance*—Only 23 of the 41 organizations with QIO contracts have a board finance committee, only 15 reported that they have an audit committee, and only 8 reported that they have a strategic planning committee. Thus there appears to be a need for increased attention to these important areas of board responsibility to provide adequate oversight and strategic direction to QIO management.
- *Overall responsibility*—In addition to financial oversight and strategic guidance, the QIO board should be responsible for assessing the overall performance of the CEO and senior staff, as well as the accomplishment of defined goals and priorities.

Physician-Access or Physician-Sponsored QIOs

Outmoded Requirement

The legislative requirement that QIOs be physician-access or physician-sponsored organizations was intended to assure physicians that their clinical work would be reviewed by their peers on the basis of local practice standards. Although certain clinical assessments and case reviews still require medical expertise, the physicians need not be local because quality of care is now defined according to evidence-based national guidelines and standards rather than local patterns of practice. The committee concludes that this requirement is now outmoded and unnecessarily limits the competition for QIO contracts from other entities.

Limited Competition

The committee finds that few entities other than out-of-state QIOs have been serious competitors for QIO core contracts in the past or are expected to compete for the 8th SOW, given the wide and complex assortment of required tasks and structural requirements. Other entities that are not physician-access or physician-sponsored organizations might have the capacity to perform all or portions of that contract (see Chapter 3 for further discussion of "other entities"). Yet there has been a history of very limited competition for QIO contracts, and there have been few opportunities to replace QIOs that did relatively poorly or that failed on their previous contract:

- All but two of the QIOs in the 7th SOW held their state's contract under the 6th SOW.
- Fully 70 percent of the 7th SOW contractors were also contractors under the 1st SOW.

- No outside entities bid against the previous QIO for three of the seven state contracts opened for competition for the 7th SOW.
- As of the end of the 7th SOW, five contracts had been recompeted and one was to be; there were no competitors for three of five contracts (personal communication, S. Pazinski, November 14, 2005).

Conflicts of Interest

Federal regulations for QIOs are designed to foster impartiality and to prevent conflicts of interest between members of the QIO board and the health care providers whose care is the focus of the QIO assessment through case review (see Chapter 7). These regulations contribute to a perception of neutrality and respect for the QIO, as well as acceptance of its quality improvement and case review tasks, among the provider community and beneficiaries. They also mean that the QIO boards have derived limited benefit from the involvement of executives from the provider community, such as hospital CEOs whose hospitals might come under the review of a QIO.

Under the 8th SOW, organizations that hold QIO contracts are not permitted to contract with providers in their state(s) for technical assistance or to review services for Medicare beneficiaries that are similar to the assistance or services they provide under the QIO contract. Although some providers and insurers in some states may wish to purchase additional QIO services beyond those supported by Medicare funds, the QIO is not allowed to negotiate such a contract (personal communication, D. Schulke and T. Ketch, American Health Quality Association, June 30, 2005). This prohibition appears to be based on a perception that lucrative contracts with the QIO could influence relations with certain providers and the review of their cases. The potential for such conflicts appears less likely now, however, given the decreased emphasis on case review and sanctions since the early days of the Professional Standards Review Organization program. There is clearly a market demand for the additional services of some QIOs, and under its current level of funding, the Medicare QIO program is unlikely to meet fully the future need for technical assistance with quality improvement. The committee finds that many QIOs have demonstrated a capacity to develop external revenues (not from CMS) and extensive relations with providers and provider organizations within their own states. At least 15 QIOs receive more than half of their revenues from sources other than the core contract. The committee concludes that if the case review functions were no longer maintained within each QIO, the need for this contracting prohibition might be eliminated. Reasonable controls, however, would be necessary to prevent favoritism in the QIOs' selection of recipients of their technical assistance with Medicare quality improvement.

Confidentiality Restrictions

The attitudes of the early predecessors to the QIOs and physician pressure have generated strict confidentiality restrictions on the QIOs' treatment of clinical data. The committee concludes that these restrictions protect the privacy of providers and are not well suited to the current need for transparency, public reporting, and consumer access to information (Gaul, 2005). The restrictions also constrain the use of data on quality measures to support the quality improvement process. These restrictions were established mainly through regulations, and the secretary of DHHS could make policy changes consistent with Health Insurance Portability and Accountability Act (HIPAA) regulations without the need for new legislation (personal communication, T. Jost, Washington and Lee University School of Law, December 21, 2004).

Consistent with CMS's concerns regarding the use of data and protection of providers, CMS required that for this study, the committee use measurement data on the performance of each QIO only in the aggregate for the nation as a whole, or deidentify the data to protect the QIOs. The IOM had never requested access to physician or patient data, which would have required protections. The committee finds that the program's lack of transparency concerning its key contractors is incompatible with the broader trends within Medicare and the health care system to disclose providers' quality measures through public reporting.

OVERSIGHT OF THE QIO PROGRAM[3]

CMS has the challenge of managing the QIO program in the field, as well as integrating it into the operational responsibilities of the Medicare program. The main oversight functions required of the CMS Quality Improvement Group, which runs the QIO program, include the following:

• Operation of complex data processing and communications systems for the program
• Management and evaluation of QIO core contracts and contracts for QIOSCs, special studies, and support contracts
• Strategic planning needed to ensure the continued usefulness of the QIO program to the Medicare program

Chapter 13 describes the various communications and management mechanisms used by the QIO program and its data systems.

---

[3]Most of the information in this section was drawn from the committee's site visits, telephone interviews, and web-based data collection tool.

Data Processing and Communications

Communications among the QIO Central Office, the Regional Offices, and the QIOs are maintained through e-mails, list serves, restricted and public websites, and electronic reporting tools. To some extent, the QIOs are expected to operate in the virtual world, and they are encouraging providers to move in that direction as well. Training for CMS staff and programs, including QIO staff, is conducted over the Internet; communities of practice stay in touch with monthly conference calls; and meetings are video broadcast across the country to minimize travel. Some of these mechanisms do not work as well as the QIOs would like: CEOs claim that the frequency of conference calls makes it impossible to participate every time; that they do not receive policy memoranda and other necessary guidance promptly; and that reporting systems, such as those for case review and program activities, are difficult to use.

Management communications among CMS Project Officers, QIOs, and CMS Contract Officers are particularly problematic. A QIO can be caught between two different interpretations of an issue, and the interpretation of the Contracts Office has priority. The CMS Project Officer provides routine guidance to the QIO and often serves as a communications link when policy questions arise. While the Project Officer may request an activity outside the scope of the QIO contract and beyond the budget, however, the Contracts Office may subsequently refuse to consider a contract modification.

The Standard Data Processing System supports the communications tools mentioned above, as well as the flow and processing of data from medical records. It is key to the QIO program, and 63 percent of the QIOs rated the value of the system as excellent or good, although some QIOs mentioned the need to update the system and integrate it with their own equipment. It will be important for QIO and CMS staff to be closely involved with national and regional initiatives concerning data exchange, to understand strategic policy issues related to health information technology, and to keep their software and hardware current. The main concern QIOs expressed is that the data reported through the Dashboard section of the QIONet internal CMS website and used to monitor the progress of the QIOs' quality improvement efforts often are not timely (see Chapter 13). Although there is some conflicting evidence about the value of rapid data feedback (Beck et al., 2005), the QIOs and providers frequently stressed the usefulness of real-time data for quality improvement and for the care of specific patients.

As CMS increases the measures required for public reporting by hospitals and physicians, the challenges to the Standard Data Processing System will increase. (CMS conducts much of the processing of the data for nursing home and home health care measures.) The committee concludes that the growing volumes of data, the expanded numbers of data sources, the increased need for the timeliness of data processing, and the interest in user-friendly data reports for different stakeholders will exert pressures on the current system. At the same time, the transition to electronic health records may reduce the demand for data abstraction, increase the need for data-auditing services, and improve the timeliness of the data. Long-range planning for these changes is essential to smooth operations and should include an array of people with detailed operational expertise early in the process. The implementation of a national system for quality measurement and reporting will have an additional impact on the demand for data processing and other activities (IOM, 2006). The committee recognizes, however, that full implementation of both electronic health records and the new national public reporting system will take time. Therefore, paper-based tools that can be used prospectively, as opposed to chart abstraction, will also be important. With DHHS fully supporting providers' move to the use of electronic health records, as well as electronic communications, Medicare could serve as a guide to the future if its data systems keep pace with the transition.

QIO Contract Management and Evaluation

CMS's day-to-day management of each QIO contract is a major responsibility of staff in the Regional Offices, who perform detailed on-site assessments at 9 and 18 months into the contract period and in the interim keep in touch with the QIOs to which they are assigned. However, most of a QIO's performance rating for contract renewal is based on data on providers' performance on quality measures and complex formulas, with separate calculations for each task. The increased complexity of tasks in the 8th SOW led to a significantly more complicated set of formulas and incentive awards than those in the 7th SOW (see Chapter 10). The absence of an overall evaluation plan, guidance, and program priorities has created a situation in which each of CMS's Government Task Leaders designs the evaluation formulas for his or her own tasks in the SOW. The formulas do not draw upon consistent time frames, goals, or definitions. The resulting complexity makes it difficult to construct a coherent overall assessment of a QIO. It is unclear, therefore, whether these formulas adequately assess "improvement" and "quality," and the committee finds that the program's system for evaluating the QIOs requires further development to enhance its effectiveness. As recommended in a 1994 IOM letter report, staff with expertise and experience in program evaluation, as well as outside assistance, are needed to design formative and summative evaluations of the QIOs and to contribute to the design of contract performance reviews (IOM, 1994).

The complex method for evaluating the contract performance of QIOs under their core contract is in sharp contrast to the limited, relatively simple methods used in the 7th SOW to assess the performance of the QIOSCs, QIOs conducting special studies, and organizations carrying out support contracts. Although these contracts are assessed for timeliness and completeness of deliverables and spending, CMS relies primarily on the judgments of the Project Officers. It may be noted that contracts for QIOSCs, special studies, and program support accounted for almost one-third of the total apportionment for the 7th SOW. The value of these expenditures is diminished by the lack of a comprehensive listing of these various contracts and summaries of their contents and results, which are thus not diffused throughout the quality improvement community. Although many of the support contracts are related tangentially to the QIO program, QIOs may be unaware of those contracts or of a special study that is under way and would be of interest to them. CMS is in the process of developing a management and accountability plan to better administer all of its contracts. Few details were available as of this writing, however, and implementation of the plan remains to be seen.

One factor that may have contributed to the previously discussed limited competition from other entities for the 8th SOW was the timing of submission of proposals for the core contract. The request for proposal was released on April 1, 2005, and the deadline for submission of proposals was April 15, 2005, before the SOW was final and the full amount of funds available was known. An official version of the 8th SOW was issued on May 20, 2005, but some elements were still under discussion within DHHS and the Office of Management and Budget that could have required future and unknown modifications to the SOW. In the first contract round, the QIOs were required to submit their bids before the release of the final SOW, and the bids had to be based on a draft SOW and spending estimates. Major revisions to the 8th SOW were made on November 4, 2005, well past the beginning of the new contract period. Because late revisions can affect QIO staffing and work schedules, QIOs reported that the timing has been frustrating and has hampered their ability to prepare for the start of the new contract (personal communication, D. Schulke and T. Ketch, American Health Quality Association, June 30, 2005). Additionally, delayed releases may deter organizations with no previous experience in holding a QIO contract from bidding because of the inadequate amount of time to prepare.

During the committee's site visits and telephone interviews, several QIOs indicated that the 3-year length of the contract is also a problem. They believe this period of time is insufficient to obtain data describing the initial impact of their quality improvement projects and to allow them to adjust their interventions and later be remeasured for their contract performance evaluations. Given the experience with the preparation for the 8th

SOW, as well as the increased expectations of this SOW, it appears that CMS would also benefit from a longer contract period.

Strategic Planning

Two positive signs concerning policy planning for the QIO program suggest to the committee that CMS is moving in the right direction. First, the Quality Improvement Group has initiated a long-range planning process to better position the program 12 years into the future. Although some strategic planning discussions have recognized the importance of coordinated care and crosscutting issues in improving the overall safety and quality of care, representatives of hospitals, home health care agencies, physician practices, and nursing homes have not had opportunities to meet to discuss appropriate measures and mechanisms for tracking a patient being released from one facility and placed in another. Much of the internal strategic planning process has focused on individual tasks and separate Government Task Leaders; the external planning process with stakeholders has followed the same pattern of separating each of the four main health care settings. The committee concludes that implementation of the new Part D prescription drug benefit and therapeutic pharmacy strategies offers important opportunities for QIOs to focus on the coordination of care across provider settings. Strategic planning separately for different providers and care settings is inconsistent with future measures of quality and performance that will be encouraged by the national performance measurement and reporting system recommended by this committee (IOM, 2006).

Another positive sign concerning strategic planning is the rejuvenation of the CMS Administrator's Quality Council and its staffing by the Quality Team. This management structure could give the QIO program an opportunity to integrate its activities with those of other CMS functions, such as public reporting, in the early planning stages. The council has adopted a vision of the QIO program—"the right care for every person every time"—and has made it the vision of the whole agency. The Quality Council is coordinating the development of a number of quality-related projects and presented a Quality Improvement Roadmap to guide the agency's ongoing quality-related work. The current roadmap is more a listing of projects and strategy options than a guide with priorities. Nonetheless, the QIOs are identified as having a major role in one of five major strategies: "assisting practitioners and providers in making care more effective, particularly including the use of effective electronic health systems" (CMS, 2005b:13). Given the commitment throughout CMS to improving the safety and quality of care nationally, the QIO program could play an important part in carrying out this strategy.

The committee concludes that thorough evaluations of the impact of the QIO program as a whole and of the effectiveness of specific quality improvement interventions, based on the articulation of clear and well-defined goals and priorities, would provide useful input to the long-range strategic planning process. Evaluations of QIO efforts in physician offices will be particularly important since the QIOs have had relatively little experience in that provider setting, and there is little evidence of what approaches are most successful in stimulating major system changes.

SUMMARY

While there is evidence that the quality of care for Medicare beneficiaries has been improving, the evidence concerning specific quality improvement efforts, the overall impact of individual QIOs, and the impact of the QIO program in the aggregate is limited and inconclusive. Nevertheless, the committee considers the QIO program to be a potentially rich resource as the health care system moves toward the increased use of performance measurement and pay for performance. The QIO program has shown considerable adaptability over its 35-year history. It currently has a strong foundation of quality improvement experts in each state; a network of collaborative relationships with providers and stakeholders; and a national infrastructure to support data collection, reporting, aggregation, and auditing, as well as research to further the development and the use of quality measures. To make more effective use of these valuable resources, however, a major restructuring of the program is needed. In Chapters 4 and 5, the committee presents its recommendations and rationales for these changes. First, however, Chapter 3 presents a discussion of the changing health care environment and new functions that will affect QIOs and other organizations conducting similar activities. It reviews the committee's first report and how implementation of that report's recommendations concerning the establishment of a national system for performance measurement and reporting will likely affect the QIO program. The chapter also examines other entities that might compete to perform the needed functions.

REFERENCES

Beck C, Richard H, Tu J, Pilote L. 2005. Administrative data feedback for effective cardiac treatment: AFFECT, a cluster randomized trial. *Journal of the American Medical Association* 294(3):309–317.

Bradley EH, Carlson MDA, Gallo WT, Scinto J, Campbell MK, Krumholz HM. 2005. From adversary to partner: Have quality improvement organizations made the transition? *Health Services Research* 40(2):459–476.

Chu LA, Bratzler DW, Lewis RJ, Murray C, Moore L, Shook C, Weingarten SR. 2003. Improving the quality of care for patients with pneumonia in very small hospitals. *Archives of Internal Medicine* 163(3):326–332.

CMS (Centers for Medicare and Medicaid Services). 2002. *7th Statement of Work (SOW)*. [Online]. Available: http://www.cms.hhs.gov/qio [accessed April 9, 2005].

CMS. 2004. *The Quality Improvement Organization Program: CMS Briefing for IOM Staff*. [Online]. Available: http://www.medqic.org/dcs/ContentServer?cid=1105558772835& pagename=Medqic%2FMQGeneralPage%2FGeneralPageTemplate&c=MQGeneral Page [accessed December 26, 2005].

CMS. 2005a. *Best Practice Methods Special Study: Report of First Year Scan of QIO Inpatient Practice*. Unpublished. Baltimore, MD: Centers for Medicare and Medicaid Services.

CMS. 2005b. *Quality Improvement Roadmap*. [Online]. Available: http://www. medicaldevices.org/public/issues/documents/CMSMedicareroadmap.pdf [accessed December 26, 2005].

Daniel DM, Norman J, Davis C, Lee H, Hindmarsh MF, McCulloch DK, Wagner EH, Sugarman JR. 2004. A state-level application of the chronic illness breakthrough series: Results from two collaboratives on diabetes in Washington state. *Joint Commission Journal on Quality and Safety* 30(2):69–79.

Dellinger EP, Hausmann SM, Bratzler DW, Johnson RM, Daniel DM, Bunt KM, Baumgardner GA, Sugarman JR. 2005. Hospitals collaborate to decrease surgical site infections. *The American Journal of Surgery* 190(1):9–15.

Gaul GM. 2005, July 26. Once health regulators, now partners. *Washington Post*. p. A1.

Gould BE, Grey MR, Huntington CG, Gruman C, Rosen JH, Storey E, Abrahamson L, Conaty AM, Curry L, Ferreira M, Harrington KL, Paturzo D, Van Hoof TJ. 2002. Improving patient care outcomes by teaching quality improvement to medical students in community-based practices. *Academic Medicine* 77(10):1011–1018.

IOM (Institute of Medicine). 1994. *An Assessment of the HCFA Evaluation Plan for the Medicare Peer Review Organization*. Washington, DC: National Academy Press.

IOM. 2000. *To Err Is Human: Building a Safer Health System*. Kohn LT, Corrigan JM, Donaldson MS, eds. Washington, DC: National Academy Press.

IOM. 2001. *Crossing the Quality Chasm: A New Health System for the 21st Century*. Washington, DC: National Academy Press.

IOM. 2002. *Leadership by Example: Coordinating Government Roles in Improving Health Care Quality*. Corrigan JM, Eden J, Smith BM, eds. Washington, DC: National Academy Press.

IOM. 2004. *Keeping Patients Safe: Transforming the Work Environment of Nurses*. Page A, eds. Washington, DC: The National Academies Press.

IOM. 2006. *Performance Measurement: Accelerating Improvement*. Washington, DC: The National Academies Press.

Jencks SF, Huff ED, Cuerdon T. 2003. Change in the quality of care delivered to Medicare beneficiaries, 1998–1999 to 2000–2001. *Journal of the American Medical Association* 289(3):305–312.

Jha AK, Li Z, Orav EJ, Epstein AM. 2005. Care in U.S. hospitals—the hospital quality alliance program. *New England Journal of Medicine* 353(3):265–274.

Jost TS. 2005. *Racial and Ethnic Disparities in Medicare: What the Department of Health and Human Services and the Centers for Medicare and Medicaid Services Can, and Should Do*. National Academy of Social Insurance Study Panel on Sharpening Medicare's Tools to Reduce Racial and Ethnic Disparities. Washington, DC: National Academy of Social Insurance.

Kiefe CI, Allison JJ, Williams OD, Person SD, Weaver MT, Weissman NW. 2001. Improving quality improvement using achievable benchmarks for physician feedback: A randomized controlled trial. *Journal of the American Medical Association* 285(22):2871–2879.

Leatherman S, McCarthy, D. 2005. *Quality of Health Care for Medicare Beneficiaries: A Chartbook.* New York: The Commonwealth Fund.

Marciniak TA, Ellerbeck EF, Radford MJ, Kresowik TF, Gold JA, Krumholz HM, Kiefe CI, Allman RM, Vogel RA, Jencks SF. 1998. Improving the quality of care for Medicare patients with acute myocardial infarction: Results from the Cooperative Cardiovascular Project. *Journal of the American Medical Association* 279(17):1351–1357.

National Health Policy Forum. 2004. *Quality Improvement in Maryland: Partnerships and Progress.* Washington, DC: National Health Policy Forum.

NCQA (National Committee for Quality Assurance). 2005. *The State of Health Care Quality Report: Industry Trends and Analysis.* Washington, DC: National Committee for Quality Assurance.

NORC (National Organization for Research at the University of Chicago). 2004. *Final Report: Physician Meetings on Take-Up of Electronic Health Records.* Unpublished. Washington, DC: National Organization for Research at the University of Chicago.

Orlikoff JE, Totten MK. 2005. The pros and cons of board compensation. Does the promise justify the means? *Healthcare Executive* 20(1):46–48.

Qualis Health. 2004. *HCQIP Improvement Methodologies Survey Results.* Seattle, WA: Qualis Health.

Rollow W. 2005. *QIO Program: Update and Policy Considerations.* PowerPoint Presentation to the Committee on Redesigning Health Insurance, June 13, Washington, DC.

Westat. 2005. *Survey for Provider Satisfaction with Quality Improvement Organizations.* Unpublished. July 1. Rockville, MD: Westat.

3

Performance Measurement, Quality Improvement, and Other Entities

CHAPTER SUMMARY

This chapter summarizes the key points of the committee's first report, Performance Measurement: Accelerating Improvement *and reviews the functions of the performance measurement and reporting system proposed therein. It also examines alternative organizational structures for quality improvement and potential roles for the QIO program and other capable organizations in government and the private sector.*

The legislative mandate for the Institute of Medicine's (IOM) evaluation of the Quality Improvement Organization (QIO) program requested an overview of the program and an assessment of the program's impact (see the introduction to this report). The committee assumes that another question is implicit in that mandate: On the basis of the QIO program's past performance, what should its role be in the future? The committee believes examining a program's past is of particular value in considering changes that should be made in the future. It should also be noted that the committee's judgments about future roles for the QIO program are based on certain expectations regarding the changing health care environment. Those expectations derive from the committee's work on the two other studies in the IOM's Redesigning Health Insurance project—on performance measurement and payment incentives (also described in the introduction to this report). The first section of this chapter summarizes the case for an organized performance measurement and reporting system, along with the recommendations made in the committee's first report, *Performance Measurement: Accelerating Improvement* (IOM, 2006). The second section examines the potential roles for the QIO program and other organizations in the new health care environment of the future. The committee's report on payment incentives will be published in 2006.

82

THE NEED FOR AN ORGANIZED PERFORMANCE MEASUREMENT AND REPORTING SYSTEM

The introduction to this report and the *Performance Measurement* report document serious problems with the quality of health care in the United States: substantial variations in provider performance among both individual and institutional providers; substantial variations in provider performance by the patient's geographic location, race or ethnicity, and insurance status; high error rates; and high and rising costs. The gap remains wide at present between the level of performance called for in the IOM's *Quality Chasm* report (IOM, 2001) and envisioned by the committee and the care that is provided (IOM, 2001). A congressional mandate separate from that for the present study, Section 238 of the Medicare Prescription Drug, Improvement, and Modernization Act of 2003 (P.L. 108-173), requested that the IOM consider how the application of two key strategies within the health care environment—public reporting and payment incentives—can be used to promote quality improvement. Both mandates were assigned to this committee. These two strategies, together with quality improvement initiatives, can influence the way care is delivered. The committee believes these strategies have the potential not only to improve the quality and increase the value of care delivery, but also to improve overall health outcomes. Implementation of these strategies will require the use of performance measures. Indeed, a performance measurement system can provide support and guidance for the formulation of national priorities and goals and for quality improvement strategies to achieve those goals. Moreover, a common performance measurement infrastructure is needed to support the efforts of private and public insurance plans to realign incentives.

Many performance measure sets are currently used for quality improvement in the health care delivery system, creating unnecessary burdens on providers and confusion among consumers and purchasers. A multitude of organizations have created their own quality measures for purposes specific to their particular needs, leading to an uncoordinated proliferation of measures. Those efforts have contributed to a "nonsystem" of performance measurement. In cataloging more than 800 measures, the committee found many of the measure sets to be duplicative, with slight differences in the specific details of the numerator or the denominator. Public reporting methods also vary greatly, with little evidence on how best to present the data to the public and on what impact the reports have on health care delivery.

Efforts have been made to harmonize the various measures. For example, those used in the QIO program are generally consistent with some of the common measure sets, and the Centers for Medicare and Medicaid Services (CMS) has been collaborating with the relevant associations to eliminate the slight differences in specifications among measures used for various purposes in the Medicare program. Measurement remains incomplete, however, failing to address important aspects of the health care system. For example, measures of efficiency, equity, and patient-centeredness are less developed than measures of effectiveness. Processes of care are measured more frequently than structures and outcomes. Also, the measures used cover a disparate set of clinical conditions and populations. As a result, current measures are not robust enough to support the strategies of performance measurement and reporting and payment incentives.

Regardless of one's political persuasion—whether one believes the health care system should be primarily publicly run, governed by the free market, or governed by a mix of the two approaches—it is generally recognized that coherent and comprehensive performance measurement and reporting are fundamental to achieving better-quality care and represent a public good. Such a system should ultimately include data from all payers, all patients, and all providers. Strong national leadership is needed to create such a public good; it has not evolved spontaneously and is unlikely to develop without effective public guidance.

The committee believes an organized system is necessary to align all current measurement efforts and to accelerate the diffusion and pace of performance measurement and reporting. Many issues innate to the measurement of performance—such as risk adjustment to account for differences in patient populations and the severity of cases from one provider to another and adjustment for patient compliance—would be difficult to address adequately outside of such an organized system. Because performance measurement and reporting are a public good and would serve a broad and diverse audience, investment from society in general should be considered. In sum, the committee believes the chaos that characterizes the current nonsystem inhibits the rate of improvement in health care quality, and that strong federal leadership is necessary to create a system for measurement and reporting that can achieve the vision of the *Quality Chasm* series of reports.

A National System for Performance Measurement and Reporting

In the *Performance Measurement* report, the committee recommends the establishment of a new, independent governing board, the National Quality Coordination Board (NQCB), to be housed as an independent entity within DHHS. This recommendation reflects and builds upon a history of earlier efforts to establish a national performance measurement and public reporting system, including recommendations of the Strategic Framework Board and the Advisory Council for Health Care Quality. (Chapter 2 of *Performance Measurement* reviews in detail previous attempts in the

United States and other countries to establish such a system.) The committee envisions the NQCB as working with and not supplanting existing stakeholder groups from both the public and the private sectors to ensure that all of the following functions of a high-performing system for measurement and reporting are carried out:

- Specification of a purpose and aims for American health care
- Establishment and prioritization of short- and long-term national goals
- Designation or development and promulgation of standardized measures
- A guarantee of adequate data collection, validation, and aggregation
- Establishment of public reporting methods responsive to stakeholder needs
- Identification of a research agenda for the development of new measures
- Evaluation of the impact of the overall system

The work of the NQCB will need to be grounded in sound, scientific evidence. The board should be given adequate funding and contract authority, should have structural independence, and should be free of undue influence from special interests in completing its tasks. It should also have standards-setting authority and external accountability. Its members should have substantive expertise, should have experience gained in the field, and should be able to guide existing organizations with ongoing efforts that address its goals and functions. The collaboration of stakeholders will contribute to an organized national system that, although not a solution in and of itself, has great potential to accelerate improvements in health care quality for the entire health care delivery system.

The NQCB as envisioned by the committee will harmonize and refocus measurement and reporting efforts for three main purposes: accountability, quality improvement, and population health. With respect to accountability, the committee believes performance measurement and reporting should support patients' decisions in choosing providers, as well as give purchasers information to aid in the selection of providers and the development of health insurance networks. Quality oversight organizations should be able to use these data in their accreditation and certification activities. Performance data should also support decisions on the quality improvement interventions to be undertaken in provider settings. In addition, the data and analyses of the NQCB should inform stakeholders about how well the system is functioning in addressing population health issues, such as access to health care, disparities in health care, and health promotion.

Key Functions of the NQCB

Certain functions essential to the new system, such as the definition of goals and priorities, should be carried out by the NQCB itself at the national level; other functions can be performed by various organizations and agencies, with national coordination provided by the board. Specification of the board's purpose and aims is the first step in creating the new system (see Figure 3.1). This should be done at the national level, along with the establishment and prioritization of national goals for the delivery of quality health care. Without a set of priorities, efforts will not be targeted efficiently to the areas of greatest need. On the other hand, the development of national priorities and goals for the health care delivery system, similar to those developed in the *Healthy People* series of reports in the public health system, is not meant to stifle local innovation. In fact, the committee recommends that innovation and achievement of local priorities in pursuit of the national goals be encouraged, recognizing that such local efforts can help improve current approaches to quality measurement.

The promulgation of standardized measures built upon the measures currently in use or under development is another key function of a high-performing measurement and reporting system. The NQCB could begin by endorsing a minimum set of such measures for use by all providers in ambulatory care, acute care, health care plans, and long-term care settings; for the treatment of end-stage renal disease; and for longitudinal measurement of health outcomes and health care costs for a given condition or patient. To this end, the committee identified a starter set of measures drawn from current leading measure sets developed or used by such programs as the End Stage Renal Disease program in Medicare; the Leapfrog Group; the Agency for Healthcare Research and Quality's National Quality and Disparities Reports; the Ambulatory care Quality Alliance; the National Committee for Quality Assurance's Health Plan Employer Data and Information Set (HEDIS); CMS's Nursing Home Compare and Home Health Compare; the Hospital Quality Alliance; and the Consumer Assessment of Healthcare Providers and Systems' (CAPHS) health plan, hospital, and ambulatory surveys of consumers' views on health care they received (see Table A.3 in Appendix A). The measures in this starter set will need to be defined with consistent specifications and detailed elements. They will also need to be updated periodically to reflect advances in performance measurement. The continual evaluation of the measurement and reporting system, including feedback from providers and users of the data, will contribute to the updating and refinement of the measures.

As noted above, the committee's review of existing performance measures revealed both duplication and gaps. The gaps included important aspects of the health care system not adequately measured (limited scope), a

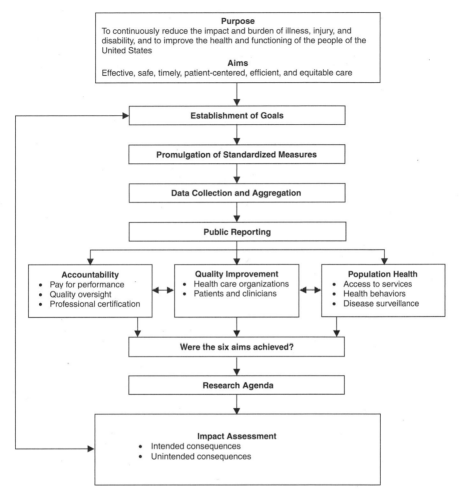

FIGURE 3.1 Functions of a national system for performance measurement and reporting.
SOURCE: *Performance Measurement: Accelerating Improvement*, adapted from Strategic Framework Board (McGlynn, 2003).

time window too narrow for the assessment of health care delivery, a provider-centric rather than a patient-centric focus, and a narrow focus of accountability (see Table 3.1). To address these gaps, the committee identified four approaches for improving performance measurement and reporting:

- *Comprehensive measurement*—Through comprehensive performance measurement, aims and conditions not being adequately measured will become apparent.
- *Longitudinal measurement*—Longitudinal measurement examines the quality of services as patients move through the delivery system over time and across settings of care. For example, longitudinal measures would be necessary to follow a patient through an episode of care or for 30 days after hospital discharge.
- *Individual-level, population-based, and systems-level measurements*—Individual-level, population-based, and systems-level measurements assess how well the delivery system is providing care to individuals and populations (by geographic location, race or ethnicity, or some other designation).
- *Shared accountability*—All providers treating a patient should share responsibility for the patient's health outcomes.

TABLE 3.1   Gaps in Current Performance Measure Sets

Gap	Relevant Design Principles	Description
Limited scope of measurement: Few measures of patient-centered care, equity, or efficiency. Few measures for children or those at the end of life. Many important conditions unrepresented in measures.	*Principle 1:* Comprehensive measurement	A performance measurement system should advance the core purpose of the health care system and foster improvements in all six aims identified in the *Quality Chasm* report (IOM, 2001): safety, effectiveness, patient-centeredness, timeliness, efficiency, and equity.
Narrow time window: Most measures focus on a single point in time and do not assess care across settings.	*Principle 3:* Longitudinal measurement	Standardized performance measures should characterize health and health care both within and across settings and over time.
A provider-centric focus: Current measures focus on existing silos of care (e.g., physician's office, hospital).	*Principle 7:* Individual patient-level, population-based, and systems-level measurement	Measurement and measures should assess the health and health care of both individuals and populations and the many systems within which care is provided.
Narrow focus of accountability: Most measures focus on an individual provider's actions.	*Principle 8:* Shared accountability	Measurement should not be constrained by the absence of a current, identifiable, single responsible agent.

SOURCE: IOM (2006).

To the extent that measures are useful at all levels of the health care system and relevant to all stakeholders, reporting is likely to be less burdensome to providers, and improvement efforts are more likely to be successful. Also, performance measurement will be more efficient and timely if data used to calculate measures are, to the extent feasible, generated in real time and as a byproduct of patient care processes rather than collected retrospectively. While real-time data collection and reporting can be done either electronically or manually, it will require changes in procedures for many providers. The committee recommends that the performance measurement and reporting system be implemented rapidly, but without overwhelming providers. Technical support to providers will be essential.

Performance measurement and reporting require various related functions, such as data collection, validation, and aggregation. The committee does not specify in detail the activities to be conducted or coordinated by the NQCB. Many of these activities are ongoing under the direction or operation of various public and private organizations across the country, including the QIO program. The committee recognizes the importance of current stakeholders in the new system that will be coordinated through the NQCB. The committee also recognizes that its focus has been on roles for CMS in the performance measurement and reporting system. This is the case because the Medicare program has implemented a public reporting system, is moving ahead with the development of payment incentives, and is such an important purchaser of services; because the studies' mandates relate to the federal program; and because CMS sponsored the studies carried out by the committee. Although the committee does not define specific roles for CMS and its relevant programs under the new system, leaving the formulation of such details and their implementation to the NQCB, it does anticipate a strong collaborative role for CMS given its expertise and current responsibilities. The discussion of various activities and organizations that follows in this chapter is meant to be illustrative, not to provide a work plan for the new board.

The committee foresees increased requirements for providers to report on performance measures in the future because of calls for greater accountability. These requirements will place an increased burden on providers even if all reporting requirements are aligned. Providers will need assistance in minimizing this reporting burden. The validation and aggregation of data will require substantial investments. The NQCB will need to determine the optimum means of carrying out these functions and the organizations best suited to performing them, whether at the local or national level. A robust system for the development, maintenance, collection, validation, and aggregation of performance measures will facilitate reporting for purposes of improving the quality of health care.

The continued advancement of performance measurement and reporting will depend on a research agenda. The NQCB, working with stakeholders, should develop an agenda for addressing the gaps noted above, as well as other systemic needs. The formulation of such an agenda will require work in four specific areas: development of new measures, resolution of methodological issues, determination of the best methods of reporting so the data can be used by consumers, and assessment of the overall impact of the system. It will be essential as well to monitor the system for any unintended, negative consequences, such as adverse selection and inappropriate data manipulation.

The committee realizes that the establishment of a functioning NQCB and a national measurement and reporting system and the achievement of the board's performance goals will not be accomplished overnight. Nevertheless, it is essential to the health care system and to the health of the U.S. population that such a national system be established. During the transition, while the NQCB is being established and a performance measurement and reporting system is being implemented, it will be especially important for CMS to play a strong leadership role in coordinating the goals and measures of its programs with those developing nationally within the new system and to support the necessary infrastructure.

FUNCTIONS OF THE NATIONAL QUALITY COORDINATION BOARD AND IMPLICATIONS FOR QIOs

This section reviews the various functions likely to be carried out in some fashion by the NQCB and the national system for performance measurement and reporting it establishes, potential contributions of the QIO program, and possible roles for other organizational options and other entities. The discussion here is based on the committee's recommendations in its first report, but goes further to encompass quality improvement efforts as well.

In the *Performance Measurement* report, the committee acknowledges many private and public organizations that have played significant roles in the development and use of performance measures. Chapter 2 and Appendix B of that report provide details on those organizations that are not repeated here. Many of these organizations have been working with the QIOs in developing measures, reporting on the CMS Compare websites, and providing technical assistance. The committee expects that many of these organizations will continue to perform their current functions, but under the coordination of the NQCB. If, however, any of these organizations could not or did not wish to carry out the functions required for the national system, the NQCB would have the authority to contract for those services. There may also be other services required for the national system for which additional contracts would be necessary. To the extent that contracting under the NQCB was done on a competitive basis, organizations holding QIO contracts, as well as other entities discussed in this chapter, could have an expanded role to play.

After strongly endorsing an ongoing role for CMS in the performance measurement and public reporting system, the committee considered whether CMS should have a continuing role in quality improvement, as discussed in Chapter 2. Other possible locations within the federal government could house the quality improvement program, such as the Agency for Healthcare Research and Quality, which has contributed significantly to research on quality measures and improved clinical pathways; the Veterans Health Administration, which has made dramatic improvements in care within its own system; and the NQCB, which will be directing quality measurement and reporting activities.

Moving responsibility for the quality improvement program from CMS to another federal agency offers some advantages. These include opportunities for CMS to concentrate on measurement and payment issues and to pursue a strong regulatory approach, when such an approach appears necessary, without fear of jeopardizing providers' willingness to participate in the quality improvement program. Moreover, other federal agencies might better manage the program by integrating it with their ongoing quality improvement activities.

On the other hand, the disadvantages of moving quality improvement efforts from CMS to another site also deserve consideration. The first is CMS's loss of the QIO apportionment, which supports other quality-related projects. Also lost would be the opportunity to achieve closer coordination among the offices responsible for public reporting, conditions of participation, Medicaid, the State Children's Health Insurance Program, Medicare payment, and quality improvement. The QIO program has worked closely in the past with the offices tasked with measure development and management of conditions of participation to ensure a consistent approach and to synchronize the details of the measures so as to minimize the burden on providers. Under the NQCB and the new performance measurement and reporting system, those functions will become even more important, and the QIO program's value will increase to the extent that it is able to coordinate its measurement work. Some QIOs have worked with Medicaid but at the state level, primarily on data analysis and case review, rather than on technical assistance to Medicaid providers. They serve as External Quality Review Organizations to state Medicaid programs, reviewing care provided by managed care organizations paid on a capitation basis by the state; survey consumers of that care; and perform special analyses of data collected by the state program. The potential of the QIO program's coordination with Medicaid within CMS has yet to be realized.

In the end, the committee decided it has serious reservations about moving the quality improvement program to another federal agency, for several reasons:

- The experience of the Veterans Health Administration with quality improvement is unique, based on its own management control over providers, and is not readily replicable in the private sector.
- The Agency for Healthcare Research and Quality has had little experience with running an operational program of the scale of the QIO program nationwide.
- Moving the quality improvement function would diminish opportunities for coordination within CMS, including Medicaid, and with other quality-related activities. It would also stifle the progress made through the strong efforts of the current administrator, as well as the rejuvenation of the administrator's Quality Council staffed by the Quality Coordination Team (see Chapter 13), and diminish the potential support and guidance of the NQCB.

The next issue the committee addressed was whether it would be better to allow the NQCB to manage the QIO program directly. The advantages of that arrangement would be the potential for close synchronization of QIO and NQCB priorities; the opportunity for the NQCB to have an operational arm that would reach every state; and the explicit expansion of QIO activities to cover the entire population, not just Medicare beneficiaries. In addition, the NQCB could help strengthen relationships and coordinate activities between public- and private-sector entities. Yet the committee chose not to pursue this option, for the following reasons:

- As recommended in the *Performance Measurement* report, the NQCB should not become a large federal entity assuming responsibility for the operation of all facets of the performance measurement and reporting system. Rather, the NQCB should be an independent entity that would rely, to the extent possible, upon existing stakeholder organizations, such as CMS, to perform specific functions.
- The focus and most immediate priority of the NQCB should be on performance measurement and reporting; assuming other duties for quality improvement would require additional roles and resources that could overwhelm the board's formative efforts. However, the extent to which the NQCB should and could be involved in quality improvement activities in the future is yet to be determined.
- The NQCB has not yet been established, so its assumption of the management of an ongoing federal program would be premature.

As noted above, a number of organizations have made important contributions to the development and use of performance measures. Working with these other organizations is necessary to advance the state of quality improvement, as the functions of performance measurement, reporting, and quality improvement are clearly interrelated. Coordination between the NQCB and the QIO program should therefore be explored to the extent that it can advance the goals and priorities of all these organizations. For example, such coordination could lead to more direct links between private-sector and QIO efforts. The NQCB will be working closely with private organizations—for example, the Institute for Healthcare Improvement, the Institute for Clinical Systems Integration, and such provider groups as the Physician Consortium for Performance Improvement and national specialty societies—to guide the development of performance measures. Combined with the emergence of policy levers such as pay for performance, coordination between the NQCB and the QIOs could link the QIOs more directly to these private-sector efforts to hold providers responsible for the quality of care they provide. Important relationships such as these tend not to develop by themselves. This type of coordination between the NQCB and the QIO program offers a unique opportunity that the committee believes should be explored.

The committee recognizes that the functions ultimately to be assigned to CMS by the NQCB, as well as those currently under CMS's purview through the QIO program, could be conducted by CMS directly through its own staff or, alternatively, through contracts with other private technical assistance organizations. For the QIO program, such direct operations would, of course, presume an increase in CMS's hiring ceiling and all the related administrative changes necessary to hire additional staff. The size of the agency would dramatically increase. Such an arrangement could offer several advantages:

- Given that program policy is currently set by federal staff, this arrangement would allow management to follow the entire operational process to ensure implementation of that policy.
- The federal agency would have more direct control over all activities in each state and over each employee.
- Communications among employees across the United States and between staff in each state and the policy directors and managers in the Central Office might be easier to arrange.
- Most of the QIO contracting functions could be eliminated.

However, the disadvantages of CMS running the QIO program through its own staff are more compelling:

- Hiring practices and salaries under the federal personnel system create more constraints than are faced by private organizations and could make it difficult for CMS to hire people with the necessary expertise and experience.
- The federal personnel system is relatively inflexible and does not respond as quickly as can private companies to changing program priorities and personnel needs.
- CMS has chosen to manage many other important Medicare functions through contracts with intermediaries, carriers, information technology vendors, and other private organizations, and is accustomed to various contracting arrangements.

Thus, the committee supports CMS's continuing to operate the QIO program through contractors rather than operating the program directly through federal staff.

The committee then considered whether the QIO program should continue with its current contractors, many of which have held QIO core contracts for multiple scopes of work (SOWs), or other entities should become eligible bidders. The committee believes the bidding process should be opened up for several reasons:

- The new SOW, based on the committee's recommendations, will be significantly different from past SOWs.
- Some current organizations holding state QIO contracts may excel at case review, but may be less successful at providing technical assistance for quality improvement, the focus of the next SOW.
- Some organizations holding QIO state contracts that have excellent technical assistance programs may want to expand to neighboring states where regionally organized activities would be appropriate.
- Some other entities may be better positioned to perform the tasks of the QIO core contract than are current QIO contractors.

The same rationale generally applies to other contracts in the QIO program, such as contracts for QIO Support Centers (QIOSCs), special studies, operation of the data system, and general program support.

It should be noted that the committee's discussion of this issue relates to that portion of the legislative mandate for the QIO study in Section 109 of the Medicare Prescription Drug, Improvement, and Modernization Act of 2003 (P.L. 108-173(d)(1)(D)) which calls for a review of "the extent to which other entities could perform such quality improvement functions as well as, or better than, quality improvement organizations." By definition, only those organizations that meet the requirements to compete for QIO core contracts do so, and bidding for QIOSC contracts and special studies is open only to organizations that hold a QIO contract. In the few instances in which there has been competition for a QIO contract, it has generally come from an out-of-state QIO. No other entities (private businesses or government agencies) are performing the same range of functions carried out by the QIOs under the SOW for the core contract with Medicare or meet the structural and organizational requirements to become a QIO. Therefore, no direct evidence exists as to how and how well these other organizations might perform those same functions, and it is impossible to judge whether in the future, some other entities might do a better job than the QIOs. Thus, the committee interpreted this request from the Congress to mean an examination of other organizations that could possibly assume the functions now performed by QIOs.

The QIO program has functioned as a closed system of contractors with relatively little change from one SOW to the next. The committee's recommendations in Chapters 4 and 5 are designed to open up the contracting process in the QIO program to more competition and to encourage participation by new and different organizations. There should be opportunities for competition not only for the core SOW for each state, but also for QIOSC contracts, special studies, and support contracts that might be used to promote quality improvement and sustain functions for the NQCB. CMS should take advantage of existing federal contracting mechanisms to select the best bidders efficiently.

Thus, the committee envisions the QIO program as providing QIO core services in each state through contracts with the best-qualified organization bidding on each state's contract. Given the committee's recommendations in the following two chapters that include eliminating QIO requirements for physician access or sponsorship, changing board representation, and limiting QIO functions, other entities in addition to organizations currently serving as QIOs might be expected to be well positioned to bid on the core contracts. Of course, the anticipated funding level of future QIO contracts will also affect the amount of competition.

Rather than limit federal contracting to what the QIO program has done in the past, the committee considers here hypothetical and potential contracting options for CMS and, possibly, the NQCB that would allow them to offer technical assistance to providers for performance measurement, quality improvement, and various other services to support the national system for performance measurement and reporting. As mentioned above, the present discussion of activities is at a general level because the precise functions of the NQCB and the national system it will coordinate have yet to be detailed and established. Nevertheless, many of the salient activities or their elements are now under way, although they are not occurring in a coordinated fashion. For the purposes of this discussion, the committee assumes that the NQCB, CMS, and other stakeholders will define the specific functions to be performed under the contract, invite bids for contracts to perform the necessary activities, and choose from among the various bidders. In this context, collaboratives and other quality improvement methods, whether conducted by QIOs or other organizations, often have not been rigorously examined; the body of peer-reviewed evidence on these efforts is small, and it shows mixed effectiveness.

The committee expects there will be an important need for technical support to providers for quality improvement in each state. Many of the other functions related to the national performance measurement and reporting system, however, may be conducted more efficiently at the regional or national level. Of the general tasks discussed below, some should probably be carried out in each state and should therefore be part of the QIO core contract. Both organizations that hold existing QIO contracts and other entities might choose to bid on future QIO contracts. Contracts for other functions not part of the core contract in each state likewise might attract bids from some QIOs and other entities. Finally, certain functions might appropriately be funded by the QIO program from its Medicare apportionment at the national level. A significant portion of the apportionment for the QIO program has traditionally been spent on projects and activities related only tangentially to the QIOs and could continue to be used to support functions related to quality improvement under the guidance of the NQCB. The following are examples of functions that could support the national system for performance measurement and reporting:

• *Data collection*—All types of providers nationwide need assistance with the collection and reporting of performance measures. Because performance data come from medical charts, administrative claims, registries, and electronic health records, and because providers have different levels of sophistication in the use of those types of records, assistance will be necessary to ensure that the data reported are uniform. The QIOs have worked with providers in various health care settings through improvement collaborative interventions and other technical assistance efforts. QIOs also have helped hospitals responding to the reporting efforts of the Hospital Quality Alliance to collect accurate data efficiently. The collection of uniform data is integral to any quality improvement effort, and technical assistance will be needed in each state to promote the reporting of measures, particularly by those providers ill equipped to staff such services internally or unable to purchase them. Therefore, the provision of such assistance should remain part of the QIOs' core contract. Even so, either in addition to or instead of QIO assistance, many providers rely on other entities, including private businesses, consultants, and professional associations, for assistance with data collection and reporting (see Table B.1 in Appendix B).

- *Data validation*—After data have been reported and aggregated into performance measures, it would be useful to review the original data with each provider to ensure that they validly reflect what is intended, and that all providers understand how to interpret and compare their own performance with overall provider performance as determined through the aggregated data. It would also be useful to offer the provider suggestions for improvement. Although this would be a natural core task for the QIOs, it is beyond the current scope of the QIO program to reach every provider. Other organizations having good working relationships with providers, such as state and national professional societies and private vendors of data services, would also be able to assist the NQCB with data validation. Other such entities, for example, HealthShare and THA, a subsidiary of the Texas Hospital Association, might bid on this data validation task in their own states if the NQCB decided to let state-level contracts for measure validation (see Table B.1 in Appendix B).

- *Data aggregation*—The NQCB will need data aggregated at the national level and at various other geographic levels, as well as down to the patient level, for analysis and reporting purposes. Whether one or more data repositories will be needed has yet to be determined. Currently, the QIO program supports a private data repository that serves the needs of the QIOs as well as those of the Hospital Quality Alliance's public reporting program (see Chapter 11 for more detail on public reporting of data). The QIO program also supports secure data communications systems that can be used for data transmission. Some private organizations, such as Medstat and the RAND Corporation, also have large data repositories and data aggregation capabilities (see Table B.1 in Appendix B). Even if the NQCB decided that data aggregation functions should be a public responsibility, it might choose to contract for some of the related activities, either through the QIO program or with one or more of the private entities profiled in Appendix B.

- *Data auditing*—The accuracy of performance data will become increasingly important as more providers participate in a coordinated reporting system and as financial rewards and public recognition are based on the data collected. Although the QIOs have conducted case reviews in the past and are capable of data auditing, the data-auditing function is inconsistent with their role of providing technical assistance to promote quality improvement and with their collaborative relations with the provider community. The committee believes regulatory functions such as data auditing should not be handled by the QIOs, but should be consolidated and conducted at a level higher than the state. A QIO might thus choose to bid on a contract covering a different region without jeopardizing its own provider relations. Other organizations are performing such functions as well.

• *Public reporting*—The NQCB's reputation as an independent public body will be important when it issues national reports on the findings obtained from the evaluation of performance measures. Ideally, the measures in the National Healthcare Quality Report prepared by the Agency for Healthcare Research and Quality would be congruent with those of the NQCB, and the functions and goals of the two reports would be coordinated or integrated. The QIOs have experience with tailoring performance data to the needs of their states. They might fruitfully help consumers interpret and make use of the national reports of individual provider performance data to inform their choices of providers and treatments, and help providers identify general areas of care that may be in need of improvement. Undoubtedly, many professional societies and other entities will also use the public reports for their own members and clients. It may be noted that for providers to focus on specific, actionable internal efforts, other, more detailed and preferably real-time data will be necessary in addition to the publicly reported global data.

• *Improvement of performance*—Once baseline performance measures in various domains are available, the committee believes CMS should expect all providers participating in the Medicare program to improve the quality of their services. The committee recognizes that many providers do not have the internal resources (staff expertise and funds) to make the necessary changes for quality improvement, but if they are given free technical assistance, they can make greater progress. This has been an important role for the QIOs, particularly during the last decade, and in the future should become their primary focus so they can handle the expected demand from those providers requesting assistance. Many providers also rely on internal quality improvement staff and other organizations to assist with quality improvement efforts, and are more likely to use those resources once public reporting and payment incentives become more common.

• *Promotion of population health*—In their core contracts, the QIOs have had responsibility for promoting some activities at the provider level to improve the health of populations, and this responsibility continues in the 8th SOW. In the context of the QIO program, specific activities include a focus on minorities and underserved populations. QIOs have also been charged in the 7th and 8th SOWs to increase rates of mammography and immunization and decrease rates of tobacco use, measures that help providers promote public health (see Chapter 8). QIOs tend to collaborate with many state and local stakeholders in specific campaigns. Although other sections of CMS are involved with educating beneficiaries directly, resources from the QIO program at the national level could be directed toward the support of national, state, and local campaigns if the NQCB were to decide that such support was necessary to achieve the goals it has delineated.

• *Evaluation of the system*—The NQCB will need feedback on how the performance measurement and reporting system is working, when unintended consequences have been detected, when problems with the collection and submission of data by providers are detected, or when there are difficulties with the measures themselves. Such feedback is necessary for continuous improvement of the system. The QIOs, along with the resources available in each state, are a good source of this information, and this function could be built into the QIO core contract. Other evaluations of the system that might target operations in a sample of states could include participation by the relevant QIOs as necessary.

The committee identified companies currently working on functions related to those listed above for various clients and gleaned relevant information from the organizations' websites (see Table B.1 in Appendix B). These companies are merely examples, but they do indicate the level and quantity of experience potentially available to CMS and, ultimately, the NQCB. In addition, several university health policy and research centers and professional associations have relevant capabilities. It is unlikely that any of these organizations have had experience with the full range of functions in the current QIO core contract, but some may offer unique and relevant areas of expertise.

One organization suggested as an obvious "other entity" that could operate the QIO program is the Institute for Healthcare Improvement. However, the institute's business model does not appear to be suited to the expanded growth necessary for this organization to provide direct services within each state; rather, its management prefers to work through the QIOs to extend the organization's impact. Similar limitations may apply to other organizations described in Table B.1 of Appendix B. Collaboratives and other quality improvement efforts, whether conducted by QIOs or other organizations, have often not been rigorously examined; the body of peer-reviewed evidence is small, and it shows mixed effectiveness.

It was not feasible within the scope of this study to conduct assessments of the performance of the various organizations listed in Table B.1. In fact, because the activities of these other entities are so varied, it would be virtually impossible to compare or rate them. It was also impossible to compare the performance of these organizations with that of the QIOs since none have performed the same set of functions on a similar scale. Thus the committee does not endorse any of these organizations and can make no judgment about their expertise or suitability for specific tasks. The NQCB and CMS would have to use competitive contracting processes to choose the organization—a QIO or some other entity—that appeared to be most appropriate for a particular task. The committee cannot predict which organizations among those listed in Table B.1 might bid or which would be most appropriate for a given task.

Once the recommendations in Chapters 4 and 5 have been implemented and competition for QIO core contracts is no longer limited in practice to existing QIOs, there will be opportunities for these and other organizations to compete for contracts to provide QIO core services and other services related to the performance measurement and reporting system. It will be up to CMS and the NQCB to define the specific tasks to be accomplished, ensuring that the tasks in the QIO core contract promote the goals of the national performance measurement and reporting system, and to determine how to assess the bids and bidders. When evaluating proposals, CMS might consider the following criteria:

- The value of preexisting relationships with providers and other stakeholder organizations
- Relevant experience
- The technical expertise and demonstrated capacity of the bidder's staff
- Staff turnover
- The creativity of the bidder's proposal
- The feasibility of the proposal
- Evaluations or references from current and recent clients
- The financial health of the organization
- The composition of the governing board and its processes for ensuring accountability

To some extent, the amount of competition for a contract will depend upon how CMS and the NQCB decide to structure the tasks in the contract—what needs to be done on the ground in each state, what functions can be performed regionally or nationally, and how CMS and the NQCB will organize their management and oversight functions. CMS and the NQCB will need to consider the complexities of contract management and how to streamline the number of contracts and contractors that could result from restructured tasks. The more narrowly defined functions are, the more likely it is that there will be increased competition involving new entities.

On the basis of the committee's perception of the history of the QIO program, its findings and conclusions about the program's current operations, and its view of a future health care system that includes a national performance measurement and reporting system and performance incentives, recommendations for the QIO program are offered in the next two chapters. Chapter 4 focuses on the QIOs' key tasks, and Chapter 5 on how the QIOs' structure can be strengthened and how CMS's oversight and management capabilities can be improved.

REFERENCES

IOM (Institute of Medicine). 2001. *Crossing the Quality Chasm: A New Health System for the 21st Century*. Washington, DC: National Academy Press.

IOM. 2006. *Performance Measurement: Accelerating Improvement*. Washington, DC: The National Academies Press.

4

Improving Quality and Performance Measurement by the QIO Program

CHAPTER SUMMARY

This chapter examines approaches that can be used to help Quality Improvement Organizations (QIOs) and health care providers fulfill the Centers for Medicare and Medicaid Services' vision of providing "the right care for every person every time" through a focus on quality improvement and performance measurement. The committee recommends that the emphasis of the QIO program be redirected to increase its immediate impact and to align its role with expanding efforts at performance measurement and pay-for-performance programs, as well as the eventual implementation of a national performance measurement and reporting system.

As discussed in Chapter 2, the quality of health care for Medicare beneficiaries has gradually been improving over time. Health care providers are more likely to follow recommended guidelines for the treatment of many of the most common conditions affecting the elderly, although significant gaps in quality remain for many measures. To some extent, these improvements may be the result of changes in accreditation, Conditions of Participation, and professional recertification requirements, as well as efforts of Quality Improvement Organizations (QIOs) to improve quality.

Safety remains problematic, however, despite the attention resulting from an earlier Institute of Medicine (IOM) report (IOM, 2000; see also Bleich, 2005; Leape and Berwick, 2005), and the need for improvements in the quality of health care is still urgent and great (IOM, 2001; McGlynn et al., 2003). We are now at a point in time when many important pieces of the quality puzzle are coming together, creating a unique opportunity to make rapid progress toward achieving the purpose of health care articulated in 1998 by the President's Advisory Commission on Consumer Protection and Quality in the Health Care Industry (1998:1) and endorsed by this committee: "The purpose of the health care system must be to continuously reduce the impact and burden of illness, injury, and disability, and to improve the health and functioning of the people of the United States."

Key components of a major quality improvement strategy are now emerging throughout the health care system:

- The federal government is taking the lead in developing a national health information infrastructure and promulgating data standards.
- The Centers for Medicare and Medicaid Services (CMS) is creating partnerships with other government, health professional, and consumer stakeholder groups (such as the Centers for Disease Control and Prevention, the Agency for Healthcare Research and Quality, the Nursing Home Quality Initiative, the Institute for Healthcare Improvement, and the American College of Surgeons) to develop measures and new initiatives designed to promote quality (CMS, 2005b).
- A coalition of stakeholders, working as the Ambulatory Care Quality Alliance, has proposed a set of quality measures that can be used to monitor the ambulatory care provided by physicians. The Hospital Quality Alliance has similarly convened groups and hospitals to report publicly on performance measures. These alliances were formed independently by private organizations to accelerate advances in quality.
- Fully 98 percent of prospective payment system hospitals now report core measures voluntarily to Medicare.
- Public reporting of quality measures in CMS and the private sector has increased and expanded (see Table A.3 in Appendix A).
- Voluntary reporting procedures by hospitals have evolved to form a national system for the collection and analysis of data on safety mistakes under the Patient Safety and Quality Improvement Act of 2005 (P.L. 109-41).
- Medicare is implementing demonstrations of payment systems that reward quality performance by health care providers.
- Congress is moving aggressively to consider new payment proposals that encourage performance improvement.
- Many private payers are collecting data on quality measures, making some of these data public, and paying providers on the basis of their scores on these measures.

The convergence of these key components represents an opportunity to enhance the quality of health care provided through the Medicare program and nationwide. However, this convergence will not come about on its own. As proposed in this committee's first report, *Performance Measurement: Accelerating Improvement* (IOM, 2006), a national infrastructure—the National Quality Coordination Board (NQCB)—is needed to help coordinate quality improvement activities in both the public and private sectors. Such activities will involve quality improvement experts across the country who can help collect, aggregate, and interpret data, as well as offer technical assistance to providers in implementing the internal system changes required to improve quality (IOM, 2006). The committee sees the QIO program as ultimately operating synergistically with the NQCB. However, the committee's recommendations for the QIO program are not tightly linked to the NQCB because the former is an ongoing operational program, while the latter has yet to be created, and its precise structure and direction cannot be predicted.

Quality measurement and improvement are not easy and will take time; the development of a coordinated infrastructure for quality improvement is a first step. Providers will need help with developing the capacity to measure performance and incorporating quality improvement activities into their practices. Small groups of physicians and solo practitioners, as well as institutional providers lacking quality improvement staff and expertise, are particularly likely to need assistance. QIO executives (in the committee's interviews and site visits), providers, and purchasers say that they expect the demand for technical assistance from providers to grow dramatically (personal communication, F. deBrantes, General Electric, May 13, 2005).

The QIO program is the only public infrastructure devoted to quality improvement with resources on the ground in every state, as well as with electronic communications systems and expertise for transmitting, aggregating, validating, and analyzing quality measurement data. Other organizations have some capacity to offer technical assistance to promote performance improvement efforts. For example, a number of private organizations offer assistance through conferences, consulting, collaborative activities, and web-based programs, primarily for hospitals and ambulatory care settings (see Chapter 3 and Table B.1 in Appendix B). While some of these private programs are free and available to certain types of providers, they generally are not accessible to all providers across the country, particularly those who cannot afford the costs or the time associated with registering for and traveling to national meetings. The QIOs are able to provide local guidance for providers in their own states without charging for the service—a unique capability in that they can not only assist with quality improvement in general, but also address local concerns regarding the implementation of generally accepted quality improvement techniques.

As discussed in Chapter 2, the evidence base regarding the effectiveness of health care quality improvement interventions in general and the contributions of the QIOs to improvements in the health care settings that serve Medicare beneficiaries in particular is limited (see also Chapter 9). While the committee recognizes that evaluations of an ongoing, operational program are complex and that it is difficult to produce conclusive results, more evidence could have been generated by the program over its 35 years of operation. Neither the U.S Department of Health and Human Services (DHHS) nor CMS has made evaluation of the impact of the program and of quality improvement interventions a priority for the QIO program. Greater emphasis should be given to such assessments in the future. To conduct appropriate evaluations that can be used to compare results, the QIO program must have clear priorities and goals for such evaluations.

Uncertainty about the past impacts and future success of the QIO program makes it difficult for the committee to decide on an appropriate future role, if any, for the program. The lack of evidence for attributing improvements to QIO efforts does not mean, however, that QIOs have had no impact on the quality of health care. Moreover, it is clear that a large need exists to help providers improve their quality of care and that the QIOs can help meet this need. Therefore, the committee concludes that if the QIO program were repositioned and strengthened to fulfill its potential, it could support provider efforts to improve the quality of care received by Medicare beneficiaries and help support a national performance measurement and reporting system. The committee believes the absence of QIOs would be a significant loss for emerging quality improvement efforts, and that if such a program did not exist, CMS would need to create one to fulfill its obligation to ensure that all beneficiaries receive high-quality health care. In addition, the committee believes the program's national support centers, external support contracts for data and communications services, and funds for research and development should all be focused on the new national system for performance measurement and quality improvement (see Chapter 3). Thus, the committee recommends that CMS redirect the emphasis of the QIO program such that the technical assistance role of the QIOs is their highest priority and the primary focus of all program resources. Moreover, periodic evaluations should assess the program's impact on the quality of health care services received by Medicare beneficiaries (see Recommendation 7 in Chapter 5 for a discussion of the recommended evaluations). The remainder of this chapter details the committee's specific recommendations for focusing the QIO program on quality improvement and performance measurement.

TECHNICAL ASSISTANCE FUNCTIONS

Recommendation 1: The Quality Improvement Organization (QIO) program must become an integral part of strategies for future performance measurement and improvement in the health care system. The U.S. Congress, the secretary of the U.S. Department of Health and Human Services (DHHS), and the Centers for Medicare and Medicaid Services (CMS) should strengthen and reform

key dimensions of the QIO program, emphasizing the provision of technical assistance for performance measurement and quality improvement. These changes will enable the program to contribute to improved quality of care for Medicare beneficiaries as they move through multiple health care settings over time.

- Quality improvement should embrace all six aims for health care established by the Institute of Medicine (IOM) (safety, effectiveness, patient-centeredness, timeliness, efficiency, and equity).
- QIO services should be available to all providers, Medicare Advantage organizations, and prescription drug plans.
- QIO services should emphasize hands-on and other technical assistance aimed at building provider capacity as needed by each provider setting, such as:
  - Instruction in how to collect, aggregate, and interpret data on the measures to be used for internal quality improvement, public reporting, and payment.
  - Instruction in how to conduct root-cause analyses and deep case studies of sentinel events or other problems.
  - Advice and guidance on how to bring about, sustain, and diffuse internal system redesign and process changes, particularly those related to the use of information technology for quality improvement and those that promote care coordination and efficiency through an episode of care.
  - Enhancement of and technical support for the direct role of providers in beneficiary education as an integral component of improved care, better patient experiences, and patient self-management.
  - Assistance with convening and brokering cooperation among various stakeholders.

Technical assistance for quality improvement encompasses a multitude of activities beyond interventions focused on the redesign of systems or the use of new techniques (see Chapter 8). In the course of their quality improvement interventions over the past few years, for example, QIOs have helped providers collect, aggregate, and interpret data from medical records and other sources to determine the immediate changes resulting from those interventions. Under the 7th scope of work (SOW), QIOs offered all hospitals, home health care agencies, and nursing homes assistance with the collection and interpretation of data, as well as with efforts to improve on the measures reported to CMS for use on the websites made available to the public for comparing the quality of care offered by different providers. QIOs also helped hospitals with the reporting of the data. This experience in working with providers to collect data and with the media and the public to interpret those data will be good preparation for offering the types of assistance that will be needed as performance measurement and reporting expand under a national system, and as providers become more strongly motivated to reform their internal systems and processes to ensure better-quality care. The committee anticipates that the rapid changes it envisions in performance measurement and reporting and in payment for performance, as well as the evolution of a national performance measurement system, will increase interest in quality improvement interventions among some providers who have not participated in such interventions to date and who may need significant hands-on technical assistance.

The Conditions of Participation, the Joint Commission on Accreditation of Healthcare Organizations, and the recertification requirements of many specialty societies require competency activities that focus on quality improvement and patient-centered care. According to a survey by the Commonwealth Fund, however, only 34 percent of physicians are actively involved in systems redesign for quality improvement, and only 33 percent receive data on the quality of the care they deliver (Audet et al., 2005). Yet a study of physician practices and their use of common care management processes (guidelines, registries, physician feedback, and case management) for the chronic conditions of diabetes, asthma, congestive heart failure, and depression showed that only 1 percent used the common management process for each condition, although about half used the process for at least one condition (Casalino et al., 2003). Clearly there is substantial room for improvement. In telephone interviews, QIO executives suggested that the provision of support for those providers who have been reluctant to adopt quality improvements would likely be more labor-intensive than QIO efforts to date and would present a challenge to the QIOs, but that these providers may need help the most.

The adoption of electronic health records by providers is key to the implementation of a national performance measurement system and the full datasets recommended by the committee in the *Performance Measurement* report (IOM, 2006). A few QIOs gained experience assisting physician practices with the adoption of health information technology and with the redesign of their office systems during the 7th SOW under the Doctor's Office Quality–Information Technology project. Most QIOs performed only a small trial of this work at the end of the 7th SOW, however, and all QIOs began this function in earnest only under the 8th SOW. The committee anticipates that the QIOs in some states will have difficulty acquiring staff with the necessary technical skills in computerized information systems, and that it may be better for them to subcontract with a regional or central entity that could provide this expertise. The QIO's own staff could then focus on the system redesign and quality aspects of the implementation of information technology in the physician office setting, with physicians obtaining guidance from local professionals who can customize the QIO's advice to the situation in their offices.

Other important QIO activities related to technical assistance for quality improvement include cooperation with local stakeholder organizations for general educational information, promotion of coordinated care across settings and time, and support for providers in their direct education of individual beneficiaries, all of which can contribute to the larger goal of more patient-centered care. While the committee recommends that the QIOs focus on helping providers engage and educate beneficiaries, not on providing direct education to individual beneficiaries or patients, this recommendation is in no way intended to diminish the importance of beneficiary education as an aspect of patient-centered care. Indeed, the committee believes beneficiary education is an essential part of any physician–patient relationship, as well as any quality improvement approach, and should be included as appropriate in all quality improvement interventions. QIO support for this function may include materials for direct education by the provider, mailings or other such materials offered by the provider to patients, and coordination with efforts of consumer-focused community coalitions. QIOs should also help providers improve the patient-centeredness of the care they offer by supporting beneficiaries in becoming more responsible for their own care and by using consumer surveys to guide their practice patterns. The Center for Beneficiary Choices within CMS is responsible for providing direct outreach and answering individual beneficiaries' questions on their rights under the Medicare program. QIOs should focus on quality improvement and performance measurement activities aimed at improving health outcomes and on related activities that contribute to patient-centered care while the Center for Beneficiary Choices strengthens its direct contacts with beneficiaries.

The scale of demand for technical assistance may surpass the capacities of the QIOs if they do not develop tools and procedures that can be used to assist greater numbers of providers more efficiently. Internet-based seminars and other forms of web-based communications could expand the QIOs' reach, and structured, self-administered toolkits might help providers progress in some technical areas with fewer personal contacts from the QIO. The QIOs will have to determine what types of assistance need to be personal and designed for a specific provider's situation and what assistance can be delivered to groups of providers or applied by the provider internally. CMS should not delay exploring and testing alternative approaches to technical assistance, such as train-the-trainer programs; electronic programs that can reach larger audiences effectively; and other improvement tools used in the private sector, such as shared decision-making programs for particular preference-sensitive care choices. Collaboration and alignment of priorities will be essential to meet the demands of the future.

Another way QIOs can help achieve improvements more efficiently is by convening providers to share best practices. The QIO Support Centers are an important locus for efforts within the QIO program (see Chapter 5). But it is important to note as well that providers associated with the QIO program work with a patient population that goes beyond the Medicare population and also includes patients from commercial health plans. Many of these plans are also making efforts to improve quality and value for their patients, creating another logical source for knowledge transfer. QIOs should, as appropriate, coordinate with groups at both the local and national levels to determine the best approaches to improving quality.

QIO SUPPORT FOR QUALITY IMPROVEMENT EFFORTS

Recommendation 2: QIOs should actively encourage all providers to pursue quality improvement and should assist those providers requesting technical assistance; if demand exceeds resources, priority should be given to those providers who demonstrate the most need for improvement or who face significant challenges in their efforts to improve quality. CMS should encourage and expect all providers to continuously improve the quality of care for Medicare beneficiaries.

Considering the large gap that exists between the quality of health care received by Medicare beneficiaries today and the level of care they should be receiving, the committee strongly believes that all providers in every setting should participate in formal efforts to improve the quality of the services they deliver (IOM, 2001; Casalino et al., 2003; McGlynn et al., 2003). Some providers, such as teaching hospitals and large group practices, have the staff and expertise to devote to internal quality improvement efforts. Many other providers do not have internal quality improvement programs and may support staff participation in formal programs run by private firms or the QIOs.

Currently, provider participation with QIOs is completely voluntary. During the committee's site visits and interviews, most QIO chief executive officers (CEOs) said they favored the voluntary nature of the program, recognizing that readiness for change and motivation are important aspects of an effective quality improvement effort (see Chapter 8). They asserted that working with opinion leaders and early adopters helps diffuse change. Although the committee recognizes that readiness for change and motivation are important factors in the quality improvement process, this does not change the committee's belief that all providers should be actively seeking ways to improve the care they provide and need to take responsibility for their actions.

Providers who volunteer for participation with QIOs may be at any level of performance, including those already performing at a high level and those with problems who are motivated to seek improvement. If a provider is performing poorly but resists efforts to effect change, the QIO or other quality improvement expert currently has little recourse. With the onset of such initiatives as pay for performance and public reporting, however, many more providers will likely seek help with improving the quality of the care they deliver (personal communication, F. de Brantes, General Electric, May 13, 2005). CMS should establish priorities to guide the QIOs in selecting providers to participate in technical assistance interventions should demand exceed the resources available and too many providers request assistance. Ideally, there should be sufficient funding to include early adopters and opinion leaders along with more needy providers, and to cover the extra QIO time and effort that may be required to assist some participants. As part of its evaluation of the QIO program, CMS might seek to identify those characteristics of providers that make them most receptive to and successful in QIO quality improvement interventions. The evidence base concerning early and late adopters of quality improvements is currently quite limited and provides little guidance. Recommendation 8, presented in Chapter 5, is aimed at allowing QIOs to charge providers or seek additional funds for quality improvement to expand their reach beyond the Medicare core contract, thus enhancing the mix of providers receiving assistance.

QIO BOARD AND ORGANIZATIONAL STRUCTURE

Recommendation 3: Congress and CMS should strengthen the organizational structure and governance of QIOs to reflect the new, narrower focus on technical assistance for performance measurement and quality improvement. Congress should eliminate the requirement that QIO governing boards be physician-access or physician-sponsored, while also enhancing the boards' ability to provide oversight and direction.

- **Congress and CMS should improve QIO governance by requiring (1) broader representation of all stakeholders on QIO boards, including more beneficiaries and consumers with the requisite training and executive-level representatives of providers; (2) expansion of the areas of expertise represented on QIO boards through the inclusion of individuals from various health profes-**

sional disciplines, group purchasers, and professionals in information management; and (3) greater diversity of quality improvement professionals on QIO boards through the inclusion of experts from outside the health care field and beyond the local community.

- QIO boards should strengthen their committee structures and consider development plans for individual members, implementation of annual performance evaluations, and annual assessments of the board as a whole as well as plans for its improvement.
- Organizations holding QIO contracts should include on their websites a listing of members of their boards of directors, along with information on the compensation provided to those members and the chief executive officer.

Until the recent revelations about QIO board payments, the governance of QIOs had not received much attention, but that situation is rapidly changing (Gaul, 2005). There is now a greater interest in board accountability and transparency, an interest that extends to corporate governance generally in both the for-profit and not-for-profit sectors. Although the Sarbanes-Oxley Act (P.L. 107-204) mandated changes in for-profit boards, several organizations, such as Independent Sector, the Aspen Institute, and Board Source, have focused on strengthening the governance of not-for-profit organizations.

The current physician domination of most QIO boards results in unbalanced representation that fails to include all the players needed to achieve effective quality improvement interventions (see Chapter 7). For the patient to become the focus of care delivery, greater participation of beneficiaries at all levels of the quality improvement process is required. It is unrealistic to expect a single beneficiary to shift the direction of a board heavily dominated by providers (personal communication, D. G. Schulke, October 18, 2005).

Most QIO boards would also benefit from broader representation of individuals from the various health care professions, individuals at the executive levels of various provider organizations, and individuals from outside the health care field with expertise in information management and oversight as well as quality improvement. In addition, a more formal, systematic, and clearly defined evaluation of the performance of individual board members and overall board performance would likely stimulate stronger board governance (Tyler and Biggs, 2005; McDonagh, 2005; Middleton, 2005; Orlikoff, 2005). In preparation for such board evaluations, it would be helpful to provide ongoing training and development to enhance the board's effectiveness as a team. Moreover, as transparency is an important aspect of performance measurement and quality improvement, information on board members should be made transparent to the public and readily available on each QIO's website.

From the beginning of the QIO program, contracting organizations have been required to have formal physician-access or physician-sponsored status (see Chapter 7). This requirement has contributed to the overall predominance of physicians on QIO boards. Local peer review has been based on local standards of care, defined implicitly by local physicians, and is now considered obsolete. This holdover legal requirement should be changed. Removal of this requirement might also facilitate increased competition from other entities when QIO contracts are opened for bids.

RESPONSIBILITY FOR COMPLAINTS, APPEALS, AND CASE REVIEWS

Recommendation 4: Congress and CMS should develop mechanisms other than those already in place to better manage complaints and appeals of Medicare beneficiaries, as well as other case reviews. The QIO in each state should no longer have responsibility for handling beneficiary complaints, appeals, and other case reviews for payment or other purposes.

- Reviews of beneficiary complaints regarding the quality of care received are critical and should be a top priority for contractors that treat the beneficiary as their primary client. CMS should consolidate the review functions into a few regional or national competitive contracts or determine the most appropriate agencies with which to contract for the purpose in each state.
- To handle beneficiaries' appeals and other case reviews more efficiently, CMS could contract at the national or regional level with a limited number of appropriate organizations, such as fiscal intermediaries or individual QIOs. This devolution of responsibilities would allow QIOs to concentrate their resources on quality improvement efforts with providers.

The QIOs will need to focus on quality improvement if they are to meet the expected increase in demand for technical assistance among providers discussed above. Earlier incarnations of the QIO program focused on case review to identify and punish egregious outliers. In the 7th and 8th SOWs, the balance shifted toward a greater emphasis on quality improvement activities and less responsibility for complaints, appeals, and case reviews.

During the committee's site visits, it became clear that the QIOs are not comfortable with the combined roles of technical assistant and regulator;

the provider community holds a similar view (NORC, 2004; Bradley et al., 2005). In the interest of attracting participants to their quality improvement programs, the QIOs could favor collaborating with providers over disciplining them, and could be less aggressive in their handling of complaints. Moreover, the pressure on QIOs to maintain or improve their relationships with providers may grow under the 8th SOW, in which the weight of hospital satisfaction ratings increases to 25 percent of the QIOs' evaluation scores for the hospital quality improvement task (CMS, 2005c). Indeed, the number of QIO recommendations for sanctions against physicians and hospitals stemming from beneficiary complaints has dropped from an annual average of 31 to an annual average of 1 over the last 20 years (Gaul, 2005). During the 8-year period from 1986 to 1994, QIOs recommended 278 sanctions against providers, whereas from 1995 to 2003 they recommended only 12.

Beneficiary Complaints

The recommendation to shift the review of beneficiary complaints from the QIOs to other entities does not imply any diminution of Medicare beneficiary rights and protections. It is merely meant to transfer responsibility for handling complaints from the QIOs to other agencies at the state, regional, or national level. This shift should be effected for several reasons. First, the committee is recommending that the quality improvement and performance measurement functions become the focus of the QIOs, but these technical assistance activities are incompatible with a strong regulatory function. Hence, the two functions should be separated. Second, the number of complaints reviewed by QIOs nationwide is surprisingly small— approximately 3,000 during fiscal year 2004, or about 1 for every 14,000 beneficiaries (Gaul, 2005; Rollow, 2005). Yet many beneficiaries may be unaware of their local QIO and its complaint review function, even though the contact information for all QIOs is listed in the Medicare handbook.

Another reason to support this shift of functions is that a plethora of other organizations and agencies charged with investigating medical complaints might handle the complaints of Medicare beneficiaries if given the funds normally spent by the QIOs on complaint reviews. Some of the organizations may have greater visibility among consumers than others. Internet searches for "[state] medical complaints" produce a variety of organizations, such as the state department of health or state department of insurance, the nursing home ombudsman for the state, the state medical society, and usually the QIO. Some QIO websites prominently feature information on how consumers can submit complaints, but others do not. Internet searches, moreover, do not necessarily make obvious which agency is most appropriate for handling a particular consumer complaint.

Beneficiary complaints should be reviewed under a contract that recognizes the beneficiary as the primary client. CMS and the QIOs themselves, as mentioned during the committee's site visits, currently recognize providers as the primary client of the QIO program (CMS, 2004). Again, working collaboratively with providers and investigating their activities within a single contract can create an inherent conflict of interest for the QIOs. Aside from assigning the complaint task to an agency that considers beneficiaries as the primary client, the ability of a contractor to perform these reviews effectively needs to be considered. Data on QIO activities related to beneficiary complaints are limited (see Chapter 12). Overall, QIO surveys of complaints revealed high levels of beneficiary satisfaction with the complaint review process but much lower levels of satisfaction with the outcomes of the reviews.

A study by the Office of the Inspector General of DHHS in 2005 revealed difficulties with CMS's beneficiary call centers (primarily 1-800-MEDICARE) (DHHS, 2005). The study found that 84 percent of callers were satisfied overall, but 44 percent had experienced problems with accessing information, while 24 percent had been unable to receive some or all of the information they sought. The study also raised questions about CMS's oversight of the accuracy of the information received. Two reports of the Government Accountability Office in 2004 likewise showed problems with both 1-800-MEDICARE and Medicare carrier call centers (GAO, 2004a,b). A July 2004 study found that only 4 percent of 300 policy-related calls made to carrier call centers had yielded correct and complete answers. Similarly, a December 2004 study showed that only 61 percent of 420 callers to 1-800-MEDICARE had received accurate answers; the remaining answers either had been inaccurate or could not be provided. These studies also suggested a need for improved oversight by CMS (see Chapter 11 for further discussion). The above problems may not be unique to CMS. Overall, however, the provision of confusing or incomplete information and the lack of a central location where beneficiaries can lodge complaints needs to be examined, with the aim of serving the best interests of Medicare beneficiaries. In the interest of these beneficiaries, the complaint process should be handled separately from the QIO core contract.

Under the 7th SOW, a new option of mediation was offered to beneficiaries under very limited circumstances (see Chapter 12). As of July 2004, only 15 states had completed at least one mediation under this new option (Rollow, 2005). While this option is too new for its costs and value to be assessed, the mediation procedure could be shifted to the agency that assumes responsibility for conducting complaint reviews should Medicare determine that the process is valuable.

The committee suggests that before determining where best to lodge the complaint review function, CMS examine the various national and regional options for complaint review, as well as the agencies available for complaint review in each state, the patterns of state responsibilities and delegation of responsibilities for health care complaints or case reviews, and the effectiveness of different agencies in handling complaints. Among the entities considered should be state health departments and the state Survey and Certification agencies, which already contract with CMS to conduct certain functions for the Medicare program, including the review of all quality-related complaints for nursing homes.

Beneficiary Appeals

Recommendation 4 does not imply any reduction of the rights or protections of Medicare beneficiaries in appeals. In the past, both DHHS and the Social Security Administration were involved in the appeals process (GAO, 2005). Because of concerns about poor coordination, however, a section of the Medicare, Medicaid, and SCHIP Benefits Improvement and Protection Act of 2000 (BIPA) (P.L. 106-554) calling for reforms to the appeals process was enacted in December 2000. Additional reforms were included in the Medicare Prescription Drug, Improvement, and Modernization Act of 2003 (P.L. 108-173), including the transfer of all Medicare appeals activities to DHHS by October 2005. (See Chapter 12 for more information on BIPA appeals.)

Typically, when a service is denied or proposed for termination, the beneficiary receives a written notice explaining the appeals process. During fiscal year 2004, there were 8,168 expedited appeals and another 3,084 retrospective appeals. Private insurers review similar appeals, which are handled through routine administrative procedures. The fiscal intermediaries for Medicare might be the type of organization that could logically conduct such reviews because they are familiar with the benefit structure and limitations on services. Because expedited reviews require the availability of a full range of specialists who are on call 24 hours a day, 7 days a week and decisions are now based primarily on national standards of care, it would be more efficient to consolidate the review process for those cases at the regional or national level instead of having each QIO support the full range of on-call physicians for relatively few reviews. The review process is usually based on a review of records, which are faxed or delivered overnight; they could as readily be sent to a regional office of the intermediary as to an in-state QIO. Just as oversight of the appeals process has been consolidated into one federal agency (DHHS), then, the appeals process itself may best be carried out at the regional or national level (see Chapter 12 for detail on the appeals process).

Hospital Payment and Other Case Reviews

The QIOs have continued to conduct a substantial number of case reviews concerning hospital payments and a smaller number of reviews in a variety of different categories, although the overall volume of these reviews has been much reduced over the years of the program (see Chapter 12). The QIO program annually screened and abstracted a random sample of approximately 38,000 hospital claims during the 7th SOW, the mean payment error rate at the beginning of the 7th SOW was 4.33 percent (CMS, 2005a). Most payment errors in the hospital setting were found to be related to inappropriate admissions. Overall, CMS data show that over- and undercoding mistakes tend to cancel each other out (Rollow, 2005).

QIOs conducted 46,000 other types of case reviews, mainly for hospital care, in fiscal year 2004 (Rollow, 2005). The value of each of these types of reviews should be carefully assessed to see whether it exceeds the costs of the review process. Such a study should consider the numbers of cases reviewed in each category, the net payment savings identified by the QIOs, QIO and abstraction expenditures for each review, and other administrative costs for processing the cases according to the QIOs' recommendations. The funds ultimately collected from providers and the deterrent effect of the reviews, if any, should also be encompassed by such a study. On the basis of the study results, the various case categories and the numbers of cases could perhaps be pared down and better targeted before CMS determines whether case review services need to be continued under contract separately from the QIO core contract. Reviews for cases with relatively low volumes should be dropped. For example, from October 2002 to September 2004, QIOs performed only 14 reviews for the presence of an assistant at cataract surgery, and all of those cases were approved (personal communication, S. Blackstock, April 29, 2005).

If a few regional case review contracts were put up for competition, Medicare's fiscal intermediaries, other private-sector entities, and possibly organizations holding core QIO contracts might bid on those contracts. It would be possible for an organization with particular skill in case review holding a QIO core contract to win a contract that covered states where the organization did not offer technical assistance for quality improvement. Thus, a QIO could maintain its independence and focus on quality improvement with local providers without being perceived as threatening because of its regulatory activities.

In the committee's site visits and telephone interviews, QIO executives mentioned two aspects of their case review functions that are of particular value to them. First, some executives mentioned that through case review, they have discovered quality problems common to more than one provider and amenable to correction through a quality intervention. However, a new entity conducting case reviews could be charged with seeking such opportunities and could perform similar analyses of its data for this purpose. Because the contractor would review cases from multiple states, it would be able to identify a pattern unique to one state that the state-based QIO might not recognize as aberrant. The use of national guidelines by out-of-state reviewers should minimize any tendency to favor local practice patterns. Detection of deviant patterns would also be enhanced with the implementation of a national performance measurement and reporting system. Additionally, QIOs would still be able to perform root-cause analyses in the course of their technical assistance activities and in response to patterns revealed through national case reviews or requests from providers perceiving internal problems. QIOs could still help providers with their corrective action plans by performing these analyses and assisting providers with the implementation of any changes necessary as a result of problems detected by outside contractors.

A second indirect benefit of conducting case reviews cited by QIO executives is that the QIOs contract with a substantial number and proportion of physicians in their states to conduct the reviews. As a result, a significant number of local physicians are aware of the QIO and its activities, and the QIO can communicate directly with these physicians about quality issues. Some QIOs rely on their contracted physician reviewers to help promote their improvement interventions and serve as informal liaisons to the rest of the provider community. The committee is cognizant of the value of these relationships with providers for some QIOs. The committee suggests that such informal relationships be maintained, but shifted to focus on using these providers to lead the implementation of performance measurement activities in outpatient office practices and to encourage the adoption of health information systems.

The committee recommends that the QIOs focus solely on quality improvement and support for performance measurement for three reasons:

- QIOs experience inherent conflicts in carrying out regulatory responsibilities while partnering in quality improvement activities with the same providers.
- The budget for the 8th SOW provides too little funding for the QIOs to accomplish the full range of mandated technical assistance activities while achieving transformational change.
- Most important, technical assistance for activities related to quality improvement is the highest priority, and the infrastructure of the QIO program is best positioned to provide that assistance. Other organizations could assume the responsibility for complaints, appeals, and case reviews.

With the QIOs focusing all of their energies on quality improvement and performance measurement activities, it may be hoped that progress on quality improvement measures will be more substantial for all providers. Whether QIOs will be able to meet the challenges of the future, however, will depend in part on how CMS manages the program. Adequate evaluations of the accomplishments of the QIO program as a whole and of individual interventions will also depend on CMS management. The results of those evaluations should influence future program directions and funding, if any. These issues are addressed in the next chapter.

REFERENCES

Audet AMJ, Doty MM, Shamasdin J, Schoenbaum SC. 2005. Measure, learn, and improve: Physicians' involvement in quality improvement. *Health Affairs* 24(3):843–853.

Bleich S. 2005. Medical errors: Five years after the IOM report. *Issue Brief (Commonwealth Fund)* 830:1–15.

Bradley EH, Carlson MDA, Gallo WT, Scinto J, Campbell MK, Krumholz HM. 2005. From adversary to partner: Have quality improvement organizations made the transition? *Health Services Research* 40(2):459–476.

Casalino L, Gillies RR, Shortell SM, Schmittdiel JA, Bodenheimer T, Robinson JC, Rundall T, Oswald N, Schauffler H, Wang MC. 2003. External incentives, information technology, and organized processes to improve health care quality for patients with chronic diseases. *Journal of the American Medical Association* 289(4):434–441.

CMS (Centers for Medicare and Medicaid Services). June 2004. *The Quality Improvement Organization Program: CMS Briefing for IOM Staff*. [Online]. Available: http://www.medqic.org/dcs/ContentServer?cid=1105558772835&pagename=Medqic%2FMQGeneralPage%2FGeneralPageTemplate&c=MQGeneralPage [accessed December 26, 2005].

CMS. 2005a. *QualityNet Dashboard*. [Online]. Available: Private Network [accessed April 13, 2005].

CMS. 2005b. *Quality Improvement Roadmap*. [Online]. Available: http://www.medicaldevices.org/public/issues/documents/CMSMedicareroadmap.pdf [accessed December 26, 2005].

CMS. 2005c. *8th Statement of Work (SOW)—Version #080105-1*. [Online]. Available: http://www.cms.hhs.gov/qio [accessed November 4, 2005].

DHHS (U.S. Department of Health and Human Services, Office of Inspector General). 2005. *Medicare Beneficiary Telephone Customer Service*. Washington, DC: U.S. Department of Health and Human Services.

GAO (U.S. Government Accountability Office). 2004a. *Medicare Call Centers Need to Improve Responses to Policy-Oriented Questions from Providers*. Washington, DC: U.S. Government Printing Office.

GAO. 2004b. *Accuracy of Responses from the 1-800-MEDICARE Help Line Should Be Improved*. Washington, DC: U.S. Government Printing Office.

GAO. 2005. *Medicare: Concerns Regarding Plans to Transfer the Appeals Workload from SSA to HHS Remain*. Washington, DC: U.S. Government Printing Office.

Gaul GM. 2005, July 26. Once health regulators, now partners. *Washington Post*. p. A1.

IOM (Institute of Medicine). 2000. *To Err Is Human: Building a Safer Health System*. Kohn LT, Corrigan JM, Donaldson MS, eds. Washington, DC: National Academy Press.

IOM. 2001. *Crossing the Quality Chasm: A New Health System for the 21st Century.* Washington, DC: National Academy Press.

IOM. 2006. *Performance Measurement: Accelerating Improvement.* Washington, DC: The National Academies Press.

Leape LL, Berwick DM. 2005. Five years after To Err Is Human: What have we learned? *Journal of the American Medical Association* 293(19):2384–2390.

McDonagh KJ. 2005. The changing face of healthcare boards. *Frontiers of Health Services Management* 21(3):31–35.

McGlynn EA, Asch SM, Adams J, Keesey J, Hicks J, DeCristofaro A, Kerr EA. 2003. The quality of health care delivered to adults in the United States. *New England Journal of Medicine* 348(26):2635–2645.

Middleton EG Jr. 2005. Priority issues for hospital boards. *Frontiers of Health Services Management* 21(3):13–24.

NORC (National Organization for Research at the University of Chicago). 2004. *Final Report: Physician Meetings on Take-Up of Electronic Health Records.* Unpublished. Washington, DC: National Organization for Research at the University of Chicago.

Orlikoff JE. 2005. Building better boards in the new era of accountability. *Frontiers of Health Services Management* 21(3):3–12.

President's Advisory Commission on Consumer Protection and Quality in the Health Care Industry. 1998. *Quality First: Better Health Care for All Americans—Final Report to the President of the United States.* Washington, DC: U.S. Government Printing Office.

Rollow WC. 2005. *The Medicare Quality Improvement (QIO) Program 7th SOW and Results.* PowerPoint Presentation to the Committee on Redesigning Health Insurance, June 13, Washington, DC.

Tyler JL, Biggs EL. 2005. Getting a grip on governance. *Frontiers of Health Services Management* 21(3):37–42.

5

CMS Oversight of the Operations and Management of the QIO Program

CHAPTER SUMMARY

This chapter focuses on the Centers for Medicare and Medicaid Services (CMS) and its oversight of the operations and management of the Quality Improvement Organization (QIO) program, including communications among the various program participants, data processing, strategic planning, and program evaluation and funding. CMS's current management is examined from two perspectives: the first considers how CMS could improve the operations of the QIO program in the short term; the second is a longer-range perspective that considers how CMS and the QIO program might fit into the operations of a national performance measurement and reporting system once it is fully implemented.

The Centers for Medicare and Medicaid Services (CMS)—specifically the Quality Improvement Group, which manages the Quality Improvement Organization (QIO) program—has undertaken considerable discussions regarding tools and methods the Medicare program can use at the national level to enhance the quality of care received by both Medicare beneficiaries and other patients (Rollow, 2005; personal communication, W. Rollow, CMS, July 7, 2005). Likewise, long-range issues related to better quality measurement and reporting, such as the expansion of public reporting and implementation of pay-for-performance methods, are being discussed at various levels within CMS (CMS, 2005; McClellan, 2005). The Quality Improvement Group is planning, under the guidance of a consultant, well beyond the 8th scope of work (SOW) to consider the role of the QIOs 12 years into the future, during the 12th SOW (W. C. Rollow, unpublished data, 2005; Rollow, 2005). With a horizon of 2017, it can be tempting to assume that major changes, such as the universal adoption of electronic health records (EHRs), will reduce or eliminate certain current problems.

The committee encourages both short- and long-range planning. It also cautions, however, that managerial and organizational problems of current concern should be tackled now instead of being deferred until potential intervening changes occur. At the same time, near-term actions should be undertaken with the aim of moving the health care delivery system closer to the long-range goal of producing the right care every time for every person.

The recommendations presented below reflect three basic themes voiced to the committee by many sources throughout this study: (1) the need to improve the processing and availability of quality-related information at all levels throughout the operations of the QIO program; (2) the need to manage the program better to increase the likelihood of quality improvements; and (3) the need for evaluations to determine what quality improvement methods do and do not work and under what circumstances, to assess the overall performance of individual QIOs, and to assess the impact of the QIO program overall on the quality of health care. Fundamental to each of these themes is the need for adequate funding, which is addressed in the committee's final recommendation.

DATA PROCESSING

Recommendation 5: The secretary of DHHS and CMS should revise the QIO program's data-handling practices so that data will be available to providers and the QIOs in a timely manner for use in improving services and measuring performance.

- CMS should initiate a comprehensive review of its data-sharing systems, processes, and regulations to identify and correct practices and procedures, including abstraction of medical chart data, that restrict the sharing of data by the QIOs for quality improvement purposes or that inhibit prompt feedback to the QIOs and providers on provider performance.
- The QIO program should support the processes of national reporting of performance measures, data aggregation, data analysis, and feedback.
- The secretary of DHHS should allow and encourage the sharing of medical claims data when the sharing of such data is not precluded by the privacy protections of the Health Insurance Portability and Accountability Act, as well as the sharing of more detailed complaint-resolution data with complainants.
- CMS should work toward the ultimate goal of integrating more care data from all providers and public and private payers to create both records of patient care over time and population-level data.

- Independently of the core QIO contract, CMS should be responsible for ensuring and auditing the accuracy of the data submitted by providers that participate in the Medicare program. Providers should be accountable for the validity and accuracy of the quality measurement data they submit. The QIOs should supply providers with technical assistance to improve the validity and accuracy of the data collected.

Data Processing for Quality Improvement Interventions

The QIO program needs to receive and provide timely data on quality indicators for use by the QIOs and providers during quality improvement interventions. Because the program relies on pre- and postintervention measurements both to provide feedback to the participating providers and to enable CMS to evaluate the QIOs' performance during the 8th SOW, timeliness is critical. The current 3-year contract cycle is relatively short, given the time needed to start up new interventions and the remeasurement deadline for judging contract performance. For example, data presented by CMS on accomplishments under the 7th SOW show that the periods between pre- and postintervention measurements may be as short as 12 months for hospitals. It will be difficult to demonstrate rapid transformational changes during the 8th SOW, particularly because the QIOs need time to adjust to the SOW's new tasks and late release. The feedback loop to all participants in an intervention becomes too slow to provide guidance on the techniques that work or that need to be adjusted to achieve better results within the 3-year period of a SOW (see Chapter 13). Also, some providers value real-time data feedback to improve care for specific beneficiaries.

Now that CMS publicly reports data on hospitals, nursing homes, and home health care agencies on at least a quarterly basis, relatively current data are available for a very limited set of measures at a frequency greater than that in the past. A rapid expansion of the measures included in the publicly reported measure sets, as envisioned in the committee's first report, *Performance Measurement: Accelerating Improvement* (IOM, 2006), would increase the amount of timely data that could be used for technical assistance, as well as for QIO performance assessments. Much of the publicly reported data represents all of a provider's patients, regardless of payer, and that approach should eventually be expanded to all provider settings. Until the number of measures collected for public reporting is increased, CMS should give priority to speeding up the process of data feedback and should ensure prompt data processing for future publicly reported measures.

Methods for collecting data from paper records in physician offices need to be improved. In physician practices and facilities lacking EHRs, QIOs could help with the testing and use of paper-based templates or flow sheets that could be used to collect encounter and performance data in real time during provider contact with the patient. Properly designed, such documents could be cost-effective for entering data into electronic databases, could be less time-consuming than retrospective chart abstraction, and could serve as a guide for clinicians at the time of service. Retrospective chart review can also be a valuable tool for research and should not be ignored.

At the same time, it is important to consider how the growing use of EHRs and the electronic transmission of the data from those records could enhance the ability of QIOs to offer technical assistance to physicians. The centralized development of tools that physician offices could use independently would aid in the acquisition and use of health information technology and would perhaps help the QIO program reach a larger audience. Some physicians who are already using EHRs could also use specially designed tools on their own to produce aggregated data and analyses to guide their quality improvements efforts, as well as to facilitate the redesign of their practices to take advantage of the EHRs. This would in turn allow the QIOs to concentrate on providers that have less capacity for adjusting to the new technology and a greater need for guidance, and would benefit from the experiences of other providers. With the expectation that many small physician offices will require hands-on assistance with the adoption of health information technology and that many thousands of practices may request assistance with office redesign, new methods to fill the need must be developed.

Confidentiality of QIO Data

There are currently three potential key audiences for QIO data on provider performance:

- *Providers*—both those participating in QIO projects who need to measure their own progress from the baseline and all providers who need benchmarking data to see how they compare to their peers. In general, providers tend to show an interest in publicly reported data, and many are motivated by the reporting of these data to improve their performance (Hibbard et al., 2005).
- *Consumers and beneficiaries*—those who may want to compare the performance of providers on more measures than the handful now publicly reported and, if QIOs continue to have a role in case review activities, complainants who want to understand the details of their case.
- *CMS*—which needs data for assessment of the performance of the QIOs and providers and for case review, complaints, and appeals. In addition to highlighting specific providers that have quality problems or that provide high-quality care deserving of recognition by a payment incentive,

the performance data could highlight clinical or geographic areas in need of quality improvement.

Beneficiary Confidentiality

Even before a national performance measurement and reporting system is implemented, more data will begin to flow through the health care system and will receive increased scrutiny as reporting of measures expands. Greater openness needs to be balanced with the maintenance of protections for patients, particularly with the growing use of data from patient records. It will be essential to include strong safeguards in communications systems to protect the confidentiality of those records. Results of a national consumer survey show that two-thirds of the American public and nearly three-quarters of members of racial and ethnic minorities are concerned about the privacy of their personal health information (CHCF, 2005). The current QIONet Exchange, designed for the transmission of clinical quality data in the QIO program, is also used for the hospital public reporting program because it is secure and is compliant with the mandates of the Health Insurance Portability and Accountability Act. To maintain the confidence of beneficiaries, it is essential that any new communications systems or expansions of existing systems used for clinical reporting include similar safeguards. Precautions concerning access to data at geographic or provider levels will also need to be taken when the sample or cell size is small enough to permit identification of individual patients. A national performance measurement and reporting system will need to ensure patient confidentiality for all data on measures and providers at the same time that it promotes the transparency of the data.

Greater flexibility in the use of case data is also important for tracking the quality of services received by a patient during an episode of care or over a longer period. Longitudinal data that can be tracked across various providers or settings and linked to a patient identifier are essential to promoting improved care.

Provider Confidentiality

The current confidentiality requirements of the U.S. Department of Health and Human Services (DHHS) prohibit QIOs from sharing their data—such as those collected within a quality improvement collaborative, used in case reviews, or derived from a complaint or appeal—with providers other than the source of the data unless the source agrees to their use. These confidentiality requirements also constrain the QIOs from sharing all but a minimum of information with complainants on how their cases were resolved. Complainants may receive notice only of whether their care met professionally recognized standards; they may not receive information on what if any actions were taken as a result. If the physician withholds consent, the QIO cannot release the physician's name or other details to the complainant (Gaul, 2005). Consumers do not have access to data identifying sources and providers by name because of the same issues of confidentiality; CMS also has limited access to QIO data. (The publicly reported data from hospitals, nursing homes, and home health agencies are considered CMS data, not QIO data, and thus are not subject to the same confidentiality restrictions.)

The current QIO confidentiality restrictions are not necessary or supportable in the current era of public reporting and are incompatible with the aim of a national performance measurement system and the goal of CMS to serve multiple audiences with a transparent system. The committee recognizes the need to balance concerns about malpractice with the importance of limiting the discoverability of QIO data. Because the QIO legislation gives the secretary of DHHS the authority to set confidentiality standards by regulation, new legislation for this purpose is not necessary (personal communication, T. Jost, January 7, 2005). Thus the secretary may establish new regulations that increase the transparency of QIO data and the ability to share those data. (See Chapter 7 for more detail on confidentiality issues.)

Ensuring the Accuracy of Reported Data

Many current public reporting efforts rely on the QIO program, its Clinical Data Abstraction Centers, and its national Data Warehouse at the Iowa QIO to edit, validate, aggregate, and store the reported data (personal communication, W. Matos, CMS, July 7, 2005; personal communication, J. Kelly, M. Krushat, and W. Matos, CMS, October 25, 2004; personal communication, M. B. McClellan, June 24, 2005). The Data Warehouse, originally designed for QIO data, has grown to accommodate the public data from hospitals for all payers and will need to grow further as the reporting of performance measures expands. (See Chapter 13 for more detail on data issues.)

Although public reporting reduces the need for separate abstraction of data from patient records within the QIO program for some settings, CMS has an increased responsibility to audit the data that are reported to ensure their accuracy. Use of the data on quality measures for payment as well as public reporting purposes increases the incentives to manipulate the system and the need for accuracy. Although the data-auditing function will be crucial, there is no need for it to be a responsibility of every QIO. In fact, it would be better for the QIOs not to have this added regulatory function, as conflicts of interest could arise. Exercising this function could jeopardize the QIOs' collegial relationships with providers in their states and their ability to conduct quality improvement interventions with providers, who participate as voluntary partners. Moreover, in the interest of maintaining good relations with providers, QIOs might be less than zealous in carrying out their regulatory auditing function. In addition, there does not appear to be a strong reason for conducting audits comparing reported data with data in case records at the state level. A national or regional contractor could conduct such reviews. Private organizations and QIOs with strong auditing capacities could compete for such contracts, with the QIOs precluded from conducting audits in states where they offer providers technical assistance for quality improvement.

On the other hand, measure validation (consultation with providers on their initial submissions of data on new measures to ensure that the data accurately represent what is intended) is an important function the QIOs could appropriately handle. Because the QIOs have staff available in each state, they could meet with providers, particularly those in small practices or those that serve as safety net providers, to help them interpret their data before the data are publicly posted and to gather comments concerning any possible problems with the data.

Decisions about the level at which the data repository should be established under a national performance measurement and reporting system—national or subnational—will have to be made as part of the strategy for that system. In any case, the system will have to be able either to accumulate data at the patient level and aggregate them to the local, state, and national levels or to do the reverse: accumulate the data in a national repository, with the ability to break them down to lower levels of aggregation for analyses, such as tracking patients across states and time.

QIO PROGRAM MANAGEMENT

Recommendation 6: CMS should establish clear goals and strategic priorities for the QIO program. Congress, the secretary of DHHS, and CMS should improve their management of the QIO program as necessary to support those goals, especially by enhancing contracting processes for the QIO core contract and QIO Support Center (QIOSC) contracts; integrating the program's core, support, and special study contracts; and improving coordination and communication within the program.

- **CMS should provide the QIOs with a coherent and feasible scope of work that sets forth clear priorities for quality improvement and performance measurement.**

- CMS's priorities and planning efforts should focus on integrating QIO collaboration with various types of providers to improve the coordination of patient care across multiple settings.
- To prepare for the 9th scope of work, CMS should consider conducting a national survey of the main provider settings (nursing homes, home health agencies, hospitals, outpatient physician practices, end-stage renal disease facilities, prescription drug plans, and pharmacies) to determine specific unmet needs for technical assistance. Such information might be complemented by information from focus groups conducted with a mix of representatives from the various settings.
- The QIO core contracts and the QIOSC contracts should include incentives aimed at promoting a broader transfer of knowledge concerning successful quality improvement interventions and more rapid improvement.
- The QIOs should have the resources they need to conduct at least one locally initiated quality improvement project on the basis of demonstrated need and the design and evaluation criteria established by CMS.
- Congress and CMS should change the contract structure for core QIO services for the 9th scope of work:
  - Strong incentives and penalties that reward high performance and penalize poor performance should be included. CMS should encourage sufficient competition for the core contracts to permit the selection of a QIO contractor on the basis of contractor-proposed interim and final performance measures and goals. During the contract period, there should be less process management of internal QIO operations by CMS.
  - Congress should permit extension of the core contract from 3 to 5 years to allow for the measurement, refinement, and evaluation of technical assistance efforts and the achievement of transformational goals.
  - There should be greater competition for each new contract. CMS should consider previous experience and performance as a QIO among the selection criteria; demonstrated capacity to support quality improvement on the part of any eligible organization should predominate.
  - Performance periods should be consistent. All QIOs should begin and end the contract cycle on the same date so the planning, implementation, and evaluation of each scope of work can be applied nationally.

- A timetable should be established for goal setting, program planning, and funding processes for the core QIO contracts. The schedule should ensure that new scopes of work are issued in a timely fashion, and that contracts and funding levels are developed and finalized so as to allow sufficient time for QIOs and competing organizations to prepare in advance for the new contract without major program and staff disruptions.

- CMS should award QIOSC contracts several months in advance of a new QIO contract cycle to allow for the preparation of tools and materials for QIO use, definition of the required tasks and deliverables that will serve the QIOs and the Government Task Leaders, and inclusion of explicit methods for assessment of the contractor's performance. Congress and CMS should allow entities other than QIOs with expertise in quality improvement to bid on QIOSC contracts; familiarity with QIO work, the capability to carry out the work, and experience in performing the required functions should be appropriately weighted when the bids are assessed.

- The QIO core contract and contracts for special studies, support services, and QIOSCs should all reflect the explicit goals and priorities of the program.

- CMS and the Agency for Healthcare Research and Quality should establish ongoing mechanisms for sharing quality improvement knowledge and research results, especially through QIOSCs.

- CMS should take steps to improve coordination and communications within the QIO program and with QIOs. In particular, the roles and responsibilities of and communications among Project Officers, Contract Officers, Government Task Leaders, Scientific Officers, and QIO executives and their staff should be clarified.

  - CMS should build self-assessment, transparency, clearer communications, and continuous quality improvement into the daily workings of the team overseeing the QIO program, just as the QIOs expect providers to do.

  - The contracting function should be subordinate to and support the program management and business functions.

  - Ongoing program evaluations (see Recommendation 7) should provide guidance for the continuous improvement of program management, coordination, and communications.

Priorities

Whereas the 7th and the 8th SOWs included a multiplicity of different tasks, subtasks, and performance measures and suffered from a lack of priorities, the 9th SOW should be clearly focused on quality improvement and related activities to support a national system for performance measurement and reporting. At the same time, it will be important to indicate priorities within that narrower focus. Future QIO contracts will need to be more coherent and should include clearly stated priorities for QIO activities and precise goals for the SOW overall.

Current quality improvement tasks are subdivided and evaluated by provider setting; there needs to be a new priority on improving care across provider settings. As the single largest purchaser of health care in the United States, the Medicare program spent more than $295 billion in benefit payments in 2004 to care for 41.7 million beneficiaries. Among the population over age 65, 84 percent have at least one chronic condition, and 62 percent have two or more such conditions. Transitions in care from one provider setting to another are particularly important for individuals who are chronically ill. The growing need for chronic care among the Medicare population and the implementation of the Medicare Part D prescription drug benefit make a crosscutting perspective particularly important. For example, the continuity of drug therapies as a patient transitions from the hospital to his or her own home or a nursing home could be tracked as new data became available from the Part D benefit. Such tracking of the data would provide an opportunity for the QIOs to integrate the clinical aspects of care, as well as encourage multidisciplinary collaboration (Schulke, 2004).

Cross-site coordination should build on the initial efforts made under the 8th SOW and should feature more prominently in future contracts. The need for quality improvement interventions that follow the patterns of patient care delivered by a variety of providers in the community will increase as a national performance measurement and reporting system implements measures that cut across settings of care, monitor patients over time, and include composites from more than one provider. The QIOs will be challenged to broaden their thinking about service delivery and to convene providers from hospitals, nursing homes, home health agencies, and outpatient physician practices to work together on filling the gaps in care that occur when a patient is between settings, a gap through which too many patients now fall. The program should also help the health care system meet the challenge of transforming relationships between patients and clinicians, as well as within health care organizations. Many safety and quality problems, often resulting from poor documentation and communication, occur during the handoff of patients from one setting to another—a point illustrated by beneficiary complaints, each case of which generally requires the review of more than one set of provider records (CMS, 2004).

Provider Surveys

It is difficult to plan nationally for the technical assistance projects that are needed and will be well received by providers without knowing basic information about providers' internal capacities for quality improvement and measurement work: what they have done in the past and are currently doing internally, what assistance they are purchasing externally, and what gaps remain with which the QIOs could be helpful. Gathering this information could be viewed as basic market research to identify potential clients and their needs. Provider surveys addressing the above questions might serve multiple purposes beyond a basic needs assessment for QIO assistance. For example, they could become part of an effort to track quality improvement trends and serve as a mechanism for identifying and describing best practices. Although it is unlikely that such a survey could directly contribute to measurement of the impacts of the QIOs' efforts, it could provide a picture of the context within which the QIOs operate. In addition to surveys of each provider setting, it would be useful to conduct some focus groups that included a mix of providers to help identify needs for crosscutting quality improvement interventions.

Knowledge Transfer and Local Creativity

Given the strong need for evaluation of quality improvement interventions (as will be discussed further in Recommendation 7), it should be possible to identify various improvement methods, successful projects, and failures. QIOs should be encouraged to share their unsuccessful efforts and their best practices, and to transfer that knowledge broadly both within the QIO community and to other organizations, such as commercial health plans and provider organizations seeking to improve quality at the local and national levels. One type of incentive for knowledge transfer that might be offered to the QIOs is giving them permission to develop their own locally designed projects. In addition, similar incentives should be provided to encourage the publication of articles on quality improvement. For example, the evaluation formula in the contract for the 8th SOW provides a bonus point for QIOs that publish reports on their payment review projects (see Chapter 10). Alternatively, all QIOs performing at a high level or meeting interim goals could be rewarded for their performance on a local project.

Group award fees are built into the contract for the 8th SOW (see Chapter 13) in an attempt to encourage QIOs to share and cooperate toward a mutual goal of improvement. The 8th SOW also allows four QIOs to develop a local nursing home project instead of meeting the requirements delineated for the nursing home task (see Chapter 8). This incentive for top performers could also be made available for projects in other settings. If additional resources were not available to support local projects, one local project could be substituted for one of the required projects. In any case, QIOs must receive approval from CMS for such local projects, whose design must include a thorough evaluation. Consideration should be given to coordinating the local projects of several states in such a way that they could be compared in a single evaluation; this might prove to be a useful testing ground for new approaches to quality improvement.

QIO Contract Reforms

When the next SOW is developed, all contracts should be put up for bid. Because the 9th SOW will be significantly different from the 8th SOW, one cannot assume that organizations currently holding QIO contracts will be best suited to carrying out the new functions. Other entities that meet structural, staffing, and conflict-of-interest qualifications should be allowed and encouraged to compete. Without the requirement to have a physician-sponsored or physician-access designation (see Recommendation 3), new entities might choose to respond to a request for proposals. Moreover, a SOW with a more limited range of functions focused on quality improvement might entice other entities to compete. The degree of competition generated might also reflect the amount of money expected to be paid for the services; other entities might not be interested in bidding on proposals if they did not expect to be adequately remunerated. With open competition for all state core contracts, more-successful contractors might bid on and win contracts to provide QIO services in more than one state, as happens now on a limited basis. Thus, more regionally based contractors might be able to offer services in several states, especially where doing so would be geographically efficient. (See Chapter 13 for further detail on the bidding process.)

The QIO core contract should include rewards and penalties for contractors on the basis of their performance. With increased competition, CMS should expect bidders to propose rates of improvement they believe they can achieve on given measures above the minimums set by CMS, and should offer financial rewards for those contractors that reach their goals and impose penalties for those that do not. Doing so would provide stronger incentives for QIOs to accelerate improvements.

Under a contract providing incentives for high performance (instead of focusing on process management), QIOs would be allowed more flexibility in their intervention methods with less oversight of their daily activities. Although such flexibility was discouraged in the past because of the inability to compare results across states, increased emphasis on formal evaluations of individual interventions (see Recommendation 7) would allow better comparisons, especially for determining the effectiveness of various quality improvement techniques. Therefore, QIOs would be able to focus on achieving the desired result. This approach would also align the QIO program with the focus on defined quality improvement goals in the national system for performance measurement and reporting.

Extension of the QIO contract period from 3 to 5 years would allow more time for providers to implement quality improvements and measure the results, as well as to receive feedback and adjust their quality improvement efforts accordingly. With a longer contract period, CMS should perform more interim monitoring of the progress of the QIOs. CMS should also arrange the contract cycle so that all QIOs receive contracts for the same time period. QIO boards should be held accountable for the operations of their organizations and should be involved in monitoring performance. Shifting all QIOs to the same time frame for contracting rather than continuing with the current situation of three rounds of contracting staggered over 6 months should streamline QIO evaluations and some other management functions, as well as improve CMS's ability to compare performance results among QIOs. Effective management planning would be necessary to process 53 contracts concurrently and to prevent other potential work-flow bottlenecks. It would be necessary to plan monitoring functions carefully to ensure that they could be completed fairly with limited staff from the Regional Office. (See Chapter 13 for additional discussion of contracts.)

Planning for the 9th SOW should move expeditiously to avoid the delays and uncertainties of the process for the 8th SOW. As discussed in Chapter 2, the release of the 8th SOW, expected in the late summer of 2004, was delayed until the spring of 2005, and significant changes were made as late as November 2005. Much of the delay appeared to be related to internal departmental debates and budgetary discussions. Because these discussions would need to occur only every 3 or 5 years if the QIO contracts were extended as proposed by the committee, it would be helpful for the program office to establish an ongoing dialogue with the key parties to keep them informed of current program progress, as well as CMS's thoughts about the next SOW. Explicit planning and drafting of each SOW should begin early enough to permit its timely release by CMS so that QIOs will have adequate time to prepare for the SOW, including program planning and staffing. Mindful of the time needed to prepare adequately for a new SOW and the fact that this report will be released after the start of the 8th SOW, the committee formulated most of its recommendations with a view toward the 9th SOW rather than recommending many hasty, major revisions to the 8th SOW.

QIO Support Centers and Other Contracts

The intent of the QIO Support Centers (QIOSCs) is to serve QIOs as national technical resources, and QIOSCs are often expected to offer training programs for QIO staff and prepare materials all QIOs can use to carry out their tasks. Therefore, the QIOSCs need a head start on each new SOW. In particular, it is important that they have materials ready for the QIOs when the new contract period begins. (See Chapter 7 for detail on QIOSC structure and Chapter 13 for discussion of QIOSC contracts.) This is a particular challenge for QIOSCs that have not conducted special studies or served in this capacity in the past, and it could be a problem for experienced QIOSCs as well if the substance of the QIO tasks should change significantly. Having the next SOW well defined before the current contract is completed would allow CMS to contract for QIOSCs a few months before the commencement of the SOW. Doing so would become feasible if the QIOSC contract were opened to other entities with the requisite expertise. Currently, only QIOs may act as QIOSCs; therefore, QIOSC contracts cannot be awarded until the bidders know they have received a QIO core contract.

The QIOSCs sometimes face competing demands to serve the QIOs that need assistance, as well as the Government Task Leader. The QIOSC contract should define in more detail, to the extent feasible, the specific tasks expected of the QIOSC for each audience and the measures to be used for evaluating its performance.

CMS should consider including in the new SOW for the QIOs and QIOSCs the development of national resource teams. These teams would enable QIOs to work collaboratively with multistate providers to promote quality improvement by reducing the barriers encountered by corporate providers operating in more than one state. This task should be based on a thorough assessment of the Corporate Nursing Home Collaboratives, operated through the Nursing Home QIOSC and the Colorado Foundation for Medical Care during the 7th SOW. This task coincides with the above-discussed need for CMS and the QIO program to consider more of the crosscutting issues of health care delivery.

The Quality Improvement Group in CMS administers not only the QIO core contracts and QIOSC contracts, but also other contracts with QIOs and other organizations that are intended to support the QIO program and quality improvement in general, as defined more broadly within the Medicare program. These other contracts would have greater synergistic value if better tracking and management systems were in place to oversee them and ensure their coordination with program priorities. (See Chapter 7 for more detail on contracts.) For example, if the QIOs had a list of all the special studies and the QIOs holding the contracts for those studies, they might use this list as both an indicator of expertise on a topic and a guide to the topics under study. CMS should coordinate with other entities, such as the Agency for Healthcare Research and Quality, to facilitate ongoing discussions of research results. QIOSCs are one mechanism through which this knowledge transfer could readily occur.

Management Relations

The development of a new and substantially different SOW presents an opportunity for CMS to assess the different roles, responsibilities, and communications systems that will be needed for all QIOs to accomplish the new tasks. To ensure a smooth transition to the new SOW, all participants will need to understand CMS's priorities and policies, as well as those of a national performance measurement and reporting system as it develops. Perhaps some of the lessons QIOs learn in working with providers to improve their communications across various health care settings could be applied to better link the many offices within CMS that are involved with processing QIO contracts and working with the contractors. Given the number of personnel involved in running the QIO program, CMS should seek to clarify the roles of all these individuals in light of the defined priorities of the SOW. (See Chapter 13 for further detail on CMS management.)

QIO PROGRAM EVALUATIONS

Recommendation 7: CMS should develop four types of evaluation to assess the QIO program. CMS should conduct three of these four types of evaluation internally to assess QIO performance against predetermined goals and priorities at the following levels: (1) the program as a whole, (2) individual QIOs with respect to the core contract, and (3) selected quality improvement interventions implemented by QIOs. DHHS should periodically commission the fourth type of evaluation—independent, external evaluations of the QIO program's overall contributions.

- The QIOs should be learning organizations, continually improving the assistance they offer to health care providers. CMS should develop explicit benchmarks for use in ongoing measurement of progress on the effectiveness and costs of the program.
- CMS should form a technical expert panel to offer ongoing guidance on the design of the three types of internal CMS evaluations, including options for identifying optimally performing QIOs, as well as methodologies for attributing quality improvements to the QIO program's interventions.

- CMS should ensure that evaluations of the effectiveness of quality improvement interventions are conducted. The committee suggests that CMS should use the most rigorous evaluation designs practicable, including randomized controlled trials. This approach should also contribute to CMS's overall program evaluation.
  - Evaluations should include concurrent, qualitative descriptions and assessments of the nuanced nature of the QIOs' role in quality improvement interventions and the roles of other players.
  - As appropriate, evaluations should be stratified among provider settings and across states and regions.
  - CMS should assess the cost-effectiveness of each type of intervention to assist with the allocation of resources.
- The secretary of DHHS should allocate adequate funds from the QIO apportionment to carry out, on an ongoing basis, both internal and external evaluations.

Evaluation of Progress Toward Goals

As discussed in Recommendation 6, CMS must set explicit overall goals and priorities for the QIO program, in part because goals are needed to create a robust evaluation plan for determining achievement. These goals should be considered in conjunction with those already established that also focus on enhancing health, such as those set for the public's health by *Healthy People 2010* (HHS, 2000) and the *National Healthcare Quality Report* (AHRQ, 2004), when applicable. Evaluation of the program's success in achieving those goals, as well as its overall impact, has been largely ignored, and the focus has remained on evaluation of QIO contract performance alone. Although contract evaluation is needed, CMS must initiate plans to evaluate the QIO program as a whole and the effectiveness and impacts of individual intervention approaches.

Levels of Evaluation

Four levels of evaluation are important. The first is evaluation of the program as a whole to help prove its value and efficiency in the arena of health care quality improvement. As noted above, explicit goals against which the program can be evaluated must be set by CMS. This level of evaluation should be focused not only on determining the success of the program in improving quality overall, but also on such factors as CMS's oversight of the program's management and operations and the effectiveness and value of the support services provided within the program. Without such program-level evaluation, it is difficult to justify a specific apportionment and budget.

Second, it is important for CMS to assess the performance of individual QIOs because under a performance-based contract, the QIOs are compensated for achieving specific results. It is necessary to understand which QIOs are excelling across all their quality improvement tasks, not just in a particular provider setting. Thus evaluations must be used to determine the success of individual QIOs in achieving the results delineated in their contracts. The results of such assessments can help CMS judge the bids for future QIO contracts. These evaluations can also contribute to setting the bar for success. For example, if some QIOs are able to achieve much higher levels of improvement, it may be that other QIOs could achieve the same levels of improvement if encouraged to do so through knowledge transfer, goal setting, and other methods. To the extent appropriate, QIO boards should be involved in the monitoring and evaluation of their respective organizations.

Third, evaluations of the QIOs are linked to the need for CMS to incorporate requirements for rigorous intervention study designs into the QIO contract. For example, approval of local projects could be contingent on plans to compare the results with those of other QIO projects. With a variety of QIOs carrying out different quality improvement interventions, CMS is uniquely positioned to determine which intervention methods lead to higher levels of quality improvement. The QIO program should be viewed as a learning enterprise that fosters constant improvement, innovation, and transfer of knowledge.

Finally, periodic evaluations of the QIO program as a whole should be performed by an external entity to provide an independent point of view and valuable information for CMS on the systems design and operations management aspects of the program that need improvement. Such external evaluations should also address the overall impact of the program.

CMS may choose to contract with others for assistance in all or a portion of its internal evaluations. When appropriate, CMS should collaborate with universities or others skilled in study design and evaluation to develop the strongest evaluative designs possible. CMS should also appoint and use an ongoing technical expert panel to provide guidance on the design of its internal evaluations and of future SOWs to enhance collection of the necessary data. This is not the first time the IOM has recommended an overall evaluation of the QIO program. In its 1990 report *Quality Assurance in Medicare*, the IOM mentioned the need to document the impact of the organization in each state on the quality of care (IOM, 1990). In 1994, the IOM was asked to review the evaluation plan of the Health Care Financing

Administration (the predecessor of CMS) for the Peer Review Organization program (the predecessor of the QIO program). At that time, the IOM committee recommended both formative evaluations, to learn how to improve ongoing projects, and a summative evaluation of the whole program's achievements relative to its goals and objectives (IOM, 1994). The 1994 program evaluation was not conducted, although later almost two dozen quality-of-care measures were tracked for each state over time and were summed to obtain national measures (Jencks et al., 2003). The authors could not attribute the improvements in health care quality to the QIO program. The current IOM committee reiterates the ongoing need for evaluations at both the national program level and the state and project levels.

While recognizing the challenges involved in conducting sound evaluations of quality improvements and their causes (see Chapter 9), the committee is convinced that evaluations of the QIO program must be given high priority. Not only do the technical assistance methods used by QIOs with identified participants need to be examined, but the techniques they employ to improve quality statewide also need to be reviewed. Because the QIOs spent twice as much money on statewide efforts as on identified participants during the 7th SOW, it is important to learn whether these funds were well spent and what was gained. Although studies showing how much more identified participants improved relative to other providers in the state are important in identifying certain impacts of the QIOs, they do not indicate whether statewide investments were productive. As noted above, QIOs should be charged as a part of their contract with proposing explicit plans for rigorous evaluations based on CMS guidance and methodological options. These evaluations should be part of the QIOs' interventions and should allow for formal and complete assessment of the effectiveness of those interventions.

To date, the QIOs have published a paucity of studies showing the effects of interventions on quality (see Chapter 9). Collecting data from well-designed studies of the quality improvement interventions initiated by each QIO can yield a compendium of information on the effectiveness of specific interventions in multiple states that would contribute greatly to the database on which interventions produce the best results. In addition, CMS and the QIOs should assess how different types of providers selected by various methods to participate in quality improvement projects affect the improvement achieved. In these ways, the program can help build an evidence base for determining the most cost-effective ways to improve population health. The dissemination of this knowledge should contribute to greater improvements in the future.

Types of Study Designs

Several types of studies may be considered or combined when evaluation plans are designed, and CMS should choose the strongest designs possible. CMS should take advantage of the opportunity presented by the existence of 53 QIOs, namely, a naturally occurring experiment with the potential to become a large observational study. The choice of study designs is not easy, and many complex decisions must be made. As stated above, CMS should consider the use of an ongoing technical expert panel to provide guidance on the design of evaluation plans for individual quality improvement interventions, as well as on the design of evaluations of the QIOs themselves. The methodologies that should be considered include the following:

- Randomized controlled trials
- Time series, crossover analyses
- Studies with nonequivalent control groups
- Case-control studies
- Qualitative analyses

Each of these types of design has advantages and disadvantages, which must be carefully considered before an evaluation is undertaken. One major challenge in implementing any study design concerns taking into account the voluntary nature of the program. The challenge is to separate the effects of an intervention from those due to differences in the providers seeking to participate in studies, which lead to selection bias (Campbell and Stanley, 1963; Wholey et al., 2004). Randomized controlled trials are particularly problematic for public programs such as the QIOs; nonetheless, their use should be considered as they may be suitable under specific limited circumstances. (See Appendix C for descriptions of how each of the above methodologies might be applied to aspects of the QIO program when formal evaluation plans are designed.)

QIO PROGRAM FUNDING

Recommendation 8: Congress and the secretary of DHHS should focus all QIO resources on supporting health care providers' performance measurement and quality improvement efforts. The secretary should remove from QIO core contracts funds sufficient to support case reviews, appeals, and beneficiary complaints when those functions are devolved to other organizations. The secretary should increase the remaining funds to allow for inflation, the incorporation of evaluations into all QIO work, the increased num-

bers of providers and beneficiaries being served, and the labor-intensive nature of technical assistance and quality improvement activities.

- The multiple evaluations undertaken during the 8th and 9th SOWs should guide future funding decisions, with budget increases or decreases being provided according to the evaluation findings. If the evaluations demonstrate that no positive impact is attributable to the QIO program's efforts, CMS will need to rethink its quality improvement approach and the possible benefit of transitioning funds to an alternative structure and strategy for Medicare.
- Once a national performance measurement and reporting system has been established, its priorities should help guide the funding levels and policy direction of the QIO program, recognizing that adequate funding is necessary to reach the goals set for the QIO program.
- The secretary of DHHS should ease the conflict-of-interest restriction with regard to supplementing the QIO quality improvement budgets with external funds. Given the limits of federal funding, the QIOs should be allowed to seek funds for quality improvement activities from providers and other organizations as appropriate.

The tasks confronting the QIOs during the 8th SOW are of great magnitude, and as discussed in Chapter 4, the committee expects that provider demand for technical assistance with quality improvement will increase. The committee recognizes the huge gap between what is known about quality care and the care that is delivered to most patients. It also understands that many health care providers and practitioners need help in making the changes necessary for the consistent delivery of high-quality care. The committee recognizes as well that although the QIOs should no longer be responsible for case reviews, complaints, and appeals, CMS will need to contract with other organizations to perform at least some of those functions. Thus, a portion of the current funding should be shifted out of the QIOs' budgets after the 8th SOW. During the 9th SOW, additional funds will be necessary to cover the increased demand for technical assistance from providers and extensive program evaluations. (See Chapter 7 for further discussion of funding.)

Before increased funding can be justified past the 9th SOW, however, it is necessary to assess the impacts the QIOs are having on providers at present. It would be unrealistic to expect CMS and the QIO program to perform evaluations with levels of rigor rivaling those of double-blind, randomized controlled drug trials, but certainly more could be learned about the impact of the program if evaluation were a priority. Decisions on how future funds are to be spent should be based on the results of all evaluations of the overall impact of the QIO program, the technical assistance provided for performance measurement, the specific quality improvement methods and techniques used, and which QIOs are most successful. If those evaluations indicate that the QIO program is having a significant positive impact and if there is continuing demand for technical assistance for quality improvement or new tasks are added, future funding should be increased. Information resulting from the evaluation is essential as a guide to the wise expenditure of additional funds. If the evaluations show that the program has an insufficient impact, CMS must consider other strategies for improving the quality of health care and should shift funding accordingly.

At the same time, however, it is important to recognize that adequate funding in proportion to contract requirements is necessary to accomplish the goals established for the program. In 1990, the IOM determined that investment in the QIO program was inadequate to achieve set goals (IOM, 1990). Since then, the program has added more task areas, while funding has become a smaller percentage of the overall Medicare budget (see Chapter 7). Additionally, while most of the QIOs' current expenditures for Tasks 1a–1d (quality improvement activities in nursing homes, home health settings, hospitals, and physician offices) go toward overall statewide activities, work with identified participants often incurs a higher cost per provider (see Chapter 7). For example, under the 7th SOW, QIOs worked with approximately 7.5 percent of physician offices. If demand for help increases in this provider setting, budget increases will be necessary because of the greater cost of such activities per provider in this setting (as compared with overall work with providers). At present, however, it is infeasible to estimate the budget requirements for these activities in the 9th and 10th SOWs because of a variety of unknown factors, including the scope of the increased demand, the effects of pay-for-performance and public reporting initiatives, and the possible development of more cost-effective tools for use by QIOs in reaching out to a larger number of providers.

Additional funds will also be needed to enhance the QIO program's role in supporting the implementation of a national performance measurement and reporting system and the capacity of providers to participate in the reporting of quality measures and pay-for-performance programs. Once a national performance measurement and reporting system is functioning, has established goals, and has identified additional measures for reporting, its priorities should guide the policy direction of the QIO program. Nonetheless, CMS and the QIO program also have responsibilities to the Medicare program. To the extent possible, efforts should be made to bring those responsibilities into alignment with the operation of the national performance measurement and reporting system.

Conflict-of-interest rules currently restrict QIOs from soliciting or receiving external funding from providers or grants for the provision of the same services rendered under the QIO contract (see Chapter 7). Many QIOs have already exhibited an ability to contract with non-Medicare sources for quality improvement and case review functions. These contracts are unrelated to their core contract and state providers. However, some local providers might want to contract with their local QIO for services similar to those provided by the QIO as part of the Medicare program. For example, a hospital might want to pay the QIO for extra or more intensive assistance in its internal quality improvement efforts to improve upon measures explicitly delineated in the QIO contract. In the past, the restriction on such arrangements prevented a conflict for QIOs, which would be accepting money from the same providers they might also review for any number of regulatory activities. If the QIOs' efforts were focused on quality improvement and performance measurement (see Recommendations 3 and 4), that inherent conflict would no longer exist. Additionally, increased interaction with the private sector could boost the QIOs' reputations, add to their skill sets, and enhance public–private collaboration. Nonetheless, CMS should ensure that the proportion of funds from providers and other private sources is not so large relative to the Medicare core contract that it gives the impression of a conflict of interest or impropriety. Also, QIOs need to prevent perceptions of bias toward paying contractors that might arise if resources for free assistance became scarce. Finally, by removing this restriction, more organizations with multiple lines of business might be enticed to compete for QIO contracts.

REFERENCES

AHRQ (Agency for Healthcare Research and Quality). 2004. *National Healthcare Quality Report.* Rockville, Maryland: Agency for Healthcare Research and Quality.

Campbell DT, Stanley JC. 1963. *Experimental and Quasi-Experimental Designs for Research.* Chicago: Rand McNally & Co.

CHCF (California Health Care Foundation). 2005. Executive Summary. In *National Consumer Health Privacy Survey 2005.* Bishop L, Holmes BJ, Kelly CM, eds. Oakland, CA: California Health Care Foundation.

CMS (Centers for Medicare and Medicaid Services). 2004. *The Quality Improvement Organization Program: CMS Briefing for IOM Staff.* [Online]. Available: http://www.medqic.org/dcs/ContentServer?cid=1105558772835&pagename=Medqic%2FMQGeneralPage%2FGeneralPageTemplate&c=MQGeneralPage [accessed December 26, 2005].

CMS. 2005. *Quality Improvement Roadmap.* [Online]. Available: http://www.medicaldevices.org/public/issues/documents/CMSMedicareroadmap.pdf [accessed December 26, 2005].

Gaul GM. 2005, July 26. Once health regulators, now partners. *Washington Post.* p. A1.

HHS (United States Department of Health and Human Services). 2000. *Healthy People 2010: Understanding and Improving Health.* Washington, D.C.: U.S. Government Printing Office.

Hibbard JH, Stockard J, Tusler M. 2005. Hospital performance reports: Impact on quality, market share, and reputation. *Health Affairs* 24(4):1150–1160.

IOM (Institute of Medicine). 1990. *Quality Assurance in Medicare.* Washington, DC: National Academy Press.

IOM. 1994. *An Assessment of the HCFA Evaluation Plan for the Medicare Peer Review Organization.* Washington, DC: National Academy Press.

IOM. 2006. *Performance Measurement: Accelerating Improvement.* Washington, DC: The National Academies Press.

Jencks SF, Huff ED, Cuerdon T. 2003. Change in the quality of care delivered to Medicare beneficiaries, 1998–1999 to 2000–2001. *Journal of the American Medical Association* 289(3):305–312.

McClellan MB. 2005, July 21. Statement of Mark McClellan, M.D., Ph.D., Administrator, Centers for Medicare and Medicaid Services, U.S. Department of Health and Human Services. Testimony before the Subcommittee on Health of the House Committee on Ways and Means. Washington, DC: U.S. House of Representatives.

Rollow WC. 2005. *QIO Program: Update and Policy Considerations.* PowerPoint Presentation to the Committee on Redesigning Health Insurance, June 13, Washington, DC.

Schulke D. 2004. *Opportunities for Quality Improvement Created by the Medicare Drug Benefit.* PowerPoint Presentation to the Committee on Redesigning Health Insurance, December 1–3, Washington, DC.

Wholey JS, Hatry HP, Newcomer KE. 2004. *Handbook of Practical Program Evaluation.* San Francisco: John Wiley & Sons, Inc.

Part II

━━━━

INTRODUCTION

In Part II of this report, the Committee on Redesigning Health Insurance Performance Measures, Payment, and Performance Improvement Programs presents a description of the Quality Improvement Organization (QIO) program in the 7th and 8th scopes of work (SOWs). Part I stressed the importance of looking to what needs to be done in the future to improve the quality of health care. Part II presents the basis for those recommendations and documents the current status of the program. It will serve as a resource for future examinations of the QIO program. Part II includes eight chapters that provide the information outlined below.

Chapter 6 describes the study approach. In particular, it explains the various methodologies used and the limitations encountered in accumulating information about the QIO program from stakeholders.

Chapter 7 examines the overall structure and financing of the QIO program. It evaluates the structural requirements, governance, and staffing of the individual QIOs, organizations holding QIO contracts, and the QIO Support Centers (QIOSCs). The funding for the entire program is also presented, including funding for the core contracts, special studies, and support contracts. The external activities and funding of the QIOs are also described.

Chapter 8 provides a detailed description of the technical assistance activities required of the QIOs in the 7th and 8th SOWs. First, the methods used to provide technical assistance are discussed in general, as well as how

QIOs recruit providers for these activities. Next, the chapter presents a detailed description of those activities in each setting.

Chapter 9 describes the impact of technical assistance on quality improvement and knowledge transfer. The chapter includes a literature review and considers quality improvement interventions in general and those of QIOs specifically, discusses different approaches to quality improvement, and provides an overview of knowledge transfer and its impact in the QIO program.

Chapter 10 evaluates the impact of quality improvement activities in the QIO program specifically. The detailed evaluation formulas as well as the means used to identify high performing QIOs are discussed.

Chapter 11 describes the communications and beneficiary education activities of the QIOs in the 7th and 8th SOWs. This includes the promotion of public information on websites, assistance to providers for the collection and reporting of data for public reporting, and the maintenance of toll-free help lines.

Chapter 12 describes the protective activities of the QIOs. All activities related to the review of quality concerns (including the new mediation process) as well as reviews designed to protect the integrity of the Medicare Trust Funds, such as the Hospital Payment Monitoring Program, are examined. The different categories and types of reviews and the review process are described in detail, and data that can be used to help assess their impact are presented.

Chapter 13 describes the Centers for Medicare and Medicaid Services' (CMS's) oversight of the QIO program. The structure of the QIO program as it fits into CMS's framework is first described, including the offices and the personnel involved in the management of this complex program. Next, the committee describes the various communications methods that these personnel used, including their written, oral, and electronic communications systems. The data-related issues evaluated include the various tools that CMS uses to report data and the flow of data in each of the provider settings. The manner in which the QIO and QIOSC contracts themselves are structured and awarded is then examined. Finally, the chapter discusses the overall guidance of the QIO program, including strategic planning, policy direction, program coordination, and overall program evaluation.

Part II provides a comprehensive, retrospective view of the QIO program in the 7th and 8th SOWs. The assessment presented here serves as a primary source of information about this complex program, with a description of its recent past and current status, as well as a base on which recommendations for the role of QIOs in the future of quality health care have been made.

6

Study Approach

CHAPTER SUMMARY

This chapter presents the committee's methodological approach for this study. To address the items in the legislative mandate, it was necessary to design a multifaceted study that used a mix of data collection and analytic methods, including both qualitative and quantitative analyses, rather than an experimental design. The chapter discusses each of the main data sources, including: a focused literature review, an internet-based data collection, site visits, interviews, and quantitative data requests. Finally, the research strengths and challenges are examined.

In response to the legislative mandate in Section 109 of the Medicare Prescription Drug, Improvement, and Modernization Act of 2003 (P.L. 108-173), the Institute of Medicine (IOM) formed an authoring committee, the Committee on Redesigning Health Insurance Performance Measures, Payment, and Performance Improvement Programs, to prepare three reports in a single project and a separate subcommittee to focus on the Quality Improvement Organization (QIO) study and guide the data collection and analysis. These committees included members with the necessary expertise and experience in such areas as clinical quality improvement; health economics; Centers for Medicare and Medicaid Services (CMS) management; research on organizational change, consumer behavior, and program evaluation; and the delivery of health care in physicians' offices, long-term care facilities, hospitals, academic medical centers, and integrated health care delivery systems. During the course of the study contract (April 2004 to June 2005), the members of the QIO subcommittee met three times in person and once by conference call to guide the research and data collection efforts. The main committee met seven times and gave policy direction to the research, discussed drafts, and reached consensus on the final wording of the report and its recommendations.

To discuss the items mandated by the legislation, such as an overview of the QIO program, the duties of the contracting organizations in the program, the sources and amounts of their funding, and a review of the oversight of the program, the committee needed to present descriptive data. To address the other items in the mandate, such as the extent to which QIOs improve the quality of care, the extent to which other organizations could do their duties, and the effectiveness of case review and other QIO activities, the committee needed evaluative analyses and expert judgment.

This study uses a retrospective examination of the data to present much of the descriptive information as well as to evaluate the impact of the program's efforts. Although the chapters with a retrospective view examine the data from the beginning of the Medicare quality assurance program to provide an overview, the main focus is on more recent program activities; and most data and analyses relate to the time period of the contract for the 7th scope of work (SOW), which was from August 2002 to August 2005. This study also looks at the program concurrently, because the period of the IOM study contract overlapped with the end of the 7th SOW and the beginning of the 8th SOW. The information presented in this report reflects the data collected through the midsummer of 2005 and is descriptive of the 8th SOW but does not include data reflecting the CMS and QIO work produced during the 8th SOW, which had barely begun when the report was drafted.

The unit of analysis varied, depending on the questions addressed. For example, the committee wanted to know what, if any, impact the whole program has had on Medicare beneficiaries' care and considered information reflecting the activities of all QIOs, other contractors, and CMS. Thus, the committee used aggregated data from all QIOs to examine possible national effects. When the committee examined the effects of specific quality improvement interventions on the provision of care and care outcomes, a more common focus of the published literature, the unit of analysis was often an individual QIO or a particular intervention project of one or more QIOs. The committee tried to identify the organizational and structural characteristics of the QIOs that might contribute to greater quality improvement. That is, were there characteristics of high-performing QIOs or aspects of how CMS managed them that could be identified and spread to other QIOs to help them improve the national program's overall performance? Comparisons of QIOs' structural characteristics and performance measures were necessary to attempt to answer those questions.

DATA SOURCES

The committee chose to gather data from a wide variety of sources and to compare and integrate the findings, as no one source fully covered the many facets of the QIO program and the questions being asked in the study. Fortunately, the committee found both the QIO community and CMS welcoming, willing to provide reasonable requests for data, and open and eager to talk with the committee about the program. By the end of the study, the IOM project had both personal and substantive e-mail contacts with the chief executive officer (CEO) from each organization holding a QIO contract. The main data collection methods and sources for this study included the following:

- a focused review of the literature on the impact of quality improvement and the impact of QIO efforts at quality improvement;
- data collected in 2005 from all 53 QIOs through the SurveyMonkey internet-based data collection tool;
- quantitative analyses of QIOs' relative performance on various subtasks of the 7th SOW;
- site visits by 16 committee members and IOM staff to 11 QIOs and one CMS Regional Office;
- telephone interviews with 20 CEOs from randomly selected QIOs;
- a 3-day briefing by CMS staff;
- a half-day workshop for the committee and subcommittee, including formal presentations from academic researchers as well as experts working in quality improvement in the field and comments from various stakeholders;
- access to QIONet, a CMS internal website for the QIO program that includes performance data by state on the Dashboard section;
- face-to-face interviews with CEOs and staff from certain QIOs and randomly selected QIO Support Centers (QIOSCs);
- a focus group discussion with 11 QIO CEOs;
- specific requests for data from CMS staff;
- many formal and informal discussions with the staff of the American Health Quality Association (AHQA; the national organization representing all QIOs) and the attendees at their functions (mainly QIO staff);
- informal discussions with representatives of consumer and beneficiary organizations and various providers;
- data collected from presentations and question and discussion sessions; the observation of interactions among QIO and CMS staff; and information from the informal questioning of attendees at AHQA's annual technical conference and other national meetings, CMS's annual QualityNet Conference, and miscellaneous smaller meetings; and
- suggestions from committee and subcommittee members and reviewers of businesses and other organizations performing QIO-like functions ("other entities").

It is noteworthy that the committee gained knowledge of and insight into the QIO program through multiple sources, all of which could not be fully referenced in the text. The committee attempted to indicate the main source of information throughout the report, as appropriate. Each of the formal research approaches is briefly discussed below.

FOCUSED LITERATURE REVIEW

The committee searched for an understanding of how quality improvement interventions with health care providers influence the quality of health care, and it examined literature chosen from two sources. (The committee's previous report, *Performance Measurement: Accelerating Improvement*, addressed quality improvements resulting from the availability of health care quality data for providers and the public reporting of such data [IOM, 2006].) First, the committee extracted the majority of studies from a bibliography compiled by AHQA in August 2004. This bibliography lists more than 600 studies that either were conducted in partnership with a QIO, used QIO data, or were written by an author affiliated with a QIO. Potential biases may have existed in the selection of the studies for the bibliography and the methods by which they were conducted. Although most articles in AHQA's bibliography refer to clinical treatment options for Medicare patients and descriptions of the QIO program, the committee focused on a smaller subset of studies that examined QIO approaches to improving the quality of health care. Articles were selected from AHQA's bibliography on the basis of their titles by use of an internal reliability check by two members of the IOM staff.

The committee found most of the remaining studies by the use of Medline searches, performed in November 2004 for articles published in the previous 5 years, using the following medical search headings: "quality improvement," "effectiveness," and "intervention." In addition, the committee evaluated a selection of studies to supplement the evidence base for outcome measures, collaborative studies, audits and feedback, and evaluations of the QIO program published from November 2004 through July 2005. The committee chose studies from references in previously selected studies and by searching the Cochrane Database of Systematic Reviews and the Agency for Healthcare Research and Quality systematic reviews. These studies did not focus specifically on QIO activities and are part of a broader literature on quality intervention. It would be impossible to know whether the health care providers in those studies had prior knowledge of or had participated in various QIO efforts. The literature review is discussed in more detail in Chapter 9, and a summary of selected studies on quality improvement is provided in Table A.1 in Appendix A.

The committee categorized the studies obtained from the literature review on the basis of the strength of the research methodology (see Table A.2). In general, the results and the lessons learned from randomized controlled trials outweighed those from studies with nonexperimental designs. However, the committee recognized the value of observational and qualitative studies for identifying major themes from past interventions and considered them useful starting points for understanding the impacts of the previous interventions.

WEB-BASED DATA COLLECTION

In 2005, the committee, along with a consultant, Allyson Ross Davies, used software on the SurveyMonkey.com platform to design a two-part data collection instrument, collect responses from all organizations holding one or more QIO contracts for the 7th SOW, and export raw data for analysis using SAS software. The main committee and the QIO subcommittee developed draft content. Key staff at CMS and AHQA and a CEO of an organization holding multiple QIO contracts for the 7th SOW reviewed a draft of the data collection instrument for clarity, terminology, user friendliness, and duplication of ongoing data collection efforts. The committee selected the SurveyMonkey platform because of both the ease of online questionnaire design and the familiarity of the QIO community with this survey platform. Both CMS and AHQA actively encouraged the QIOs to fully participate in this data collection effort.

The committee assured the respondents that they would remain anonymous, and SurveyMonkey guaranteed the secure transmission of responses through the use of Secure Sockets Layer encryption. The consultant exported raw data from the SurveyMonkey website for analysis, at which point she closed the data collection instruments and deleted them from the site. She did not share raw data with IOM staff, the committee, or CMS. The consultant presented only deidentified, aggregated information about the organizations to the project's main committee and the QIO subcommittee. This report includes only deidentified and aggregated data.

Content of Data Collection Instrument

Part 1 of the data collection instrument obtained information from each of the 41 organizations holding one or more QIO contracts for the 7th SOW. The questions in Part 1 focused on organizational structure; boards of directors or trustees; and financial information, which was related to both the QIO contract(s) and other business lines, when relevant.

Part 2 requested separate data on the 7th SOW from each of the 53 QIOs. Background questions focused on factual information about the organization that held the QIO contract(s), its business in the state(s) in which it held the QIO contract(s), and related topics. Other questions were related to staffing; staff qualifications, skills, and capabilities; the composition and experience of the leadership team; the organization of work; ratings on selected aspects of the working relationship between the QIO in the state, district, or territory and CMS (both the Central and the Regional Offices); the ratings of other services (e.g., the Standard Data Processing System and QIONet) provided by or for CMS to the QIO community; and perspectives on the "best" QIOs (overall and by task area).

With a few exceptions for text-based answers, the questions offered fixed-choice response categories, and an answer was required before the next question was presented on the screen. Respondents were asked to select a substantive answer whenever possible; a "don't know/prefer not to answer" response was offered as a backup.

Approach to Data Collection

The committee e-mailed a memorandum to the CEOs of all organizations holding QIO contracts for the 7th SOW. In that memorandum the committee requested the cooperation of the CEOs in overseeing completion of both portions of the online data collection instrument; provided instructions and links to the online questionnaires; and offered to provide assistance, if needed, by e-mail or telephone. A 4-week response period was offered for each part.

Completion Rates and Missing Data

All 41 organizations holding one or more QIO contracts for the 7th SOW completed Part 1 within the response period, representing a 100 percent response rate. Missing data rates were very low; only 2 of 41 organizations consistently selected the "don't know/prefer not to answer" response category, and those responses were chiefly for questions in the section on financial data.

For Part 2, 52 of 53 QIOs provided data, representing a response rate of slightly greater than 98 percent. Again, missing data rates were very low; only 2 of the 52 respondents selected the "don't know/prefer not to answer" category, and this was generally done for questions asking about current or planned lines of non-QIO business and some of the rating items.

QUANTITATIVE ANALYSES OF QIO PERFORMANCE

The committee conducted analyses of the QIOs' performance, based on the scores that CMS constructs to assess contract performance, to determine why some states and provider settings show greater improvement on given measures. The committee attempted to correlate the QIO scores with variables such as performance on other quality improvement subtasks, spending per beneficiary, contract round, QIO region, and provider satisfaction. The analyses and findings are discussed in Chapter 10.

VISITS TO QIOs

The budget limited this study, in that it did not allow the committee or IOM staff travel to all the QIOs. To gain a firsthand understanding of a QIO and to reach as many different QIOs as possible with a minimum of travel, committee members and staff visited either their local QIO or one that was in an area to which travel for other purposes was planned. In total, 16 committee members and staff visited 10 different QIOs in person and an 11th one by telephone. A semistructured interview protocol was used during most of these visits. The questions included in the protocol concerned the strengths, weaknesses, opportunities, and threats to the QIO perceived by the QIO respondents. Note that although the visiting committee members and IOM staff used similar protocols, not all QIOs were asked the exact same questions, and often, topics arose as a result of the discussions. The text attempts to reflect the number of QIOs that mentioned specific concerns, but a less than 100 percent response rate does not indicate disagreement among those QIOs.

In addition, the QIOs generally presented key staff, such as the president, medical director, director of quality improvement, and chief financial officer, who discussed programs as well as responded to additional questions that were not part of the protocol. The site visits lasted from a couple of hours to all day or more. The visiting committee members and staff submitted written notes to the IOM after each visit, but the notes for each site visit varied substantially, depending on multiple factors, including who the visitor happened to be. In addition to the written reports, the committee discussed the highlights of most visits at committee meetings. IOM staff reviewed both the notes and the presentations to identify themes, issues of concern to the QIOs, and useful ideas for further research.

TELEPHONE INTERVIEWS

To gain more insight into the views of the executive directors of the QIOs on their programs, Cheryl Ulmer, a health services research consultant working with the committee, interviewed CEOs from 20 of the 53 QIOs by telephone during March 2005.

Selection of Participating QIOs

The committee randomly selected 20 QIOs after stratification by region and the sizes of their beneficiary populations in the following manner: (1) the committee divided the states into the four CMS geographic regions; (2) the ultimate number of states selected from each region was proportional to the number in each region (ultimately, one region had four states in the sample, two regions had five states, and one region had six states); and (3) after each state was labeled large or small on the basis of whether the beneficiary population size was above or below the median size of state beneficiary populations, the committee randomly selected two or three states from the subgroups of states with large and small beneficiary populations in each region. When a region had four or six states in the sample, equal numbers of states with large and small beneficiary populations were selected. When a region had five states, three states were selected from the states with large or small beneficiary populations, depending on which subgroup consisted of more states.

The goal was to ensure that states in each region had a chance of being selected that was proportional to the number of states in that region. Within each region, states with large or small size beneficiary populations would have a chance of being selected proportionally to the number of states with large and small populations. The committee e-mailed letters to each selected CEO in February 2005. The committee first requested a telephone interview and then outlined the general topics for discussion. These topics were primarily related to knowledge transfer. All interviews occurred between March 7 and 16, 2005.

Nature of Interviews and Questions

The committee developed an interview script with open-ended questions and then, while attending the AHQA national meeting in February 2005, conducted interviews with four CEOs not previously selected to pretest the interview protocol. Upon review of the interview notes and a discussion with the consultant, the committee developed a wide-ranging interview protocol that went beyond knowledge transfer and covered topics such as QIOSCs; the selection of identified participants; diffusion of knowledge about quality improvement activities beyond the identified participants; the pros and cons of targeting the poorest-performing providers; evaluation of the QIOs; the importance of beneficiary education, case review, and payment error functions; the impact of competition for QIO contracts; the timeliness and the quality of data; and barriers to knowledge transfer. During the interview, the CEOs raised additional topics: electronic health records, Regional Health Information Organizations, and pay for performance.

The interview protocol design primarily included qualitative questions, with priorities set among the questions, in recognition of the proposed 45-minute limit of the interview with each QIO. The detailed questions were not provided to the CEOs in advance. The primary questions were open-ended; some questions contained formal probes, but even these were open-ended and did not require a certain set of closed-ended responses. In the preinterview correspondence and on the telephone, the committee and the consultant assured the CEOs that their responses would be held in confidence, would not be taped, and that handwritten or typed notes would not go to the committee or public access file. In her analysis, the consultant deidentified information attributable to specific QIOs.

The CEOs were very responsive to the consultant. Although they were advocates for their programs and quality improvement in general, they were reflective; were willing to be adaptable to changes in the quality improvement process in the future; and had particularly strong opinions on their relationships with CMS, on which types of providers moved the field forward, on the need for further incentives to prod providers to change, and on the need for more timely and comprehensive data.

The consultant conducted each interview in one continuous telephone session, with all but two of the interviews lasting 90 minutes rather than the scheduled 45 minutes. She used the interview protocol as a guide and took thorough handwritten notes that were typewritten after the telephone interview. Because the interviews were not taped, the notes were not verbatim; but they still captured the content and the context of the directors' comments in detail. The consultant did not filter the responses during the note-taking process.

Analysis of Interview Content

The committee staff and the consultant discussed the results of the first interviews to see if there were other areas that needed to be probed. For example, in the first interviews, no one mentioned collaborative activities, but upon questioning, every QIO questioned about this in later interviews indicated their use. Similarly, although there had been no specific questions on pay for performance or electronic health records, when these topics came up repeatedly, the consultant started asking the CEOs for their views.

After the completion of all 20 interviews, the consultant analyzed the contents of her notes to identify the themes that emerged in response to each topic. She then examined each theme to determine how many QIOs addressed it to identify a denominator for calculation of the percentage of QIOs that supported a particular idea or that mentioned an issue. Deliberate quantitative analysis of the responses helps confirm the general sense that one gathers during the interviews but also helps refute strongly held opinions of a few CEOs that might not reflect those of the whole respondent group. During the interviews, however, some CEOs offered unprompted comments. Therefore, a less than 100 percent response rate does not necessarily indicate disagreement among the interviewees. (In this report the committee has indicated, where appropriate, when all CEOs were asked the same question.) The consultant illustrated themes by the use of quotes from the CEOs. If there was a minority view or an issue that might be of potential value for further research, even if it was voiced by only one QIO, it was mentioned in the analysis for consideration in case the issue came up from other data sources.

THREE-DAY BRIEFING BY CMS

The study's Project Officer at CMS, Joyce Kelly, arranged an intensive series of presentations by CMS staff, both those in the Central Office and those in the various QIO Regional Offices, that covered a wide range of elements of the QIO program. She worked with IOM staff in advance to develop the agenda, soliciting questions that the committee wanted addressed and proposing topics that CMS thought would be useful to the committee. The IOM requested discussions of issues such as Central Office oversight and direction, the roles of the Clinical Data Abstraction Centers, the role of QIOs in public reporting, the volume of complaints, and beneficiary satisfaction. The briefing provided an excellent overview and introduction to the program for the whole IOM project team. Although most of the time was consumed by the presentations, IOM staff had the opportunity to ask each speaker questions. All the materials and the PowerPoint presentations from this briefing are available on the World Wide Web (CMS, 2004).

ACCESS TO QIONET

CMS uses an internal website to facilitate confidential program communications with the QIOs and the reporting of certain types of data. This site includes the Dashboard section, which presents state-specific data, updated quarterly, on many of the measures used to evaluate the performance of each QIO under its contract with CMS. CMS arranged for the IOM to have access to the website during the course of the study, with the understanding that the data would not be used with state-specific identifiers. Many of the data used in this report to assess the impacts of the QIOs on particular quality measures came from the Dashboard section of QIONet (see Table A.3 in Appendix A for a detailed list of the measures.)

FACE-TO-FACE INTERVIEWS

The committee conducted two sets of formal face-to-face interviews for the study. In September 2004, during CMS's annual conference for QIOs, the committee interviewed staff and CEOs from five randomly selected organizations (which held a total of seven QIOSC contracts); one interview served as a pretest of the interview protocol. All organizations selected agreed to participate. The interviewers used the same script for each of the four remaining interviews, although the topic and assignment of each QIOSC were different. Questions focused on topics such as the purpose of the QIOSC, its main activities, why it was selected for a QIOSC contract, the QIOSC's key partners, how the QIOSC interacts with the QIOs and CMS, and how the QIOSC is evaluated by CMS. Detailed written notes were taken during each interview. The information gleaned from the interviews guided further research on QIOSC issues.

The committee conducted the second set of interviews on February 25, 2005, at the AHQA Annual Technical Conference in San Francisco, California. The committee selected the CEOs of the QIOs of four states from the list of those that were not randomly chosen for the telephone interviews or that were not visited by representatives of the project. The CEOs of all four QIOs agreed to participate in a 45-minute interview, which primarily concerned various mechanisms for knowledge transfer. The interviews served as a pretest of the script to be used for the telephone interviews. Committee staff took detailed written notes during the interviews.

FOCUS GROUP

The committee selected the CEOs of the QIOs of 11 states from those not already chosen for the telephone interviews or visited by representatives of the study. All 11 CEOs agreed to participate, although one CEO recommended that the medical director be interviewed as a substitute. The participants represented at least two states from each Regional Office involved in the QIO program, including both predominantly rural and predominantly urban states. Also, the committee selected states to include both those with small numbers and those with large numbers of beneficiaries and providers. The QIO subcommittee chair, a professional researcher experienced with focus groups, moderated the 90-minute discussion while committee staff took notes. The moderator used a guide that included general, open-ended questions about the direction of the program in the upcoming SOW, challenges concerning information technology–related tasks, criteria important for assessment of the value of individual QIOs, and how QIO functions might change when all beneficiaries had electronic health records.

SPECIFIC DATA REQUESTS TO CMS STAFF

It would have been extremely difficult to conduct this study without the excellent cooperation of individuals responsible for the QIO program's management. Throughout the course of the contract they have willingly responded to numerous requests from IOM, spent hours of their own time and their staff's time explaining the nuances and complexities of the program, collected data to fulfill requests, and shared their knowledge of CMS and the QIO program. For example, the committee requested a major amount of data on the budget for the 7th SOW, both by each state or QIO and as aggregated data at the national level. The budgets were broken down by core tasks and included costs for special studies and support contracts. The committee also requested information about the content of major support and special study contracts. Other requests included requests for information about organizational structures, the results of QIO evaluations, CMS staffing needs, and the timing for the transition to the 8th SOW.

FORMAL AND INFORMAL DISCUSSIONS WITH AHQA

From the beginning of the study, AHQA's staff and QIO members provided background information, technical advice, documents, and data as well as access to their meetings. AHQA's active support of the IOM project enhanced the receptiveness of its members' participation in the IOM study. Formal presentations and written documents are cited by author name, but information provided informally or confidentially is not.

INFORMAL DISCUSSIONS WITH
CONSUMER ORGANIZATIONS AND PROVIDERS

The committee conducted informal discussions with people from consumer and beneficiary organizations as well as with practitioners and individuals from provider organizations at meetings and by telephone. Time, budget constraints, and federal rules prevented the committee from performing more formal interview surveys with these stakeholders.

However, the committee did recognize that CMS contracted with Westat to conduct surveys of providers' satisfaction with QIOs. These surveys, further discussed in Chapter 10, were conducted among nursing homes, home health agencies, physicians offices, hospitals, and Medicare+Choice plans for all 53 QIOs in the 7th SOW. (For nursing homes and home health agencies, survey respondents included both identified participants and nonidentified participants.) Over 21,000 providers responded to questions about their level of satisfaction, including their impressions of the effectiveness of their respective QIOs.

The federal Paperwork Reduction Act of 1995 (P.L. 104-13) prohibits the use of a survey, interview guide or systematic data collection from 10 or more persons by a federal contractor without clearance from the Office of Management and Budget. That process can sometimes take many months. Despite the committee's desire to survey providers and consumers, it determined that would not be feasible within the time limits of the study's contract with CMS.

NATIONAL CONFERENCES AND MEETINGS

The committee gathered much information and understanding about the QIO program by attending national technical conferences held by CMS and AHQA, as well as smaller meetings sponsored by various organizations that focused more narrowly on particular aspects of the QIO program and related issues, such as public reporting of quality measures, information technology use in health care, and implementation of the Medicare Prescription Drug, Improvement, and Modernization Act of 2003 Part D prescription drug benefit. A side benefit of the meetings was the opportunity for informal conversations with the employees of QIOs from across the country. These discussions had some influence on the directions of the research and the richness of the descriptions of the QIOs, but they are not cited specifically. In addition, CMS allowed project staff to attend a strategic planning meeting and a confidential evaluation panel meeting.

SUGGESTIONS OF "OTHER ENTITIES"

Suggestions were solicited from the committee and subcommittee members and additional names were offered by the report reviewers for private businesses performing functions similar to those of QIOs. All relevant suggestions were included, even if the company currently offers only one of the related functions. Data on each company were pulled from its website for the table in Appendix B. Each business was offered the opportunity to update and verify its data. The committee tabulated the data but was unable to assess the specific capabilities or potential strengths and weaknesses of each business.

RESEARCH CHALLENGES

Given the timing of the congressional mandate, this study could not be built into the beginning of the 7th or the 8th SOW and produce the report on schedule. The 7th SOW was already well under way at the time that the legislation mandating this study was signed into law. Although the 8th SOW began before the end of the IOM's contract with CMS, it was too late to be able to collect any new data reflecting the activities of the 8th SOW and meet the study's deadline. Thus, a study design and data collection methodology for the project could not be included directly in the core QIO contracts. Although CMS instructed the QIOs to consider data requests from IOM as a separate part of their activities for the 7th SOW, it did not give them additional funds to cover their time or effort spent responding.

Given those constraints, the committee could not use an experimental design. The QIO program operates in all states, participation by providers is voluntary, and all the QIOs have essentially the same basic tasks, so randomization and the use of control groups would not have been feasible without a specially designed experiment. The program was already fully operational and would continue to function and evolve during the course of the study. A Hawthorne effect might have contributed to confounding, but it was not considered a limitation of the study. For example, the committee's assessment of CMS's oversight responsibilities was based on both retrospective and concurrent information. The fact that the U.S. Congress and the committee asked particular questions about the program could have influenced CMS management to change course or expand or reduce certain activities during the course of the study.

Another constraint that affected much of the data collection effort was the need to maintain confidentiality. To gain access to many of the data from CMS and individual QIOs, the committee agreed to report only aggregated or deidentified data so that individual QIOs could not be identified. Because state-identified data could jeopardize the competitive business situation of individual QIOs and limit their willingness to communicate on sensitive issues, the IOM agreed to maintain confidentiality at the minimum level necessary.

STRENGTH OF RESEARCH CONCLUSIONS

Although limitations to each of the various research methods used in this study existed, altogether they provided a substantial amount of data and information. The committee triangulated methods by checking the consistency of the findings obtained by the different data collection methods, such as the data collected through the web-based data collection tool, the focus group, the telephone interviews, and the site visits. Triangulation among data sources was also possible. For example, the committee compared the information about the program provided by CMS with the information provided by the QIOs.

Because more than one committee member or IOM staff member often made site visits and more than one staff person generally attended most meetings, the committee triangulated among multiple analysts. The committee members routinely compared notes and impressions after a visit, interview, or meeting and discussed their perceptions and findings.

The study puts more weight on information gathered through the SurveyMonkey web-based data collection tool, which covered all QIOs, and on data collected from the telephone interviews of a random sample of QIO CEOs than on individual interviews and informal comments, which served to strengthen consistent findings. An opinion voiced by one QIO staff member might include an important idea, but it carried more weight with the committee if multiple sources expressed similar ideas or if several different research approaches led to the same conclusions.

Each research method had limitations, and it was necessary to accept CMS program data as they were given, without auditing of the data. Nonetheless, by using so many different methods to gather data, the committee strengthened its ability to paint a more complete and accurate picture of the QIO program.

REFERENCES

CMS (Centers for Medicare and Medicaid Services). 2004. *The Quality Improvement Organization Program: CMS Briefing for IOM Staff.* [Online]. Available: http://www.medqic.org/dcs/ContentServer?cid=1105558772835&pagename=Medqic%2FMQGeneralPage%2FGeneralPageTemplate&c=MQGeneralPage [accessed December 26, 2005].

IOM (Institute of Medicine). 2006. *Performance Measurement: Accelerating Improvement.* Washington, DC: The National Academies Press.

7

Structure and Finances

CHAPTER SUMMARY

This chapter describes Quality Improvement Organizations (QIOs) and the organizations that held QIO contracts for the 7th scope of work, including their structure, governance, staffing, and finances. This is followed by discussions of the QIO Support Centers and the overall funding of the QIO program. This background material serves to give an overall general picture of the structure and financing of the QIO program.

STRUCTURE OF QIOs

The Peer Review Improvement Act of 1982 (P.L. 97-248) modified and extended existing laws and regulations to create the current Quality Improvement Organization (QIO) structure, replacing Professional Standards Review Organizations (PSROs) with Utilization and Quality Control Peer Review Organizations (PROs), later renamed QIOs (Bhatia et al., 2000; CMS, 2004b). The legislation defined the organizational basis for QIO contractors and restricted the kinds of organizations that qualify for QIO status. Although this 24-year-old statute included provisions not applicable to the current health care environment, it provided sufficient flexibility to allow significant adaptation to modern practices and issues in terms of performance criteria, standards, and the requirements of the U.S. Department of Health and Human Services (Jost, 1989). This inherent flexibility permits the use of newer definitions of quality, the expression of new concerns for patients' rights, and a changed emphasis from identifying outliers to changing systems. These changes were made, in part, to encourage providers to view QIOs as collaborative partners rather than regulatory bodies (CMS, 2004b).

Physician-Sponsored and Physician-Access Designations

To be eligible to compete for a QIO contract, an entity must meet certain criteria for designation as either a "physician-sponsored" or a "physician-access" organization (CMS, 2004b). For a physician-sponsored organization, either (1) at least 20 percent of the practicing physicians in the state are owners or members of the organization or (2) 10 percent of practicing physicians are owners or members and the organization can demonstrate that the organization represents an additional 10 percent of practicing physicians in that state. For a physician-access organization, organizations must have arrangements with licensed and practicing physicians to conduct reviews and include "at least one physician, licensed in the state, from every generally recognized specialty and subspecialty who is in active practice in your review area" (CMS, 2004c:2). An organization may not qualify for either designation if it is a health care facility, an association of health care facilities, or a health care facility affiliate.[1]

These designations retain some qualities of the QIO predecessor organizations that favored local peer review. In the past, providers objected to reviews by out-of-state providers, arguing that practice patterns differed by region. However, the evolving recognition of national standards challenges the perceived need for local review (personal communication, T. Jost, Washington and Lee University School of Law, January 7, 2005). Repeal of the requirement for this designation might encourage other entities to compete for QIO contracts. Also, QIOs may be better served by geographically dispersed reviewers, which would allow expanded representation by individuals in clinical specialties and subspecialties and allow the identification of common local practice patterns that are inconsistent with generally accepted evidence-based knowledge.

One exception may be the distinction in the practice patterns of rural providers. In these circumstances, patient care is influenced by confounding circumstances, such as geography, transportation, and the availability of medical technologies; but the practice patterns under these circumstances might be comparable among rural providers around the country (IOM, 2005). However, if the requirement for physician-sponsorship or physician-access designations were eliminated and other entities were allowed to par-

---

[1]The QIO manual defines a health care facility as "An institution that directly provides or supplies health care services for which payment may be made in whole or in part under title XVIII of the Social Security Act" (CMS, 2004c:c2p3). The QIO manual defines a health care facility affiliate as "An organization that has a board on which more than 20 percent of the members are also either a governing board member, officer, partner, five percent or more owner, or managing employee in a health care facility or association of health care facilities in the QIO area" (CMS, 2004c:c2p3).

ticipate as QIOs, there might be concerns about those organizations, which could have multiple agendas, having access to private health information of patients and providers. Currently, when a QIO contract is open for bidding, the Centers for Medicare and Medicaid Services (CMS) gives priority to physician-sponsored organizations (CMS, 2004b). The committee found, using its web-based data collection tool, that 27 of the 52 reporting QIOs identified themselves as physician sponsored and 19 said that they were physician access. (Note that four answered "both" and two said "neither," even though neither of these responses are technically acceptable for a QIO contractor.)

Organizational Characteristics

During the 7th scope of work (SOW), 41 organizations held QIO contracts for 53 individual QIO core contracts—one for each state, the District of Columbia, Puerto Rico, and the Virgin Islands. According to the web-based data collection tool, the majority of the organizations (22 of 41) were established before 1975. Thirty-five of the 41 organizations stated they were originally established for the purpose of holding a QIO contract. Only six claimed to be subsidiaries of other organizations. Seventeen organizations reported that they had their own subsidiaries. Nearly all of the organizations (38 of 41) held a not-for-profit tax status. QIOs were asked whether or not they held specific accreditations. Data on the specific accreditations are presented in Table 7.1.

Additionally, some organizations listed types of accreditations. Four reported that they were certified independent review organizations (either state or national), four said that they were licensed utilization review managers (generally by state), and three said that they were accredited providers of continuing medical education credits. Seven organizations listed other accreditations including state certifications (such as medical review organization or patient safety organization) and National Committee for Quality Assurance licenses (Health Plan Employer Data and Information Set [HEDIS] auditor or HEDIS survey vendor).

The web-based data collection tool also asked the individual QIOs about Baldrige National Quality–type awards. Although most states seem to have this type of award, most QIOs do not apply for them. Of the 52 reporting QIOs, 18 said that their state has no such award. Of the 34 QIOs in states with Baldrige–type awards, 23 have not applied for the state award, eight applied and received the award, and three applied but did not receive the award.

TABLE 7.1 Accreditations Held by Organizations with QIO Contracts for the 7th SOW

Accreditation	Number of Organizations
HEDIS[a]	4
ISO 9000	0
ISO 9001:2001	4
Six Sigma	1
URAC[b] case management	2
URAC claims processing	0
URAC consumer-directed health care	0
URAC core[c]	5
URAC credential verification	0
URAC disease management	1
URAC healthy call center	0
URAC health provider credentialing	0
URAC utilization management	11
URAC health website	0
URAC HIPAA privacy	0
URAC HIPAA security	0
URAC independent review	7
URAC worker's compensation utilization management	1
URAC vendor certification	0

NOTE: One organization anticipated achieving ISO 9001:2001 in March 2005 (shortly after data collection ended), and another had URAC core accreditation pending. HEDIS = Health Plan Employer Data and Information Set; HIPPA = Health Insurance Portability and Accountability Act of 1996; ISO = International Standards Organization; URAC = Utilization Review Accreditation Commission.

[a]HEDIS is a set of standardized measures used to compare performance of managed care plans. HEDIS also includes a consumer-perspective survey (NCQA, 2005).

[b]The Utilization Review Accreditation Commission was renamed to "URAC" in 1996 when it expanded its accreditation process. URAC sometimes does business as the American Accreditation HealthCare Commission, Inc. (URAC, 2005).

[c]One organization chose "prefer not to answer/information not available."

SOURCE: IOM committee web-based data collection tool (n = 41 organizations).

QIO Staff

In the web-based data collection tool, all 52 reporting QIOs said that their employee with the shortest length of employment had been employed for 2 years or less, and almost all (50 of 52) said that the employee had been there less than 1 year. For the longest length of employment of a single employee, responses ranged from 5 years to more than 25 years. In fact, 22

TABLE 7.2   QIO Employee Turnover Rates, 2002 to 2004

| | Percentage of turnover among QIO employees | | | | | |
| | 2002 | | 2003 | | 2004 | |
Statistic	TP	SS	TP	SS	TP	SS
Minimum	0	0	0	0	0	0
First quartile	2.56	0.03	6.12	0	5.69	0.06
Median	12.00	5.00	13.00	3.99	12.15	3.22
Mean	13.00	15.50	19.53	11.80	12.38	10.93
Third quartile	19.00	24.50	23.00	21.22	18.00	11.30
Maximum	50.00	86.00	114.00	50.00	39.00	167.00

NOTE: TP = technical or professional staff; SS = support staff.

SOURCE: IOM committee web-based data collection tool (n = 52 QIOs).

QIOs related that the longest length of employment of at least one employee was 25 or more years, and 35 QIOs had had at least one employee for more than 20 years. The reported average length of employment among all employees ranged from 1.32 to 10.00 years, with a mean of 5.97 years.

Examination of employee turnover within the QIO program is important, especially in light of the new priorities of transformational change in which the employee turnover rate is used as a measure of success. From 2002 to 2004, employee turnover rates varied greatly among both the technical or professional staff and the support staff of the QIOs. The average turnover rate for both of these categories ranged from 10.93 to 19.53 percent. (Loss of a QIO contract can account for turnover rates of more than 100 percent, which can skew average turnover rates.) The individual turnover rates reported by the QIOs are provided in Table 7.2.

QIO Leadership

In the web-based data collection tool, the chief executive officers (CEOs) of 52 QIOs rated the extent to which they believed that each of 14 "leadership competencies," derived from the National Center for Healthcare Leadership competency model (National Center for Healthcare Leadership, 2004), were represented. These competencies are collaboration, relationship building, team development, performance measurement, communication skills, change leadership, process management and organizational design, strategic orientation, innovative thinking, community orientation, achievement orientation, self-development, impact or influence, and talent development. A majority of the CEOs rated their leadership teams as demonstrating each of the leadership competencies to a "substantial" extent. This finding was particularly evident in the cluster of competencies that appear to be the most obviously related to the type of work required during the 7th SOW—collaboration, relationship building, team development, and performance measurement—with more than 88 percent of CEOs rating these competencies "substantial." For only one competence—talent development—did any CEO indicate that it was represented "not at all"; overall, this particular leadership competence is least well represented across leadership teams, with 19 of 52 QIOs rating it "modest" and only 32 of 52 QIOs rating it "substantial."

Governing Board

The governing board of a QIO is responsible for the "efficient and effective management" of its QIO (CMS, 2004c:4). When responding to the CMS requests for proposals (to bid on the QIO contract), the organization must specify how the board will oversee the management of the QIO. CMS sets minimum standards in the official request. The QIO has substantial discretion in selecting the members of its governing board and their term lengths and responsibilities. Hence, each QIO can adapt its board to the vision and requirements of its own organization.

There is one notable exception to this flexibility: the board must have at least one consumer representative. The Omnibus Budget Reconciliation Act of 1986 (P.L. 99-509) added this requirement. The consumer representative must be a Medicare beneficiary and live in the state represented by the board's organization. The consumer representative cannot be a practicing or retired physician, nor can the consumer representative be "a governing board member, officer, partner, owner of more than five percent interest in a health care facility, or managing employee of a health care facility or association of health care facilities" (CMS, 2004c:6). Additionally, the consumer representative must meet at least four of the following five criteria (CMS, 2004b):

- Experience with consumer advocacy,
- Knowledge of state organizations working on senior issues,
- Knowledge of the needs of beneficiaries and providers in their state or jurisdiction,
- Basic understanding of the Medicare program,
- Experience serving on or working with other boards or commissions.

QIOs representing states with both fee-for-service and managed care Medicare contracts must ensure the adequate representation of each. Therefore, these QIOs must have an additional consumer member (for the population not represented on the governing board) "as a permanent member of at least one appropriate committee/group" (CMS, 2004c:6). In the case of organizations holding more than one QIO contract, the consumer representative may reside in any of the states served by those QIOs. The organizations are not required to have a representative of the fee-for-service Medicare population for each state. However, a managed care consumer representative for each state (if managed care plans exist in the state) must sit either on the governing board or on a committee or group.

Overall, the demographics of the board should represent the diversity of the Medicare population in the state(s) that it serves. Additionally, no more than 20 percent of board members may be "affiliated with a health care facility or association of health care facilities located in the area of any of the following capacities: a governing member; an officer; a partner; an owner of five percent or more; or a managing employee" (CMS, 2004c:4).

QIO Board Size (7th SOW)

Data supplied by the CEOs of the 41 organizations holding QIO contracts for the 7th SOW via the web-based data collection tool showed that the allowed and the actual board sizes varied widely. The maximum board sizes permitted by individual bylaws ranged from 6 to 52 members, with a mean of 21. The actual sizes ranged from 4 to 30 members, with a mean of 17. Most organizations (32 of 41 organizations) reported that 3 years was the typical term length for board members. Just over half of the organizations (21 of 41) limit the number of board terms. Most of the boards (29 of 41) meet on a quarterly basis, with the frequencies of meetings varying for the remaining organizations. Figure 7.1 shows the distribution of the number of organizations reporting the existence of specific standing committees.

Twenty-six of the 41 organizations reported that they had one or more regular standing board committees other than those listed in Figure 7.1. In most cases, the additional committees did not have regularly scheduled meetings and were used on an ad hoc basis.

QIO Board Expertise (7th SOW)

According to the web-based data collection tool, most CEOs of organizations holding QIO contracts for the 7th SOW (30 of 37 respondents) did not anticipate the need for additional board expertise for the 8th SOW. Of the seven CEOs who foresaw such a need, three specified expertise in home health care in particular. Other responses related to more general areas of expertise, such as business or financial management.

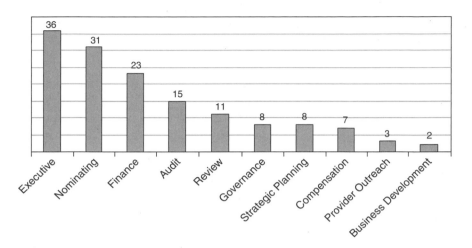

FIGURE 7.1 Numbers of QIO boards with the indicated standing committees (7th SOW).
SOURCE: IOM committee web-based data collection tool (*n* = 41 organizations).

The web-based data collection tool also requested information on the primary professional background of each board member; the organizations could report on up to 30 board members. The respondents selected the backgrounds from among 15 options. Physicians were the only professional type represented on all boards. Just less than 60 percent of these organizations included executives or managers from non-health-care-related businesses, and 56 percent included hospital executives or managers. The only other profession represented on at least one-third of the boards was nursing (41 percent). Professionals with backgrounds relevant to the tasks required in the 7th SOW other than hospital quality improvement—executives or managers in nursing homes and home health care agencies—were included on relatively few boards (28 and 2.56 percent, respectively).

Among all boards, physicians clearly dominated: 67 percent of all organizations' board members were physicians (427 of 639 board members for whom data were reported). Nurses were the second largest group, at just under 8 percent of all board members, followed by executives in non-health-care-related businesses (about 7 percent) and hospital executives or managers (about 6.5 percent). All other professional categories each accounted for less than 5 percent of board members.

Examination of the board compositions revealed that three or fewer different professional backgrounds were represented on the boards of about half of the organizations. Ten of 41 boards contained individuals with only two different types of professional backgrounds, although there was considerable variety in the second of the two backgrounds represented across the organizations (the common one being physicians). One organization's board included individuals with 11 different types of professional backgrounds, the boards of three organizations included individuals with seven different types of professional backgrounds, and the boards of four organizations included individuals with six different types of professional backgrounds. It is noteworthy, however, that the respondents were limited to choosing one background, and some board members may have had multiple relevant experiences in their professional careers.

QIO Board Members' Affiliations (7th SOW)

The web-based data collection tool requested information on the primary affiliation of each board member and showed a predominant representation of individuals from office-based practices and hospitals. The respondents selected from among 11 choices on a drop-down menu. Clinicians in office-based practice settings represented the only affiliation seen on the board of every organization holding a QIO contract for the 7th SOW. Almost 85 percent of these organizations' boards included members affiliated with hospitals. Among all boards, members affiliated with office-based practices dominated (294 of 636 board members [46 percent] for whom this information was reported). The second largest group was board members affiliated with hospitals (121 members [19 percent]).

Boards tended to have more variety in primary affiliations than in professional backgrounds. Five or six different affiliations were represented on a typical board; two boards had as many as nine different affiliations, and one board had eight. Each board had individuals with at least two different primary affiliations. Despite the potential that organizations with larger boards might demonstrate more diversity in professional backgrounds or primary affiliations, statistical analyses revealed no such relationship for the boards of these organizations. As was mentioned above in the discussion of primary backgrounds, it is noteworthy that the respondents were limited in their choices, so members may represent more than one profession or affiliation. This is notable because the QIO contract requires at least one consumer representative on each board, yet not all organizations reported a member with "Medicare beneficiary" or "consumer" as his or her primary affiliation. This indicates that some organizations have consumer representatives with other significant affiliations that they consider to be dominant over their role as a consumer representative.

QIO Board Selection, Compensation, and Evaluation (7th SOW)

Overall, at least 34 of the 41 boards for organizations holding QIO contracts for the 7th SOW had some form of involvement in either the selection or the approval of their own new board members. About half of the organizations (21 of 41) reported via the web-based data collection tool that board members are selected by or with the approval of the organization's current board. An additional 10 organizations' boards were at least partially involved in the nomination or selection process.

The data also revealed that the vast majority of board members are generally compensated in some way. Thirty-four of 37 reporting organizations provide compensation (not including travel expenses) to board members. A 2005 article in the *Washington Post* reported on the salaries and compensation for QIO board members (Gaul, 2005). The author outlined specific examples of compensation to board members of up to $45,000 each, or $250 per hour, for QIO-related activities, including one board in which 19 of the 21 board members received some form of compensation. In comparison, the article cites an estimate that nationally, only 2 percent of nonprofit groups provide financial compensation to their board members.

The web-based tool collected data on the evaluation of board performance. Those data revealed that most organizations do not regularly evaluate their boards individually or as a whole. Only 10 of 38 reporting organizations had formal mechanisms in place for the evaluation of individual board member performance. Ten of 38 organizations stated that they had mechanisms in place to evaluate the overall board performance.

Consumer Advisory Council

The QIO contract for the 7th SOW required each QIO to establish a Consumer Advisory Council (CAC) to meet at least quarterly to advise the organization on policy directions for consumer-related issues. "CAC membership must include representatives from community and business organizations. . . . More than half of the CAC members must be from organizations whose primary responsibility is protecting the interest of Medicare beneficiaries" (CMS, 2002:35). Members are chosen at the discretion of the QIO contractor. The example in Box 7.1 shows the membership of the CAC for the Health Services Advisory Group (Arizona's QIO).

Ability to Perform Case Review Activities

Organizations bidding for QIO contracts must demonstrate the ability to perform required review activities by documenting past or current experience or providing a detailed performance plan (CMS, 2004b). The

---

BOX 7.1   Health Services Advisory Group's CAC Member Organizations

AARP Arizona
ABC Coalition
Aging and Adult Administration
Alzheimer's Association
Area Agency on Aging
Arizona Academy of Family Physicians
The Arizona Center for Disability Law
Arizona College of Public health
Arizona Health Care Cost Containment System
Arizona Latin-American Medical Association
Arizona Medical Association
Arizona Rural Health Association
Consumers/Senior Community Activists
Foundation for Senior Living
Gold & Associates
Governor's Advisory Council on Aging
HSAG Board of Directors
Inter-Tribal Council Agency
State Health Insurance Assistance Program
University of Arizona College of Medicine

SOURCE: Health Services Advisory Group (2005).

---

organization must submit a document outlining its policies and procedures, including sections on rules of confidentiality, methods of information collection, the criteria used in the review process, and a mechanism for managing complaints and appeals. Additionally, the organization must provide a list of its staff and an organizational chart showing physician management of the process as well as the process for the collection of information by clinical staff. Finally, the organization must be able to demonstrate experience or an ability to analyze the medical review data (CMS, 2004b). Specific case review requirements, activities, and goals are discussed in Chapter 12. Several QIOs hold special accreditations related to case review activities (as discussed above).

Subcontracting

Data from the web-based data collection tool revealed substantial experience with the use of subcontractors for work both for CMS and for other clients among the organizations holding QIO contracts for the 7th SOW. A little more than half of the organizations (26 of 41) used subcontractors on their core QIO contract tasks or planned to use them. Additionally, 28 of 41 organizations used subcontractors (or planned to use subcontractors) for other CMS work, such as QIO Support Centers (QIOSCs) or special studies. Twenty-six reported that they used subcontractors for work for non-CMS clients.

CMS requires QIOs to meet performance planning requirements (as defined by CMS in the contract for the 8th SOW) for the tasks of the 8th SOW. Most of these requirements are based on QIO performance in the 7th SOW. If the QIO does not meet any of these requirements, the QIO must submit a written statement (a Capability Enhancement Plan) on how it plans to meet those requirements (CMS, 2005b). In the 8th SOW, CMS may require a QIO to subcontract for Task 1d1 duties (assistance with information technology implementation in the physician practice setting) if CMS determines that the QIO does not have expertise in this area.

Conflict of Interest Rules

To ensure the impartiality of case reviews and third-party independence, certain organizations cannot bid for QIO contracts (CMS, 2004b). Those excluded from bidding are health care facilities, associations of health care facilities, and health care facility affiliates. The statute also does not allow payers or their affiliates to be QIOs if other entities are available, and regulations discourage state governments from being QIOs. In most cases, CMS will exclude an organization from bidding if a member of its governing board has been sanctioned by Medicare. These conflict-of-interest rules are important because, during the site visits, the QIOs praised their independent, impartial nature, which they found to be one of their major strengths.

QIOs express concern about their ability to work outside of the QIO contract because of limitations that do not allow them to augment their QIO contracts (personal communication, D. Schulke and T. Ketch, American Health Quality Association, June 30, 2005). These restrictions prevent organizations with QIO contracts from providing services similar to those provided under the QIO contract under separate contracts with providers in the Medicare program. This restriction intends to avoid conflicts of interest that might arise if a QIO was receiving compensation for a separate contract from a provider who came under review for cases of questionable quality or other concerns.

Confidentiality Restrictions

A complex set of laws and regulations delineate the confidentiality and disclosure requirements of government-sponsored agencies, mostly imposed through 42 U.S.C. § 1320c-9, 42 U.S.C. §§ 1320c-3 and 1320c-5, and 42 C.F.R. Part 48042 U.S.C. (personal communication, T. Jost, Washington and Lee University School of Law, January 7, 2005). The Freedom of Information Act applies to federal agencies but not to QIOs. Current QIO confidentiality and disclosure rules are partially based on information presented in a 1981 Institute of Medicine (IOM) study, *Access to Medical Review Data* (IOM, 1981), which examined the policies of the Professional Standards Review Organizations, the predecessors of the QIOs. That study outlined general principles, including freedom of information, rights to privacy (for both the provider and the patient), and minimization of interference in the peer review process. The committee that wrote that report recognized the potential for harm from either erroneously damaged professional reputations or the misinterpretation of information. It also acknowledged the strong public interest in the availability of information on matters pertaining to public health and publicly funded programs, as well as the need for access to information for accountability and for consumers to purchase health care services. At that time, the committee recommended the disclosure of institution-specific information (aggregate performance data) but did not recommend that physician-specific information be revealed. The disclosure of specific information was thought to be in opposition to the philosophy of peer review—the use of root-cause analysis and improvement methodologies without penalty. With a few exceptions, all information held by QIOs is considered confidential, thereby sustaining the confidence of consumers and providers. However, many nonidentified QIO data are available.

Since publication of that 1981 IOM report, even greater efforts have been made to disclose quality data to allow consumers to make better-informed decisions about their health care, including public reporting by Medicare and some private purchasers. The U.S. Department of Health and Human Services can alter confidentiality policies without legislative action (personal communications, T. Jost, Washington and Lee University School of Law, December 21, 2004, and January 7, 2005) (IOM, 1981; CMS, 2004b).

Patients have the right to request and receive their personal information, but other specific patient or practitioner references must be omitted (personal communication, T. Jost, Washington and Lee University School of Law, January 7, 2005; CMS, 2004b). The distinction between "CMS information" and "QIO information" is noteworthy: "CMS data is the data and/or information that CMS provides to the QIO to enable it to carry out its function under this contract. QIO data is the data and/or information the QIO gathers or develops through analysis in the course of carrying out its functions under their contract" (CMS, 2004a:5). For example, CMS data include provider-level claims data that QIOs can access to identify areas in need of quality improvement or to monitor payment error rates. Examples of QIO data include information gathered through special studies or beneficiary complaint reviews. During the site visits, one QIO expressed concern that confidentiality restrictions impede its ability to assist individual providers, precluding QIO access to data that could help it better understand the individual patterns of providers. QIOs may not release any CMS information that they hold without express approval from CMS. QIO information can be released only according to general confidentiality restrictions (personal communication, T. Jost, Washington and Lee University School of Law, January 7, 2005; CMS, 2002, 2004a,b, 2005a).

QIO SUPPORT CENTERS

QIOSCs act as central resources for all QIOs on specific topic areas or for the general needs of the QIO community (CMS, 2002, 2004a). A QIOSC may provide technical information and reports, QIO staff training, and implementation materials. A QIOSC can help QIOs decide how to recruit identified participants, serve a convening function for QIOs to communicate among themselves through monthly calls and listserves, and provide other technical support as needed. By also acting as a central clearinghouse of information, the QIOSC gathers information on the experiences of individual QIOs, including best practices, change concepts, clinical techniques, and guidelines that QIOs can apply to their own interventions. However, some QIOs complain that guidance or materials from QIOSCs become available too slowly.

7th SOW

Detailed descriptions of the activities of QIOSCs will be presented throughout later chapters. Table 7.3 shows all QIOSCs in place during the 7th SOW.

8th SOW

The QIOSC system has been redesigned in the 8th SOW. During the strategic planning process in 2004, the QIO and End-Stage Renal Disease Steering Committee (see Chapter 13) decided that the QIOSC system needed to be updated because of variation in activities and performance among QIOSCs, the new missions of the QIO program, and the need to address cross issues across settings (personal communication, J. Taylor, April 29, 2005). The two main types of QIOSCs are crosscutting QIOSCs and task/topic-specific QIOSCs. The five crosscutting QIOSCs that handle issues related to provider settings or specific tasks are:

- MedQIC—the Medicare Quality Improvement Community (see Chapter 13), which maintains a public website for the quality improvement community;
  - Communications—supports all QIO communication activities;
  - Performance Improvement—provides training and support for various quality improvement methodologies;
  - Data Reports—maintains data systems to support QIO reporting activities; and
  - Measures Management—assists with the development and implementation of measures.

The topic or provider setting QIOSCs focus more specifically on certain tasks or provider settings and will use their expertise to customize the tem-

TABLE 7.3   QIOSCs in the 7th SOW

Topic Area	Name or Acronym	State
Nursing home	NH QIOSC	RI (CO is subcontractor)
Home health	HH QIOSC	MD
Hospital—heart care (acute myocardial infarction and heart failure)	Heart Failure QIOSC	CO
Hospital—infectious disease (surgical infection prevention and pneumonia)	Infectious Disease QIOSC	OK
Physician office	Physician Office QIOSC	VA
Underserved and rural	UQIOSC	TN
Medicare Advantage (Medicare+Choice)	M+C QIOSC	CA
Communications	CommQIOSC	WA and MO (MO subcontracts to WA)
Process improvement	PI QIOSC	WA
Beneficiary complaint response program (Medicare beneficiary protection)	MBP QIOSC	CA
Outpatient data	Outpatient Data QIOSC	IA
Hospital data collection Standard Data Processing System	Hospital Data Collection QIOSC	IA
	Standard Data Processing System QIOSC	IA
Quality improvement interventions and MedQIC.org	Interventions QIOSC	"Virtual QIOSC" led by IA
Hospital Payment Monitoring Program (HPMP)	HPMP QIOSC	TX

SOURCE: CMS (2002, 2004a).

plates, data, tools, etc., provided by the crosscutting QIOSCs. The 10 topic or provider setting QIOSCs are:

- Nursing home,
- Home health care,
- Hospital interventions (which includes rural hospitals; combines heart failure and infectious diseases),
- Hospital data reporting,
- Physician office (which has a coordinating role for office setting, Doctor's Office Quality–Information Technology, and the underserved population),
- Underserved,
- Outpatient data,
- Pharmacy (Task 1d3, which is related to the Medicare Part D prescription drug benefit),
- Beneficiary protection, and
- Hospital Payment Monitoring Program.

In the 8th SOW, QIOSCs support QIOs by providing tools and information, as described above for the 7th SOW. QIOSCs are expected to perform these tasks as well as interact with other QIOSCs. Additionally, satisfaction surveys will be administered to all QIOs to determine their satisfaction with the products and services of each QIOSC. In September 2005, CMS developed a draft guidebook for the QIOs on how to best use QIOSC services, including a list of the available products and contact information (personal communication, D. Chromik-Ralston, September 10, 2005). The QIOSC contractors for the 8th SOW (as of September 2005) are listed in Table 7.4.

Telephone Interviews with QIO CEOs

The following sections reflect the opinions of 20 QIO CEOs who were interviewed about their interactions with QIOSCs. The CEOs indicated that they regularly use QIOSCs and consider them valuable mechanisms for knowledge transfer, but their use can depend on a QIO's particular needs. A couple of CEOs indicated that a QIOSC is not necessarily their first stop when they are starting on a specific task, as they may have their own internal expertise.

Important Functions Performed by QIOSCs

The CEOs were asked to identify the most important functions that QIOSCs perform. Eighteen of the 20 CEOs identified specific functions and mentioned the following major categories of QIOSC activities:

- being a communications link among the QIOs (nine CEOs),
- providing a communications link to CMS on task areas (six CEOs),
- being a repository of best practices and the most current literature (eight CEOs),
- disseminating information on what is working in the field (eight CEOs),
- taking state-level experiences and standardizing models with options for local needs (four CEOs),
- developing educational and training materials and providing resource personnel (seven CEOs), and
- working on behalf of CMS and QIOs with external stakeholders (two CEOs).

TABLE 7.4   QIOSCs in the 8th SOW

Topic Area	Name or Acronym	State
Nursing home	NH QIOSC	RI
Home health	HH QIOSC	WV
Hospital—interventions	Hospital Interventions QIOSC	OK
Hospital—data reporting	Hospital Reporting QIOSC	IA
Physician office	Physician Office QIOSC	VA
Underserved	UQIOSC	TN
Outpatient data	Outpatient Data QIOSC	IA
Pharmacy (Task 1d3)	TBD	TBD
Beneficiary protection	MBP QIOSC	TX
Hospital Payment Monitoring Program (HPMP)	HPMP QIOSC	TX
Communications	CommQIOSC	WA and MO
Measures management	Measures Management QIOSC	AZ
MedQIC	MedQIC QIOSC	IA
Performance improvement	PI QIOSC	WA
Data reports	Reports QIOSC	IA

SOURCE: Personal communication, D. Chromik-Ralston, September 10, 2005.

Communications Links Among QIOs and with CMS

According to the QIO CEOs, QIOSCs open communications channels by convening QIOs using a variety of formats (e.g., monthly conference calls, listserves, web-based training), send new information to QIOs, and coordinate the efforts of the QIO so that repetitive work is not performed. The CEOs said that it is important for QIOSCs to be visible to the QIO community, have an open dialogue with all QIOs, listen to QIO needs, and be responsive in a timely manner. QIOSCs also help interpret the requests of Government Task Leaders and act as problem solvers on contract issues.

Repository of Evidence Base for Best Practices and Dissemination of Information

The CEOs agreed that the QIOSCs must be up to date in their area of expertise and should have knowledge of the evidence base for clinical medicine and performance measures as well as the application of the techniques that can be used to improve quality. The QIOSCs provide the QIOs with shortcuts to detect the techniques used in the field that have been successful and those that have not when the QIOs want to have access to such findings early on in the implementation of their tasks. An additional asset that the QIOSCs provide is to show the QIOs how to assess changes within each task.

Standardizing Models and Developing Materials

The QIOSCs operationalize the CMS vision and standardize a national model by developing consensus, helping to set priorities, and translating multiple studies and experiences into workable approaches for use by the QIOs. These approaches, however, should be able to be tailored to local circumstances. For example, an intervention in one state may require the development of bilingual materials for distribution to beneficiaries if the demographics of the beneficiary population reflects this need. Ideally, the QIOSCs develop educational and training materials and data collection tools so that each QIO does not have to perform these tasks on its own. The range of materials should be suitable for dissemination to health care professionals, quality improvement specialists, consumers, and other key groups (e.g., employers and insurers). QIOSCs also provide learning sessions on different methods for performance of the assigned tasks (e.g., breakthrough collaborative activities). The QIOSCs have resource staff who are available for consultation by telephone or who travel to the states to speak with provider audiences.

Working with External Stakeholders

QIOSCs are able to work with external stakeholders (e.g., national professional associations) and other players in the quality improvement field (e.g., the Joint Commission on Accreditation of Healthcare Organizations) in moving toward transformational change. This interaction is important because many organizations other than QIOs are also working on quality measures, and thus, the QIOs and other organizations are walking parallel paths. QIOSCs can access experts in the health care field to work on pertinent issues and to present that information to QIOs; as one CEO stated, "that degree of access would be impossible on a QIO-by-QIO basis." (source: Telephone interviews with QIO CEOs.)

Recommendations for Improvement

The QIO CEOs made specific recommendations for improving the QIOSCs, including:

- Improve the timeliness of the QIOSC response to QIOs and deal with underlying problems with CMS responsiveness and coterminous contracting of QIOSCs and QIOs on tasks (15 CEOs).
- Encourage innovation at the local QIO level with special project grants (three CEOs).
- Recruit as Government Task Leaders knowledgeable staff who have expertise in their task assignment and who are confident enough to make timely decisions in a high-profile job (11 CEOs).
- Ensure adequate QIOSC staff (two CEOs).

Need to Improve Timeliness   Fifteen of 20 CEOs specifically mentioned the need for improvement in the timeliness of the response of all QIOSCs. However, most of the reasons cited for that lack of timeliness were not due to the QIOSC itself; instead, they attribute problems to Government Task Leader control and delay (11 CEOs) and coterminous contracting with QIOSCs and QIOs (seven CEOs).

Eleven of 15 CEOs who were concerned with timeliness issues made a connection to the lack of expertise or practical experience of the Government Task Leader or the degree of control or tone set by a Government Task Leader. One CEO said, "Sometimes it is hard to know where the fault lies when a QIOSC doesn't perform well, especially when the problem is the timeliness of materials. CMS tends to delay things." Delays due to the contracting cycle relate to the difficulties that arise because the QIO and QIOSC contracts both start at the same time. This does not allow the QIOSCs to develop tools and other materials that the QIOs can use right away. These issues are discussed in further detail in Chapter 13.

Encouraging Innovation Three CEOs raised issues related to innovation or the lack of it. One CEO said that although the QIOSCs were expected to produce greater efficiency, one of the unintended consequences was that it has reduced local creativity. Two others suggested that CMS should have special funding to implement the good ideas that the QIOs propose themselves and that the QIOSC contracts should be awarded to QIOs that have demonstrated the most innovation and creativity.

Adequacy of QIOSC Staff One CEO asserted that QIOSCs tend to have two staffing models: one with staff dedicated solely to the QIOSC function and another with staff who do the QIOSC function part-time in conjunction with other QIO jobs. Another CEO commented that "the QIOs that are QIOSCs should be the strongest QIOs in the field, but in reality some of them are ones that have struggled to meet their own QIO goals."

Interviews with QIOSCs

Of the seven QIOSCs interviewed (represented by five organizations), four stated that they originally got their QIOSC contract because of previous experience (including three that were special studies or pilot programs). All saw their main focus as being the provision of support to the QIOs in their work, but they stated that the level of interaction varied according to the individual needs of the QIOs. Five of the seven QIOSCs were topic or provider setting specific, and all of these stated that the QIOs should be QIOSCs (as opposed to an outside entity) because of their intimate understanding of the QIO contract as well as their immediate acceptance and connections in the community.

FINANCES OF QIOs

QIO Program Funding[2]

For the 5th and the 6th SOWs, total apportionments (core contract, special studies, and support contracts) were $728.3 million and $1,051.0 million, respectively, for each contract period (personal communications, C. Lazarus, March 17, 2005; D. Rimel, March 3, 2006). For the 7th SOW, the estimated total obligations at the end of calendar year 2004 for the entire QIO program were $1,154.3 million. QIOs were responsible for deciding their distribution of funds across tasks and accounting for this allocation, which is subject to CMS review. During the course of the 3-year contract, the QIO had flexibility to shift funds from task to task as needed, as the contract was performance based.

As of May 31, 2005, the total apportionment for the 8th SOW is slated at $1.265 billion, a 9 percent increase over that for the 7th SOW (personal communication, D. Adler, American Health Quality Association, May 23, 2005). The estimated budgets for the 7th and the 8th SOWs are presented in Table 7.5.

However, the funds designated in the core contract for the newly required reviews under the Benefits Improvement and Protection Act (P.L. 106-554), as further discussed in Chapter 12, may not be used for any other

---

[2]Funding data are from CMS and are based on actual expenditures plus estimated obligations as of the end of calendar year 2004.

TABLE 7.5 Comparison of Estimated Budgets for the 7th and 8th SOWs

Budget Item	7th SOW Budget (millions)	Percentage of Total	8th SOW Budget (millions)	Percentage of Total
Total apportionment	$1,154.3		$1,265	
Core contract	$796.7	69.0	$860	68.0
Support contracts and special studies	$357.6	31.0	$405	32.0

SOURCES: Personal communication, D. Adler, May 23, 2005; personal communication, C. Lazarus, March 17, 2005.

area of the contract, and unused funds must be returned. Additionally, it is difficult to make a direct comparison of spending on specific areas between the 7th and the 8th SOWs because of a shift of the categories in which the spending is attributed.

Although the overall funding for the QIO program has increased with each successive SOW, Table 7.6 shows that program funding has become a smaller percentage of the overall Medicare budget since the 6th SOW.

TABLE 7.6 Comparison of Total Outlays for Mandatory Spending (Medicare) to QIO Budget

SOW	Year	Medicare Outlays (billions)	Total Medicare Outlay (per SOW) (billions)	QIO Budget (millions)	Percentage of Medicare Outlays[a]
5th	1997	$207.9	$628.2	$728.3	0.12
	1998	$211.0			
	1999	$209.3			
6th	2000	$216.0	$707.6	$1,051.0	0.15
	2001	$237.9			
	2002	$253.7			
7th	2003	$274.2	$899.1	$1,154.3	0.13
	2004	$297.4			
	2005	$327.5[b]			
8th	2006	$378.6[b]	$1,262.8	$1,265.0	0.10
	2007	$428.0[b]			
	2008	$456.2[b]			

[a]Calculations were done by the IOM committee on the basis of data from CMS and the Congressional Budget Office (CBO).

[b]Estimated outlays.

SOURCES: CBO (2005a,b); personal communication, C. Lazarus, March 17, 2005; personal communication, D. Rimel, March 3, 2006.

Core Contract

As of December 2004, estimated obligations for the core contract of the 7th SOW (Tasks 1 to 3 plus information and contractual costs) were $790.1 million, which represents approximately 68 percent of the entire QIO program budget (personal communication, C. Lazarus, March 17, 2005). (Note that the totals differ from those presented in Table 7.6 because of slight differences in the breakdowns of estimated budgets and estimated obligations prepared at different times during the 7th SOW.) The core contract funds distributed to the QIOs are indicated in Table 7.7.

For Task 1 of the 7th SOW, QIO expenditures for statewide work accounted for approximately two-thirds of the total expenditures for each of the subtasks related to the nursing home (69 percent), home health (67 percent), and hospital (67 percent) settings (CMS Dashboard, 12/19/05). In the hospital setting during the 7th SOW, QIOs only worked at the statewide level. While the majority of the total expenditures went toward these statewide-level activities, work with the identified participants was more intense with fewer providers. For example, as shown in Table 7.8, QIO work with nursing homes in the 7th SOW had a monthly cost of $170.97 for each provider in the state or jurisdiction. (This includes both

TABLE 7.7 Core Contract Obligations During the 7th SOW (as of December 2004)

Task	Estimated Obligations (millions)	Percentage of Core Contract
Task 1 (quality improvement activities)	$449.0	56.8
Task 2 (communications)	$104.2	13.2
Task 3 (case review)	$161.7	20.5
Task 3a (beneficiary complaints)	$45.5	5.8
Task 3b (Hospital Payment Monitoring Program)	$41.2	5.2
Task 3c (other case review)	$75.0	9.5
Information services	$50.4	6.4
Contractual requirements	$24.8	3.1
7th SOW total core contract	$790.1	100.0

NOTE: Calculations are approximate and were done by the IOM committee on the basis of CMS data.

SOURCE: Personal communication, C. Lazarus, March 17, 2005.

TABLE 7.8   QIO Expenditures on Tasks 1a–1d for the 7th SOW

Task	Actual Cumulative Cost (in millions of dollars)[a]	Total Number of Providers (nationwide)[b]	Average Monthly Cost per Provider (nationwide)[a,c] (in dollars)	Total Number of Identified Participants[b]	Average Monthly Cost per Identified Participant (in dollars)[a,d]
1a	89.2	16,560	170.97	2,479	350.35
1b	56.7	2,595	211.40	1,405	132.07
1c	87.3	N/A	581.48	NA	NA
1d	105.9	209,349	15.89	10,463	71.18

NOTE: NA = not applicable; N/A = not available.

[a]Data current as of August 2, 2005, calculated from cumulative QIO invoices.
[b]Data current as of October 9, 2003.
[c]Calculated as cumulative cost divided by total number of providers (nationally) divided by number of invoices.
[d]Calculated as costs associated with work with identified participants divided by the number of identified participants divided by the number of invoices.

SOURCE: CMS Dashboard (accessed December 19, 2005).

state-level and identified participant activities, and is calculated per provider for the total number of providers in the state or jurisdiction.) However, the QIOs' focused work with a subset of nursing homes cost $350.35 per identified participant, even though this work only accounted for 31 percent of total expenditures for this subtask. These data are significant since statewide work accounted for the majority of the total expenditures, but work with identified participants for nursing homes and physicians' offices had higher expenditures per provider. In contrast, in the home health setting, the cost per provider was higher for all providers statewide overall than for identified participants. In the 7th SOW, QIOs did not work with identified participants in the hospital setting.

In the web-based data collection tool, the core contract accounted for a highly variable percentage of the total revenues for each organization holding a QIO contract for the 7th SOW and ranged from 16 to 100 percent. However, as shown in Table 7.9, 17 of 39 reporting organizations related that the core contract accounted for at least 70 percent of their total revenues.

As of May 2005, the core contract budget for the 8th SOW was $860 million (personal communication, D. Adler, May 23, 2005). However, as discussed in Chapter 12, the Medicare, Medicaid, and SCHIP Benefits Im-

TABLE 7.9   Percentage of Total Revenue from the Core
Contract of the 7th SOW

Total Proportion of Revenue from Core Contract	Number of Organizations, Holding QIO Contracts for the 7th SOW
<10 percent	0
10–19 percent	1
20–29 percent	4
30–39 percent	6
40–49 percent	4
50–59 percent	4
60–69 percent	3
70–79 percent	6
80–89 percent	5
90–99 percent	4
100 percent	2

SOURCE: IOM committee web-based data collection tool ($n = 39$ organizations).

provement and Protection Act (P.L. 106-554) (BIPA) of 2000 requires QIOs to perform a new type of review (BIPA reviews) in the 8th SOW. Funding for these reviews is estimated to be $125 million for the budget for the 8th SOW (personal communication, D. Rimel, March 3, 2006). As opposed to other core contract activities, funding designated for BIPA reviews may not be reallocated to other activities. Therefore, when $125 million is subtracted from the $860 million allocation, there is, in essence, a reduction in funding for core activities during the 8th SOW.

Special Studies[3]

At CMS, the Office of Clinical Standards and Quality's Science Council formulates developmental study priorities and criteria for consideration of special study proposals (personal communication, C. Lazarus, March 17, 2005). CMS solicits proposals with a "call letter" to Central and Regional Office staff. Project Officers also send the letter to individual QIOs. Individual QIOs may propose unsolicited special studies on the basis of individual interests or state needs, but most special studies arise as a result of solicitation by CMS. When multiple QIOs submit proposals for a CMS-

[3]The information in this section was provided by CMS. Costs are estimated as of April 29, 2004.

solicited special study, the council sets the criteria for evaluation of the proposals. Final project approvals are based on priorities and review criteria, budget analysis, and an assessment of the QIO's capability. All proposals are considered and voted upon by the Special Studies Review Panel.

In the 7th SOW, as of March 2005, estimated obligations for special studies totaled $63.8 million, which represents approximately 5.5 percent of total program costs (personal communication, C. Lazarus, March 17, 2005). At that time 72 special projects were under way, and more than one state was involved in 11 of those studies (see Table A.4 in Appendix A). Twenty-seven QIOs participated in at least one special study. Of the states with special studies, seven states were involved in only one study and nine states participated in four or more special studies. Two states (Colorado and Maryland) were involved in nine studies each. The amount of funding for individual studies ranged from $10,491 for a continuing medical education project to $11.0 million for the Doctor's Office Quality-Information Technology pilot project (personal communication, C. Lazarus, March 17, 2005).

Historically, QIOs have shared the results of these studies by routine information-sharing methods (such as e-mail lists), as well as through presentations at national and regional conferences. CMS is currently developing a specific area on its internal website, QIONet (see Chapter 13), on which it will list current studies, including the topic, contact information, and periodic updates (personal communication, R. W. Nelson, June 10, 2005). In the long term, CMS is exploring options to make this information even more accessible and will provide the information at various levels of accessibility. This would allow Project Officers to monitor projects online and would also allow the public access to basic information. CMS also hopes to test other ways in which QIOs doing studies can share their information with other QIOs.

Support Contracts

Support contracts contribute to the operations of the QIO program but are not directly a part of the core contract (Tasks 1 to 4). These contracts are usually awarded to organizations not holding QIO contracts. Estimated obligations for support contracts in the 7th SOW (as of April 2004) were $243.5 million, or approximately 21.1 percent of the total QIO program budget (personal communication, C. Lazarus, March 17, 2005). In the 7th SOW, 52 support contracts (see Table A.4a in Appendix A) ranged in cost from $20,000 for a collaboration with the American Medical Association for the Doctor's Office Quality–Information Technology project to $50.2 million for the Clinical Data Abstraction Centers (personal communication, C. Lazarus, March 17, 2005). Other large contracts included $31.0

million for the Standard Data Processing System and $33.4 million for the Consumer Assessment of Health Plans Survey.

The CMS Financial Management Investment Board (FMIB) oversees certain types of spending for CMS, including the funding of the support contracts of the QIO program, and consists of one member from each office of CMS's Central Office and one member from each Regional Office. A QIO Support Small Group assists with the review and prioritization of support activities and projects at the beginning of each budget cycle (personal communication, C. Lazarus, March 17, 2005). This group consists of FMIB members along with representatives from the Central Office and the Regional Offices. Support projects are funded every 3 years, in concert with the SOW cycle. Once the priorities of the support activities are set, CMS uses the same process used in special studies to solicit proposals with call letters. This letter goes out at the beginning of each SOW and seeks projects to help meet the predetermined priorities and goals. When reviewing individual project proposals, FMIB considers how the project supports the QIO program and whether the proposed resources are appropriate. Information technology investments are considered separately under the Information Technology Investment Review Process. All proposed projects are then categorized and prioritized according to the need for funding. After a 3-year budget target is developed, the QIO Support Small Group considers the requests and proposes a plan to FMIB. The group aims to meet most of the priority needs. After FMIB approval, the FMIB chair presents the planned budget to the CMS Executive Council for final approval. Most funded projects have existed in previous SOWs and continue to support the QIO program as a whole (personal communication, C. Lazarus, March 17, 2005).

QIO Program Activities and Revenues Not Related to Core Contract

QIOs can receive funding from CMS to finance non-core contract activities, such as QIOSCs and special studies (as described above). For the 7th SOW, the estimated obligations for these activities (as of April 2004) totaled about $130.8 million, or approximately 11.3 percent of the total program budget. Of this, about $67.0 million (5.8 percent) was for activities that supported the core contract (such as QIOSCs), not including special studies or support contracts (personal communication, C. Lazarus, March 17, 2005).

Non-CMS Activities and Revenues

QIOs may serve both CMS and non-CMS clients. This section presents the results from the web-based data collection tool, which asked all 53 individual QIOs about their non-CMS work activities and all organizations holding QIO contracts for the 7th SOW about their revenues from non-CMS federal sources and nonfederal sources.

Non-CMS Activities

Aside from work on the QIO core contract and other CMS work (such as special studies or QIOSCs), many QIOs perform duties for non-CMS clients. When the 53 QIOs responded to questions on the web-based data collection tool about their work for non-CMS clients, they reported strong experience with data collection, management, and analysis; project management; and record abstraction and review. Their activities included the services indicated in Table 7.10 within and outside of their home states.

Forty-nine QIOs reported on their 3-year strategic plans for services to non-CMS clients. Of the 20 types of specific services that the QIOs were asked about (Table 7.11), all were included in the strategic plans of six or more organizations. The planned activities again showed a predominance of data-related activities, record reviews, and project implementation.

Other Federal Sources of Revenue

In the web-based data collection tool, 26 of 40 reporting organizations holding QIO contracts for the 7th SOW related that they had received no revenue from federal grants or contracts other than from CMS during the 7th SOW. Ten reported that non-CMS federal grants or contracts accounted for less than 20 percent of their total revenues, two reported that it totaled 20 to 30 percent of their total revenues, and one stated it accounted for just under 40 percent of its total revenue. During this period, only one organization indicated that it had received more than half (55 percent) of its total revenue from non-CMS federal grants and contracts.

Nonfederal Sources of Revenue

Table 7.12 details the nonfederal revenue sources for the organizations holding QIO contracts for the 7th SOW, as reported via the web-based data collection tool. State agencies, including Medicaid, were the sources of funds for many QIOs.

Total Revenue (All Lines of Work)

Table 7.13 illustrates the range of total revenues (from all sources) for organizations holding QIO contracts for the 7th SOW. The total amounts

TABLE 7.10 Services by QIOs for Non-CMS Clients During the 7th SOW

Type of Work	Number of QIOs Doing This Work in Own State	Percentage of QIOs Doing This Work in Own State	Number of QIOs Doing This Work in Another State(s)	Percentage of QIOs Doing This Work in Another State(s)
Data analysis	43	81.13	25	47.17
Quality improvement projects or consulting	40	75.47	22	41.51
Medical necessity reviews	39	73.58	29	54.72
Medical record abstraction	37	69.81	24	45.28
Independent external review	34	64.15	25	47.17
Utilization management	32	60.38	23	43.40
Data management	31	58.49	19[a]	35.85
Diagnosis-related group coding and validation	29	54.72	18	33.96
Project management	27	50.94	16	30.19
Continuing education	26	49.06	12	22.64
Health or clinical services research	25	47.17	1[b]	1.89
HEDIS-related activities	21	39.62	13[a]	24.53
Software development	21	39.62	12[a]	22.64
Claims validation	20	37.74	10	18.87
Service to public reporting efforts	17[a]	32.08	6[a]	11.32
Consumer and patient surveys	17	32.08	7	13.21
Fraud and abuse investigation	15	28.20	6	11.32
Other	14[a]	26.42	13[a]	24.53
Case management	11	20.75	10	18.87
Disease management	11	20.75	13	24.53
Health information exchange networks	10	18.87	5	9.43
Facility accreditation	8	15.09	3	5.66
Credentialing	7	13.21	4	7.55
Discharge planning	7	13.21	6	11.32

NOTE: HEDIS = Health Plan Employer Data and Information Set.

[a]One respondent selected "prefer not to answer/information not available."
[b]Eight respondents selected "prefer not to answer/information not available."

SOURCE: IOM committee web-based data collection tool (n = 53 QIOs).

ranged from less than $10 million to more than $200 million. However, the majority of reporting organizations (35 of 39) declared that their total revenues were less than $70 million, and most (28 of 39) had total revenues of less than $40 million.

TABLE 7.11   Planned Services by QIOs for Non-CMS Clients

Planned Service	Number Reporting Plans	Percentage Reporting Plans
Quality improvement projects and consulting	45	91.84
Medical necessity reviews	43	87.76
Data analysis	42	85.71
Independent external review	41	83.67
Medical record abstraction	39	79.59
Data management	35	71.43
Diagnosis-related group coding and validation[a]	35	71.43
Utilization management	34	69.39
Project management	33	67.35
Health and clinical services research	30	61.22
Continuing education[a]	29	59.18
Health information exchange network services	27	55.10
Claims validation	24	48.98
Surveys (of providers and consumers)	24	48.98
Software development	23	46.94
Disease management	22	44.90
HEDIS-related services[a]	19	38.78
Fraud and abuse investigation[a]	13	26.53
Professional credentialing services[a]	10	20.41
Facility accreditation services[a]	6	12.24

NOTE: HEDIS = Health Plan Employer Data and Information Set.

[a]For a few service types, one reporting organization indicated that its subsidiary would provide the indicated service(s) in its own state.

SOURCE: IOM committee web-based data collection tool ($n = 49$ QIOs).

SUMMARY

This chapter has discussed issues related to the overall structure and financing of the QIO program. The following are some of the main themes of this chapter, which are reflected in the finding and conclusions presented in Chapter 2:

- Some of the structural requirements are based on outdated priorities (such as the physician-access and physician-sponsored designations and confidentiality requirements) or are tied to their current case review activities (as is the case for the conflict-of-interest rules). Confidentiality restrictions prohibit sharing of data and current regulations are antagonistic to the quality improvement process.

TABLE 7.12 Sources of Nonfederal Revenue in the 7th SOW

Source	Number Reporting "Yes"	Total Number of Organizations Responding to This Question[a]
Medicaid program, own state	26	37
Other state agencies, own state	20	34
Medicaid programs, other states	14	32
Managed care organizations	12	32
Other private-sector health care organizations	12	30
Other private-sector non-health care organizations	8	34
Universities or colleges	7	28
Hospitals	7	30
State or local foundations	4	27
Local governments, own state	3	27
National foundations	3	28
Nursing homes	1	26
Physicians or physicians' groups	1	27

[a]Depending on the source, 4 to 15 organizations chose not to report on the source(s) of their nonfederal revenues.

SOURCE: IOM committee web-based data collection tool.

TABLE 7.13 Range of Total Revenues for Organizations Holding QIO Contracts for the 7th SOW

Total Revenue (millions)	Number of Organizations
< $10	4
$10–20	10
$20–30	9
$30–40	5
$40–50	1
$50–60	4
$60–70	2
$70–80	0
$80–90	1
$90–100	0
$100–200	2
>$200	1

SOURCE: IOM committee web-based data collection tool (n = 39 organizations).

- The governing boards of QIOs, in general, lack a broad representation by individuals with different areas of expertise and are especially deficient in their consumer representation. Also, the boards lack key committees likely to enhance their guidance and lack transparency about their compensation.
- Most organizations holding QIO contracts for the 7th SOW have acted as QIOs (or their predecessor organizations) for many years, with few contracts changing hands across the country with each new SOW. Almost all organizations were created to serve in this role, and almost all hold not-for-profit status. Almost every QIO had at least one staff person with a long length of employment, representing institutional and historical knowledge of the program. QIOs demonstrate substantial experience with subcontracting.
- QIOSCs serve the QIOs as central sources of information on core contract tasks, acting as a communications link to disseminate information and develop universal task materials. Overall, however, the QIOs believe that the assistance provided by the QIOSCs was not timely enough and that the QIOSCs were hindered from being innovative.
- The QIO program's budget is small relative to total Medicare spending on services (0.10 percent), and it is distributed to cover a large variety of tasks. About two-thirds of the total budget goes toward core contract activities.
- In the past, information about special studies has been relatively inaccessible to all QIOs, but CMS plans to share this information more widely in the future. CMS proposes most of the special studies; few of the special studies arise from unsolicited proposals by QIOs.
- Many QIOs perform a wide variety of services for multiple clients; these are mostly concentrated on data-related activities, record reviews, and quality improvement project implementation. However, the majority of organizations holding QIO contracts for the 7th SOW (24 of 39) said that the core contract accounted for more than half of their total revenues.

REFERENCES

Bhatia AJ, Blackstock S, Nelson R, Ng TS. 2000. Evolution of quality review programs for Medicare: Quality assurance to quality improvement. *Health Care Financing Review* 22(1):69–74.

CBO (Congressional Budget Office). 2005a. *Fact Sheet for CBO's March 2005 Baseline: MEDICARE.* [Online]. Available: http://www.cbo.gov/factsheets/2005/Medicare.pdf [accessed July 19, 2005].

CBO. 2005b. *Historical Budget Data, Table 9: Outlays for Mandatory Spending, 1962 to 2004.* [Online]. Available: http://www.cbo.gov/showdoc.cfm?index=1821&sequence =0#table9 [accessed July 13, 2005].

CMS (Centers for Medicare and Medicaid Services). 2002. *7th Statement of Work (SOW).* [Online]. Available: http://www.cms.hhs.gov/qio [accessed April 9, 2005].

CMS. 2004a. *The Quality Improvement Organization Program: CMS Briefing for IOM Staff.* [Online]. Available: http://www.medqic.org/dcs/ContentServer?cid=1105558772835& pagename=Medqic%2FMQGeneralPage%2FGeneralPageTemplate&c=MQGeneralPage [accessed December 26, 2005].

CMS. 2004b. *Quality Improvement Organization Manual.* [Online]. Available: http://www.cms.hhs.gov/manuals/110_qio/qio110index.asp [accessed May 11, 2005].

CMS. 2004c. *Quality Improvement Organization Manual, Chapter 2 (Eligibility).* [Online]. Available: http://www.cms.hhs.gov/manuals/110_qio/qio110c02.pdf [accessed May 11, 2005].

CMS. 2005a. *8th Statement of Work (SOW).* [Online]. Available: http://www.cms.hhs.gov/qio [accessed April 9, 2005].

CMS. 2005b. *8th Statement of Work (SOW)—Version #080105-1.* [Online]. Available: http://www.cms.hhs.gov/qio [accessed November 4, 2005].

Gaul GM. 2005, July 26. Once health regulators, now partners. *Washington Post.* A1.

Health Services Advisory Group. 2005. *HSAG Medicare Consumer Advisory Council Member Organizations.* [Online]. Available: www.hsag.com/cac/members.asp [accessed April 29, 2005].

IOM (Institute of Medicine). 1981. *Access to Medical Review Data: Disclosure Policy for Professional Standards Review Organizations.* Washington, DC: National Academy Press.

IOM. 2005. *Quality Through Collaboration: The Future of Rural Health.* Washington, DC: The National Academies Press.

Jost TS. 1989. Administrative law issues involving the Medicare utilization and quality control Peer Review Organization (PRO) program: Analysis and recommendations. *Ohio State Law Journal 50:* 1–71.

National Center for Healthcare Leadership. 2004. *National Center for Healthcare Leadership Competency Model.* [Online]. Available: http://www.nchl.org/ns/documents/Competency Model-short.pdf [accessed July 14, 2005].

NCQA (National Committee for Quality Assurance). 2005, June 13. *NCQA Programs: HEDIS®.* [Online]. Available: http://www.ncqa.org/programs/HEDIS/ [accessed December 29, 2005].

URAC (Utilization Review Accreditation Commission). 2005. *URAC.org.* [Online]. Available: http://www.urac.org/ [accessed December 29, 2005].

8

Technical Assistance for Quality Improvement

CHAPTER SUMMARY

During the 7th and 8th scopes of work (SOWs), Quality Improvement Organizations (QIOs) offered technical assistance to providers to help them improve their quality of care. This task (Task 1) was entitled Improving Beneficiary Safety and Health Through Clinical Quality Improvement in the 7th SOW and Assisting Providers in Developing the Capacity for and Achieving Excellence in the 8th SOW. This chapter presents an overview of this task and reviews general policy issues, including how QIOs may choose the providers they will work with intensely (the "identified participants," who work in an "identified participant group") and the modes of interaction. Next, the chapter discusses details of this task, as delineated in the contracts for the 7th and the 8th SOWs, including specific examples of projects and activities of the QIO Support Centers. Chapter 9 will discuss the impacts of these activities on clinical outcomes and the transfer of knowledge.

As technical assistants, the Quality Improvement Organizations (QIOs) use one-on-one consulting, collaborative activities, workshops, training sessions, root-cause analysis, and other techniques to assist providers with improving their health care processes and organizational systems. Budget constraints limit the degree to which QIOs can assist providers, as well as the number of organizations or individuals that they can assist within the state. Also, the presence of other quality improvement entities in the states can affect the demand for QIO technical assistance and the potential for partnering. These entities may include departments of health, state survey agencies, specialty societies, or private corporations. Although technical assistance can take many forms, the value of one methodology over another has not been determined, as will be discussed in Chapter 9.

DEFINING TECHNICAL ASSISTANCE

"Technical assistance" can have different meanings. In general, it is the process by which QIOs work with providers, managed care organizations, and other stakeholders to improve patient outcomes. Fundamentally, QIOs provide technical assistance by the following means, among others:

- detecting areas in need of improved performance;
- helping identify the root causes of problems;
- helping implement interventions and systems changes;
- teaching process improvement methodologies and promoting best practices;
- facilitating knowledge transfer;
- reducing reporting burdens on providers;
- collecting, aggregating, and analyzing data on performance measures; and
- working with stakeholders to coordinate quality improvement efforts.

RECRUITMENT OF IDENTIFIED PARTICIPANTS

Identified participants are the providers with whom the QIOs work intensely on quality improvement projects. Recruitment of identified participants is generally left to the discretion of each QIO. Provider participation is voluntary, but in many tasks the Centers for Medicare and Medicaid Services (CMS) stipulates the percentage of each provider type that the QIOs must recruit (CMS, 2002, 2005c). CMS expects the QIOs to demonstrate significant improvement in the identified participant group and, in some cases, greater improvement compared with statewide gains. These gains are evaluated by calculating the reduction in failure rate[1] (Jencks et al., 2003). Many QIOs look to their identified participant group to act as leaders for other providers in the state, especially because CMS evaluates the QIOs, in part, on the basis of statewide improvements. QIOs often recruit identified participants using a number of criteria, including readiness for change, provider volume or size, current level of quality performance, and other demo-

---

[1] A reduction in failure rate, also known as relative improvement, is the change in performance between the baseline and the follow-up (absolute improvement) divided by the difference between the performance at the baseline and perfect (100 percent) performance. The reduction in failure rate may be viewed as a crude measures of improvement, as it does not distinguish between difficulty of improving from 90 percent to 95 percent versus from 70 percent to 85 percent, both having a 50 percent reduction in failure rate.

graphics. The advantages and disadvantages of each of the methodologies related to these criteria are discussed in the next few sections.

Readiness for Change

When developing a strategy for the recruitment of identified participants, some QIOs look to the five categories derived from Rogers' theory on the diffusion of innovations. By this theory, "innovators" initiate the process by embracing new ideas. The "early adopters" are often highly regarded as opinion leaders in their communities and convince the "early majority" to adopt the innovation. Those in the "late majority" follow with adoption of the innovation because of overwhelming peer pressure. Finally, Rogers identified a group that he called the "laggards," who are the last to adopt any innovative idea or process, skeptical, and resistant to any change.

This model proposes that as innovators and early adopters embrace a new process or philosophy, the process of natural diffusion will spread ideas to the rest of the community. Because CMS evaluates QIOs, in part, on the basis of statewide improvements, QIOs may opt to target opinion leaders of the community, hoping that if these providers change their practice patterns, the rest of the community will follow, leading to greater widespread change over time. Some studies show the use of opinion leaders to be effective in changing practice patterns for specific interventions, but other studies show mixed results (Thomson O'Brien et al., 2005; Davis, 1998; Soumerai et al., 1998). In telephone interviews, many QIO chief executive officers (CEOs) expressed the value of working with early adopters: "Early adopters/willing participants are a huge resource for massive education because they have proven knowledge of how things can work."

On the other hand, QIOs might theoretically focus on the laggards who need the extra push and individualized attention provided through one-on-one relationships with QIOs. Early adopters may alter their practices on their own or with minimal assistance through other programs offered in the state. Additionally, early adopters may already be involved in other state programs and so may feel no need to participate with QIOs.

High-Volume Versus Low-Volume Providers

One theoretical methodology for recruiting identified participants is to target either providers with large patient populations (high-volume providers) or those with small patient populations (low-volume providers). By working with high-volume providers, QIOs may hope to achieve a greater impact because of the larger number of beneficiaries seen by these providers. However, others may believe that low-volume providers should be assisted first, as they are the most likely to lack the resources and staff expertise needed to investigate options, adopt change systems, and learn quality improvement techniques. In telephone interviews, one QIO CEO stated: "Critical access hospitals (small and rural) usually welcome us with open arms. In facilities with very few providers, they are often so overworked that they do not have anyone to do the quality documentation. Here, the QIO has to take more responsibility."

High Performers Versus Low Performers

QIOs may recruit participants by targeting either high performers or low performers, but this method is confounded by the difficulty in defining that distinction. In fact, in telephone interviews, many QIO CEOs expressed concern for how this distinction can be made. In theory, high performers may be either those who produce a consistent level of quality care or those who have demonstrated significant improvements from the baseline. Pay-for-performance programs or public reports may help to identify the low performers, which may help the QIOs to determine who would benefit the most from assistance. Because pay-for-performance programs provide financial incentives for improved quality, providers may be more willing to work with QIOs to improve their performance. In telephone interviews, 10 of 20 QIO CEOs independently proposed that a barrier to technical assistance is a lack of motivation of providers to work on quality. All 10 agreed that pay for performance or sanctions would be strong motivators for providers to work with QIOs. Additionally, in site visits to 11 QIOs, four raised the issues of pay for performance and public reporting as potentially strong motivators for providers to work with QIOs.

High Performers

Some QIOs prefer to work with high performers. In telephone interviews, many QIO CEOs expressed the idea that high performers are the key to the diffusion of best practices. For example, two CEOs commented, "Diffusion of quality comes from good providers spreading the word," and "When you include high performers, you get more diffusion to other patients. You are also more likely to engage specialty providers."

However, because CMS evaluates QIOs on the basis of the amount of increased improvement achieved (by calculation of the reduction in the failure rate), QIOs may have difficulty reaching contract goals when they are working with very high performers. If a provider is already performing highly, it may be more difficult to improve upon the failure rate.

Low Performers

Alternatively, QIOs may choose to recruit low performers on the basis of the opinion that low performers, by definition, are the ones who need the most immediate help. Greater absolute and relative gains in quality may be achieved by bringing the low performers up to the level of the majority of providers. QIOs may perceive that high performers are already doing well and that their limited resources are most effectively spent in the areas of greatest need. Alternatively, some QIOs encourage participation in their quality interventions by all providers and include any providers who agree to the conditions of the program. This enables QIOs to meet their participation level requirements and offer assistance to all who are willing and able to participate. In telephone interviews, all QIO CEOs said they preferred working with providers with a mix of performance levels.

Telephone Interviews: Working with Low Performers

When the QIO CEOs reacted to how a mandate to work only with the worst-performing providers would affect how they operate and what the likely outcomes would be, they stated that it would require more resources and would affect the diffusion of their quality improvement efforts statewide. The CEOs thought that providers might perceive the focus of the QIO program to be a return to weeding out "bad apples" rather than promoting quality. They also questioned how to define "worst performers" and how CMS would evaluate the QIOs.

Eighteen of 20 CEOs thought that a focus on the worst providers was not workable and has many disadvantages, such as the possibility of losing champions, diminishing diffusion of ideas, and increased investment in time and money. Only two CEOs thought that the focus on the worst-performing providers would not have much of an effect on their QIOs. However, they did qualify that by saying that the QIO might have to do more handholding of the poorer performers. Sixteen of the 20 CEOs thought that diffusion to other providers would be negatively affected if there was a focus on the worst-performing providers. Eighteen of the 20 CEOs raised the issue that poor performers barely have sufficient infrastructure for day-to-day survival, let alone quality improvement systems.

All CEOs said that the worst performers would require more financial resources per site than the other providers. They require more intensive interventions (e.g., one-on-one onsite assistance and longer periods of intervention), and they need support for data and communications systems. Some providers do not even have the components of a basic communications infrastructure, like e-mail. Funds from CMS for the direct provision of technology or the support of technology acquisition by poor performers may be necessary.

Random Selection

Another option for the recruitment of identified participants is random selection, which, to date, the QIOs have not used. This method would be useful for evaluation purposes because it eliminates selection bias (participation by the most highly motivated providers) and allows the greatest range of providers to be involved with the QIO program. Such an approach, combined with the random allocation of providers to interventions, would permit an accurate evaluation of the impact of the quality interventions. However, because participation with QIOs is voluntary, it would be impossible to enforce participation by unwilling providers who are chosen randomly. One could, however, sample with replacement, in which those providers who choose not to participate would be replaced by other randomly selected providers who agree to participate. In multiple interviews and visits, the QIO staff expressed the opinion that the willingness of the provider to participate is an important part of the success of their technical assistance work. In telephone interviews, the QIO CEOs echoed this sentiment: "Realizing that the QI [quality improvement] process is voluntary, the issue is really whether the poorest performers want to make change. If the provider has no desire to improve quality, the QIO's hands are tied unless the performance is so egregious that it requires sanctioning."

INTERACTION WITH PROVIDERS

One-on-One Consulting Versus Collaboratives

QIOs generally interact with providers through (1) individual consultation and (2) community, statewide, and national collaboratives. One-on-one consultation provides direct, specialized attention. By receiving technical assistance tailored to their needs, providers may be more likely to adopt changes. However, the development of multiple individualized relationships can be labor-intensive and cost prohibitive. This relationship can be especially complicated when many parties are involved, such as when organizations that hold contracts in more than one state work with integrated delivery networks or large nursing home chains. Even if this method leads to big changes in quality improvement, it would be in a small subset of the provider population because current budget restraints do not allow individualized assistance to every provider. On the other hand, one-on-one consulting with key providers, such as those who would act as opinion leaders, could help disseminate information as effectively.

Collaboratives can foster relationships among providers and allow the sharing of best practices, but their impacts on quality measures and health outcomes are unclear (see Chapter 9). The success of this type of interaction depends to some extent on the topic chosen, the enthusiasm of the participants, and the organization of the collaborative (Ovretveit et al., 2002). Successful collaboratives must not only have strong leadership, but the participants also must be effective leaders when they return to their practice settings. The literature shows that effective leadership is the key to organizational change (Joshi, 2000; Shortell et al., 2004; Bradley et al., 2005).

The Institute for Healthcare Improvement (IHI) developed a model for a Breakthrough Series collaborative that has been widely adapted by many organizations, including the QIO program, and has been used for many topic areas. The Breakthrough Series model creates a structured collaborative that lasts 6 to 15 months, during which the collaborative teams participate in three learning sessions (meetings in which all participants gather together to learn and share experiences), followed by three action periods (implementation of changes, tailored to local settings). Further support is provided through conference calls, Internet-based conferences, and site visits (Institute for Healthcare Improvement, 2003). Box 8.1 presents a description of the IHI's Spread Initiative, a typical example of an IHI collaborative. A detailed evaluation of the impacts of these and other methods is presented in Chapter 9.

Telephone Interviews: Collaboratives

In telephone interviews, 13 QIO CEOs talked about collaboratives. Four of the 13 mentioned the IHI model specifically, with 2 saying that they modify it because of the costs and time associated with the IHI model. Overall, QIOs widely use collaboratives, regardless of the model. One QIO CEO stated, "We have a large state geographically. We deploy collaboratives in our work in all settings. Identified participants work with collaboratives for 12 to 18 months. They come together in follow-up conferences. There is lots of learning and sharing of collected data." Another indicated, "We use collaboratives as much as possible, especially through the hospital association. We have about 60 percent voluntary participation. We use an IHI model, though [it is] less intense; IHI requires so much meeting time that we did not think that would work for our providers."

Nationally Defined Projects Versus Local Needs

As described in Chapter 2, the QIO program has undergone an evolution in which the core contract contains an increased emphasis on standard-

---

BOX 8.1   IHI's Spread Initiative

Overview

"IHI's Spread Initiative is a collaborative improvement project to help organizations establish processes and practices to spread successful change throughout their health care systems."

How It Works

"During the one-year membership in The Spread Initiative, participants will meet three times for Learning Sessions. During these sessions, IHI's expert faculty will guide participants in the development of spread goals and outcomes measures, and lead discussions about proven methods for successful spread of improvement throughout the organization. Between Learning Sessions, participants will work with IHI faculty and each other—through conference calls, a list serve, and email—and with colleagues at their own organizations to test and implement recommended changes.

Throughout the process, IHI faculty will guide organizations through the necessary steps, and will formally assess their progress on a monthly basis, providing customized feedback and guidance based on results."

SOURCE: Institute for Healthcare Improvement (2005).

---

ized national projects and less emphasis on projects related to local needs. On the site visits to 11 QIOs, 5 specifically expressed frustration with the lack of flexibility in their contracts to address local needs. Of those 5, 3 suggested the need to return to a more balanced mix of local and national projects. They suggested the possibility of substituting a local project for a national task if the QIO has successfully achieved a high level of performance on that task in previous scopes of work (SOWs), but there is concern that the high level of performance will regress if performance on the waived national task is not actively monitored. During the 8th SOW, requirements to work with underserved local populations are incorporated into part of the Physician Office Task.

TECHNICAL ASSISTANCE DURING THE 7TH AND 8TH SOWs

Over the last 35 years, the QIO program's priorities have evolved along with the environment of health care (see Chapter 1). Predecessor organizations attempted to control wasteful and ineffective practices by identifying outliers at the local level. As national standards of care gained acceptance, the QIO program developed national projects. In the 6th SOW, QIOs performed some standardized work in the hospital setting, but other projects were local in nature and differed from state to state (CMS, 1999). In the 7th SOW, all quality improvement projects in each state were standardized to achieve the same goals by use of the same measures. Projects expanded to include provider settings, in addition to the hospital: nursing homes, physicians' offices, and home health agencies (CMS, 2002). As the program progressed from a focus on cost containment to a focus on improved quality, the SOWs changed to reflect those priorities. Today, the QIO program stresses broader quality improvement in a shorter period of time. The 8th SOW looks to achieve transformational cultural and systems changes rather than the incremental changes more characteristic of the 7th SOW (CMS, 2002, 2005c). Technical assistance activities relate to five dimensions of performance defined by CMS:

- Improvement in performance measure results (such as increased rate of mammography screening in the physician's office setting),
- Improvement in clinical performance measurement and reporting (such as attaining a 25 percent level of self-reporting of expanded measures in the hospital setting),
- Systems adoption and use (such as the implementation of an electronic health record),
- Implementation of key process changes (such as implementation of an immunization assessment survey by home health agencies), and
- Changes in organizational culture (such as data collection by nursing homes on satisfaction of residents and staff).

Overall, the QIOs believe that they are extremely capable in their role as technical assistants. On the site visits to 11 QIOs, the QIO staff attributed their successes in the provision of technical assistance to positive relationships in the community (11 QIOs), internal experience and skills (9 QIOs), and a dedicated staff and a culture of quality (9 QIOs). When the QIOs were asked about challenges or threats to their technical assistance activities, 2 QIOs voiced a need for more knowledge sharing, 3 related a need for more help from Quality Improvement Organization Support Centers (QIOSCs), and 6 discussed the difficulty of engaging providers. Other issues mentioned included a lack of information and a lack of experience with communications technology, the need for funding for start-up work before the contract begins, and individual staffing problems. When the QIOs were questioned about opportunities for new areas in which the QIOs could offer technical assistance, 2 QIOs mentioned information and communications technology and 4 identified pay for performance and public reporting. One QIO recommended more crosscutting initiatives.

NURSING HOMES

7th SOW

With the release of public reports on the performance of nursing homes in November 2002 (CMS, 2004), CMS added Task 1a to the 7th SOW for QIOs to work with nursing homes. Details of the work of the QIOs on public reporting initiatives are discussed in Chapter 11. For technical assistance, CMS charged the QIOs to work with nursing homes on quality improvement projects to help improve performance on selected measures chosen from the Minimum Data Set, which was developed to assess the quality of care for both long-term and short-stay residents. The QIOs chose to work on between three and five of the following publicly reported quality of care measures:

- Decrease in pain,
- Decrease in infections,
- Decrease in pressure sores,
- Decrease in use of restraints,
- Decrease in delirium,
- Improvement in ability to ambulate, and
- Improvement in ability to perform basic daily tasks (see Table A.5 in Appendix A).

The measures were examined both at the statewide and at the individual nursing home levels. CMS expected the QIOs to partner with stakeholders such as state nursing home associations, professional societies, or local chapters of the AARP. CMS also expected the QIOs to interact with the Nursing Home QIOSC and offer quality improvement information to all nursing homes in the state. The QIOs had to enlist at least 10 percent of the nursing homes in the state to serve as members of the identified participant group (CMS, 2002). On average, the QIOs actually worked with 15 percent of the facilities in their individual states, with participation ranging from 10 percent to 100 percent (Rollow, 2005).

QIO activities included one-on-one consultations between the QIO's medical director and the nursing home's medical director, the provision of manuals on the use of restraints and on fall prevention to all directors of nursing in the state, the development of e-mail listserves with all nursing homes to share ideas, and the management of workshops with continuing education units (CMS, 2004). Several QIOs initiated innovative programs.

Health Services Advisory Group (Arizona's QIO) focused on the high performers among its participating nursing homes to determine common features and to try to replicate their successes in other locations (CMS, 2004). MetaStar (Wisconsin's QIO) evaluated innovative nursing home models around the country to better understand the implementation of resident-based models of care (CMS, 2004). The National Nursing Home Collaborative operated on a larger level by the Process Improvement QIOSC contract was held by Qualis Health through its QIO work for Washington state. In this project, 43 QIOs each worked with a subset of the participating nursing homes in their home states to improve pressure ulcer management (CMS, 2004; Eloranta, 2005). Qualis Health conducted this collaborative in the style of IHI to learn how to identify, measure, monitor, and treat pressure ulcers. The impacts of the various quality initiatives are discussed in Chapter 9.

8th SOW

In the 8th SOW, QIOs work with two groups of identified participants, in addition to their work on statewide nursing home activities (CMS, 2005c). In this subtask, QIOs focus on improving clinical performance on specific measures (as reported on the Nursing Home Compare website), setting improvement targets, and analyzing resident and staff satisfaction, which includes monitoring of workforce turnover.

Statewide

Statewide, QIOs provide assistance to any nursing home that requests assistance with their performance on clinical measures. QIOs also set statewide targets for decreasing the frequency of pressure ulcers in high-risk patients, decreasing the frequency of use of physical restraints, and helping all nursing homes set their own annual targets for these measures (and others, if desired). CMS does not define the requirements for these targets—those are left to the discretion of each nursing home. QIOs may opt to work with a subset of nursing home providers on the documentation of specific processes of care (CMS, 2005c), including:

- Skin inspection and pressure ulcer risk assessment,
- Screening and treatment for depression,
- Evaluation of physical restraint requirements or alternatives, and
- Pain assessment and treatment.

If a QIO chooses this activity, the providers must document information on 50 percent of their new admissions. For the QIO to receive credit for this

TABLE 8.1 Required Minimums of Data Transmission for Optional Statewide Work

Number of Nursing Homes in State or Jurisdiction	Minimum Number of Nursing Homes Transmitting Process-of-Care Data for QIO to Receive Credit
Up to 30	5
31–150	8
151–300	15
301–500	25
More than 500	40

SOURCE: CMS (2005c).

activity, a minimum number of nursing homes (Table 8.1) must transmit data on a monthly basis to the QIO Data Warehouse using a Nursing Home Improvement Feedback Tool (provided free by CMS) or any other compatible tool. The nursing homes must submit data for at least 14 of the months between January 2006 and September 2007, but the monthly submissions need not be consecutive (CMS, 2005c).

Identified Participant Groups

As stated above, in the 8th SOW, QIOs are working with two identified participant groups. For both groups, QIOs administer satisfaction surveys to nursing home residents and staff (CMS, 2005c). These surveys must be completed annually; therefore, successful performance includes the completion of three annual surveys of both residents and staff by at least 90 percent of the identified participants. Additionally, for both groups, QIOs collect and monitor data on the retention of certified nursing assistants and aides for at least 90 percent of the identified participants.

For the first group of identified participants, QIOs work with providers to improve upon the clinical quality of care for nursing home residents. Specifically, they strive to improve upon measures related to pressure ulcers among high-risk patients, the use of physical restraints, depression management, and pain management (CMS, 2005c). For the second group of identified participants, the QIOs work only on measures related to physical restraints and pressure ulcers.

New in the 8th SOW, CMS set specific criteria for recruitment for the two identified participant groups. Members of the two identified participant groups may not overlap. For the first group, the selection criteria include consideration of the total number of nursing homes in the state or jurisdiction (Table 8.2). CMS will ensure that the identified participants in this group are distributed across the state or jurisdiction (including rural

TABLE 8.2   Required Numbers of Participants for First Identified Participant Group in the Nursing Home Setting

Number of Nursing Homes in State or Jurisdiction	Minimum Number of Identified Participants	Maximum Number of Identified Participants
≤30	All nursing homes in state or jurisdiction (excluding providers in second identified participant group)	All nursing homes in state or jurisdiction (excluding providers in second identified participant group)
31–300	30 total nursing homes	45
>300	10 percent of nursing homes in state or jurisdiction	10 percent of nursing homes in state or jurisdiction

SOURCE: CMS (2005c).

areas). Additionally, this group must have an even distribution across the state, including rural areas. Finally, QIOs must consult with the state survey agency and local stakeholders for the selection of group participants. Confidentiality is maintained unless the provider chooses to reveal its participation.

For recruitment of the second identified participant group, a QIO must work with its respective state survey agency to identify poorly performing nursing home providers. Although CMS requires a minimum number of participants for this group (Table 8.3), it encourages QIOs to work with as many of these providers as possible.

TABLE 8.3   Minimum Numbers of Participants for Second Identified Participant Group in the Nursing Home Setting

Number of Nursing Homes in State or Jurisdiction	Minimum Number of Identified Participants
<30	1
31–300	2
More than 300	3

SOURCE: CMS (2005c).

HOME HEALTH

7th SOW

Under Task 1b, the QIOs provided technical assistance to home health agencies (CMS, 2002). The QIOs directed their efforts toward the implementation of processes for the continuous improvement of home health care quality by focusing on outcomes, a methodology known as the Outcome-Based Quality Improvement (OBQI) system. As a contractor to CMS, the University of Colorado Center for Health Services Research developed the Outcome and Assessment Information Set (OASIS) as a primary tool for the collection of outcomes data in the home health care setting. OASIS includes publicly reported quality measures related to the demographics, the physical and mental health, and the health care utilization of each Medicare patient receiving home health care (see Table A.5 in Appendix A). In 1999, CMS mandated that all Medicare-certified home health agencies start OASIS data collection and transmission (CMS, 2004).

Quality improvement work in the home health setting started as a five-state pilot project, led by the Delmarva Foundation for Medical Care, in April 2000 to see if the QIOs could work with home health agencies on the OBQI system (CMS, 2004). In the pilot, 68 percent of the agencies in the five states agreed to be trained on the OBQI system, and 76 percent of those that were trained submitted a subsequent plan of action (CMS, 2004). Plans of action outline best practices, implementation schemes, and the specific activities to be changed or monitored. CMS declared the pilot successful and added the home health care setting to the 7th SOW.

Because the home health care setting was a new provider setting for most QIOs, all QIOs had to have staff trained on OBQI techniques. QIOs then offered similar training to home health agencies in their own states. The next challenge was to get 30 percent of the trained home health agencies to select one or two outcome measures to improve upon and develop a plan of action for each measure. QIOs developed relationships with key stakeholders (such as state trade associations, OASIS education coordinators, and state survey and certification agencies), provided communications support (through listserves, teleconferences, and newsletters), and coordinated seminars and workshops (CMS, 2002, 2004). In the 7th SOW, QIOs trained about three-quarters of the agencies in their states and actively worked with about 55 percent of the agencies (Rollow, 2005). Box 8.2 presents a story about an action plan for one home health agency that worked with Health Care Excel (Indiana's QIO) on intractable pain.

BOX 8.2   Clarifying the Definition for Intractable Pain Makes the Difference

"A small hospital-based home health agency (HHA) in urban Indiana successfully used the Outcome-Based Quality Improvement (OBQI) process to improve its target outcome. After implementing a Plan of Action (POA) for Improvement in Pain Interfering with Activity, the agency achieved a rate of 32.5 percent, a statistically significant increase over its adjusted prior rate of 26.8 percent. A standard definition for intractable pain, consistent pain assessment, and appropriate interventions were important elements of the agency's quality improvement success.

"The OBQI team consisted of staff from various components of the agency, including a clinical manager, direct care staff including a physical therapist (PT), a home care coordinator, and a registered nurse (RN) who was a computer specialist. Their activities were regularly communicated to staff via staff meetings.

"The OBQI team believed that the following clinical actions were critical to their success:

• Adopting a definition for intractable pain and having all staff consistently use the same definition
• Ensuring that therapists ask patients to take their pain medication prior to exercising
• Educating staff to perform consistent pain assessment and pain rating with appropriate interventions

"The best practices implemented by the agency included:

• Patient education related to correct pain medication administration for optimal benefit
• Consistent pain assessment with correct rating by clinicians
• When the patient is in pain, the physician is contacted, within 24 hours, for a change pain medication orders
• Consistent follow-up, within 72 hours, of pain management interventions

"The OBQI team used staff training and supervision as the intervention actions to implement the clinical best practices. The team monitored the clinical documentation for a month to ensure that the staff implemented the Best Practices on the Plan of Action. Further monitoring activities included the case manager making two admission supervisory visits per month for three months to compare data gathered by the admitting discipline. They also conducted quarterly reviews of ten charts for one year."

SOURCE: Jones (2003).

8th SOW

For the home health setting in the 8th SOW, as with nursing homes, CMS defined criteria for the makeup of the identified participant groups more specific than those in the 7th SOW and presented details for the required activities more intricate than those in the 7th SOW (CMS, 2002, 2005c). The QIOs work with two groups of identified participants, in addition to addressing statewide performance. The membership of the groups—the Clinical Performance group and the Systems Improvement and Organizational Culture Change group—may overlap. Pediatric agencies and agencies with less than 10 episodes of care are excluded.

Both at the statewide level and with the Clinical Performance group, QIOs use OBQI methods to reduce the failure rate on the measure related to hospitalization for acute care as well as additional publicly reported OASIS measures (as determined by CMS) (see Table A.3b in Appendix A) (CMS, 2005c). QIOs work with home health agencies to set targets. CMS defined intricate criteria for choosing OASIS measures and for activities related to the rate of hospitalization for acute care, based on the provider's previous performance on those measures.

Statewide, the QIOs must also work with home health agencies to include influenza and pneumococcal immunizations in the comprehensive patient assessment (CMS, 2005c). The QIOs use a CMS tool to survey all the home health agencies (with a required minimum response rate of 50 percent) to determine if immunizations and follow-up activities are included in patient assessments. The QIO is charged to reach either a 50 percent relative improvement over the baseline or 80 percent performance on the inclusion of immunizations in the agencies' patient assessments.

QIOs work with the Systems Improvement and Organizational Culture Change group to focus on telehealth and culture change (CMS, 2005c). First, the QIOs help providers implement or use some form of telehealth to reduce the rates of hospitalization for acute care. Second, the QIOs administer a culture change survey related to organizational practices, including teamwork, communication, leadership, quality improvement, and patient-centeredness (CMS, 2005c). The QIOs then help the identified participants implement plans of action on the basis of the survey results.

The contract for the 8th SOW delineates selection standards for each identified participant group on the basis of the number of home health agencies in the state, not including pediatric agencies (Table 8.4). Again, the members of the two groups may overlap.

In addition, for the Clinical Performance group, selection must include specific levels of representation of small, medium, and large agencies (Table 8.5). The size designations are based on the numbers of episodes of care that each agency provides. Ten percent of the identified participants

TABLE 8.4 Required Numbers of Participants for Identified Participant Groups in the Home Health Setting

Number of Home Health Agencies	Number for Clinical Performance Group	Number for System Improvement and Organizational Culture Change Group
<14	6	2
15–25	8	3
26–45	10	4
46–65	14	5
66–90	16	6
>91	20 percent of all agencies	8 percent of all agencies

SOURCE: CMS (2005c).

TABLE 8.5 Required Sizes of Agencies in the Clinical Performance Group

Small agencies	<90 episodes of care annually
Medium agencies	91–350 episodes of care annually
Large agencies	>351 episodes of care annually

SOURCE: CMS (2005c).

must come from small agencies, 10 percent must come from medium agencies, and 15 percent must come from large agencies (CMS, 2005c). The rest of the participants may be chosen without regard to size. No similar requirement exists for the Systems Improvement and Organizational Culture Change group. The QIOs may choose up to eight additional agencies to work with on these group projects (or 8 percent of the total number of agencies for states with more than 100 agencies). These agencies may act as a substitute for one of the identified participants in the evaluation process if one of the original participants goes out of business or changes ownership.

HOSPITALS

7th SOW

The provision of QIO technical support to hospitals began in the 4th SOW (1993 to 1996). Thus, the QIOs may have long-standing relationships with hospitals and related stakeholders in their states. In the 7th SOW, the QIOs had to show only statewide improvement, as their evaluations did not involve an identified participant group. The QIOs interacted with acute care and critical access hospitals. Interventions were designed to prevent surgical infections and reduce systems failures for hospitalized patients with acute myocardial infarction, heart failure, and pneumonia. The QIOs used measures derived from preexisting clinical guidelines and scientific evidence (see Table A.3c in Appendix A). CMS chose hospital topics on the basis of the incidence of hospitalization, the rates of morbidity and mortality, and annual payments related to those diseases (CMS, 2004). Another factor was evidence showing a link between care practices and improved outcomes. In the 7th SOW, of the approximately 6,000 hospitals across the country, QIOs worked with approximately 2,400 hospitals on cardiac care, 2,000 hospitals on pneumonia, and 1,500 to 2,000 hospitals on surgical infection prevention (Rollow, 2005).

As in other provider settings, the QIOs helped providers implement quality improvement plans, provided written materials and guidelines, and gave individualized feedback. They provided much technical assistance to help hospitals collect and report data (CMS, 2004). Additionally, the QIOs facilitated collaboratives for hospitals working on the same performance measures. One example of a national collaborative is the National Surgical Infection Prevention Collaborative. Sponsored by CMS in 2003, this program allowed each QIO to select one or two motivated hospitals in the state to work on surgical site infection reduction. During the 13-month collaborative, the participating providers reduced the incidence of surgical site infections by 27 percent (CMS, 2004).

8th SOW

In the 8th SOW, QIO work in the hospital setting continues in much the same manner that it did in the 7th SOW, but the work has been divided into two subtasks: (1) all prospective payment system hospitals (Task 1c1) and (2) critical access and rural prospective payment system hospitals (Task 1c2) (CMS, 2005c).

8th SOW: Hospitals (Task 1c1)

For Task 1c1, CMS defined four strategies that can be used to improve quality of care in the hospital setting: improving performance on clinical performance measures, increasing clinical performance measurement and reporting, process improvement, and systems improvement and organizational culture change (CMS, 2005c). As in the 7th SOW, the QIOs must demonstrate improvement statewide. However, under the contract for the 8th SOW, Task 1c1 requires QIOs to also work with three groups of identified participants related to the defined strategies: the Appropriate Care Measure group, which focuses on clinical performance measurement; the Surgical Care Improvement Project group, which focuses on process improvement; and the Systems Improvement and Organizational Culture Change group (CMS, 2005c).

Statewide Performance

Statewide, the QIOs help prospective payment system hospitals report on the expanded measures set, which includes measures required by the Medicare Prescription Drug, Improvement, and Modernization Act of 2003 (P.L. 108-173), to receive the Annual Payment Update plus other measures collected by the QIOs in the 7th SOW (CMS, 2005c) (see Table A.3c in Appendix A). Reporting on the additional measures remains voluntary for hospitals; but to achieve success on this subtask, the QIOs must demonstrate that 25 percent of the hospitals statewide are reporting on this expanded set. The QIOs are available to all prospective payment system hospitals for assistance with data collection and validation. Additionally, the QIOs assist both prospective payment system hospitals and critical access hospitals to improve the validity, timeliness, and completeness of the data that they submit to the QIO Clinical Data Warehouse. Finally, the QIOs also work with hospitals statewide to improve upon the appropriate care measure and measures related to the Surgical Care Improvement Program (CMS, 2005c).

Identified Participants

The identified participants in these groups should have broad representation by size, geography, and performance level. Each group must include 15 percent of all prospective payment system hospitals and stay within a range of 6 to 36 participants (CMS, 2005c). Exceptions exist for states or jurisdictions with an inadequate number of hospitals. Additionally, Public Health Service hospitals and hospitals owned by Indian tribes may also be included under specific conditions. All identified participants in all groups (except for critical access hospitals of the Surgical Care Improvement Project group) must report on the measures required by the Medicare Prescription Drug, Improvement, and Modernization Act of 2003. The members of the three identified participant groups may overlap.

Appropriate Care Measure Identified Participant Group   The QIOs work with the Appropriate Care Measure group to improve performance on the clinical measures required by the Medicare Prescription Drug, Improvement, and Modernization Act of 2003 that address acute myocardial infarction, heart failure, and pneumonia care in the hospital setting (see Table A.3c in Appendix A). Identified participants must report on these measures to the QIO Clinical Data Warehouse. The appropriate care measure is a composite score based on how often a patient receives the care specified by all the measures. Participants must represent both hospitals that cover the distribution of urban and rural prospective payment system hospitals[2] and hospitals that cover the range of performance at the baseline on the appropriate care measure in the state (CMS, 2005c). The QIOs may do extra-credit work on this task. (See Chapter 10 for discussion of evaluation of QIO performance.)

Surgical Care Improvement Project Identified Participant Group   The QIOs assist the Surgical Care Improvement Project group to standardize processes for the following conditions (see Table A.3c for measures related to some of these):

- Surgical site infections,
- Venous thromboembolism,
- Ventilator-associated pneumonia,
- Cardiovascular complications, and
- Fistula use in hemodialysis (vascular access).

The QIOs assist hospitals with the collection of related measures for all these topic areas, but CMS will evaluate each QIO only on a subset of the measures for its contract performance evaluation. The QIOs work in conjunction with the American College of Surgeons on these activities. The work in this group is part of the project's larger national effort, and thus, the QIO must coordinate activities with the local chapter of the American College of Surgeons (if a chapter is present in the state). Hospitals must demonstrate a caseload of at least 300 annual surgical procedures to participate in this group, and critical access hospitals may count toward the required 15 percent recruitment. Additionally, the QIOs will survey End-Stage Renal Disease Networks to evaluate their satisfaction with QIO assistance in the Fistula First program[3] (CMS, 2005c). Extra-credit work is also available.

---

[2]The definition of "urban" comes from the U.S. Census Bureau's determination of Metropolitan Statistical Areas as areas with a single city of at least 50,000 residents and at least 100,000 total residents (or 75,000 total residents in New England). All other areas are considered rural.

[3]The Fistula First program is a national effort supported by CMS, the 18 End-Stage Renal Disease Networks, the Institute for Healthcare Improvement, and other key stakeholders to promote arteriovenous fistula use in hemodialysis.

Systems Improvement and Organizational Culture Change Identified Participant Group   Finally, through the Systems Improvement and Organizational Culture Change group, the QIOs engage the senior leadership of hospitals to consider the adoption of health information and communication technology, such as computerized provider order entry, bar-coding, and telehealth technologies. The QIOs act to advise, strategize, and ultimately, help hospital leadership implement plans for the use of any or all of these technologies (CMS, 2005c).

8th SOW: Critical Access and Rural Hospitals (Task 1c2)

In the 8th SOW, CMS designated a subtask for the QIOs to specifically interact with both critical access and rural prospective payment system hospitals[4] (CMS, 2005c). This is a significant change from the 7th SOW when QIOs could choose to work with rural providers under Task 1e, but were not required or incentivized to work with this specific population. Under Task 1c2, the QIOs work both at the statewide level and with an identified participant group. The QIOs in states with less than two critical access hospitals are exempt from this task. Additionally, a QIO's state must have at least six critical access or rural prospective payment system hospitals for the QIO to work with an identified participant group. If this is not the case, the QIO must get approval from the Project Officer and Government Task Leader to perform this task.

Statewide, the QIOs work with all critical access hospitals that are reporting on Hospital Quality Alliance measures to improve performance through process redesign for at least one measure (chosen by the hospital and the QIO). QIOs also help nonreporting critical access hospitals start reporting data to the QIO Clinical Data Warehouse on at least one topic for two consecutive quarters. QIOs may perform extra-credit work related to new acute myocardial infarction transfer measures or emergency department transfer measures, or both, if they become available during the 8th SOW.

QIOs also work with a Rural Organizational Safety Culture Change identified participant group. Participants may include both critical access and rural prospective payment system hospitals, with a minimum of six hospitals participating (unless a different minimum number is otherwise approved). CMS expects the QIOs to use a Rural Organizational Safety Culture Change toolkit to work with senior leaders to determine the culture of safety, including the use of the Hospital Survey on Patient Safety Culture

---

[4]For the purposes of this task, a "rural" hospital is one that is not in a Metropolitan Statistical Area (as defined earlier in this chapter).

(developed by the Agency for Healthcare Research and Quality). The QIOs will then help these providers individually to analyze the survey results. Extra-credit work is available by recruiting at least one critical access hospital to work on certain health information technology activities.

PHYSICIANS' OFFICES AND PRACTICES

7th SOW

Under Task 1d of the 7th SOW, QIOs expanded upon work begun in the 6th SOW with the implementation of quality improvement projects focused on the physician's office. In the 7th SOW, the QIOs were required to work with at least 5 percent of the physicians in the state as identified participants. On average, the QIOs actually worked with about 7.5 percent of the eligible practitioners (Rollow, 2005). Specific topic areas were care for chronic disease (diabetes) and preventive services, including cancer screening (mammography) and adult immunizations (see Table A.3d in Appendix A) (CMS, 2002).

Box 8.3 gives an example of how the Oklahoma Foundation for Medical Quality (OFMQ; Oklahoma's QIO) worked with a single physician's office to improve the rates of mammography. In this story, the Clinton Medical Clinic in Oklahoma, headed by Sharad Swami, worked with Oklahoma's QIO to increase mammography rates by 40 percent.

QIOs also supported collaboratives for Quality Assessment and Performance Improvement projects required of Medicare+Choice organizations (see the discussion of managed care later in this chapter) (CMS, 2002). The work performed in Quality Assessment and Performance Improvement projects could also fulfill the requirements for working with underserved populations (see the discussion of underserved populations later in this chapter). QIOs received individual state-level analyses of data, including county-specific and provider-level information from the Outpatient Data QIOSC, operated by the Iowa Foundation for Medical Care (Iowa's QIO). Data were not provided at the practitioner level (CMS, 2002).

8th SOW

In the 8th SOW, CMS has divided efforts with physicians' practices into three distinct subtasks:

- Physician practices (Task 1d1),
- Physician practices: underserved populations (Task 1d2), and
- Physician practice and pharmacy: Part D prescription drug benefit (Task 1d3).

BOX 8.3   Improvement Story: Mammography Scheduling Block Improves Rates

"Dr. Swami found that patients were not scheduling mammograms on their own, even with his recommendation to do so. So, his staff called the local hospital and asked for a block of time in which they could schedule his patients. The hospital radiology center was very agreeable. This program works well not just for Dr. Swami and his patients, but also for the radiology center where patients receive mammograms. They do not have to worry about scheduling these time slots since the medical center is doing it for them.

"In the physician office, the program works well because everyone is responsible for making sure that if a patient needs a mammogram, it is scheduled. Before the patient even sees the doctor, she is asked about when her last mammogram was. If it has been more than one year, one is immediately scheduled for her.

"**Intervention used:** Reserved mammography time slots at the hospital, made appointment for appropriate patients before they left the office, made reminder calls to patients the day before mammogram appointment.

"**Barriers:** Manual reminders to patient don't work, uninformed patients are less compliant.

"**Strategies to Overcome Barriers:** Worked with OFMQ to implement changes and find what works, educated staff on processes and rationale.

"**Lessons learned:** This intervention is reproducible in other settings—for example it could be used for eye exams for diabetic patients or to schedule a patient's lab work. Educating all staff on processes is key."

SOURCE: Oklahoma Foundation for Medical Quality (2005).

These subtasks combine Tasks 1d and 1e of the 7th SOW, as well as add activities related to the Part D prescription drug benefit under Medicare. The term "physician office" was changed to "physician practice" to incorporate multiple types of settings, including offices with single practitioners as well as practices with multiple physicians at multiple sites (CMS, 2005c). As with other settings, the evaluation formulas and the criteria for the identified participant groups are more detailed and complex than those in the 7th SOW.

8th SOW: *Physician Practices (Task 1d1)*

Under Task 1d1, the QIOs work statewide as well as with an identified participant group. The statewide work focuses on the promotion of quality initiatives, whereas the work with the identified participants focuses on the reliability of preventive care delivery and the effective management of chronic conditions. Additionally, the identified participants work on improving clinical performance through the use of health information and communications technologies and process redesign.

Statewide Performance   Statewide, the QIOs work with physicians' offices to improve upon clinical performance measures through the support of initiatives such as the Physician Voluntary Reporting Program[5] (CMS, 2005c). The QIOs also coordinate with state agencies working on process improvement, such as the Welcome to Medicare Visit (CMS, 2005c). As in the 7th SOW, Medicare Advantage organizations (previously known as Medicare+Choice organizations) must be included in statewide activities, and the QIOs must work with these organizations on their quality projects. In this task, the QIOs may also work with End-Stage Renal Disease Networks (upon their request) to help physicians' practices improve their rates of fistula use and immunization. Finally, QIOs must collaborate with the Medicare Management Demonstration Project as required by the Medicare Prescription Drug, Improvement, and Modernization Act of 2003 (CMS, 2005c).

Identified Participants   The QIOs assist identified participants with the use of electronic clinical information, the design of care processes for preventive care and chronic conditions (including self-management), and reporting of and improvement upon quality measures (CMS, 2005c). This area of assistance began as a four-state pilot project in the 7th SOW, known as the Doctor's Office Quality–Information Technology program, to recruit doctors' offices to adopt electronic health records (iHealthBeat, 2005). To participate in this group, a physician's practice must complete a readiness assessment form indicating its request for assistance, and the QIO must accept the form. Participants may be at different stages of technology adoption, but no more than 25 percent of the identified participants can already have a full electronic health record system in place (with some exceptions). The

---

[5]Under this CMS program, physicians will voluntarily report on quality data, receive feedback on their performance, and suggest improvements to streamline reporting requirements. As of this writing, CMS plans a January 2006 launch.

identified participant group must include, at a minimum, 5 percent of the physicians' practices in that state or jurisdiction. Additionally, CMS requires the group to be divided as follows:

- At least 40 percent of the participants must come from small practices (one to three physicians),
- No more than 60 percent of the participants may come from medium practices (four to eight physicians), and
- No more than 20 percent of the participants may come from large practices (nine or more physicians).

QIOs will continue to recruit participants throughout the 8th SOW. All identified participants must complete office systems surveys at the baseline and undergo a remeasurement. To achieve success, the QIOs must help the identified participants achieve improvements in reporting, implementation of new care processes, and adoption of clinical information systems.

8th SOW: Physician Practices: Underserved Populations (Task 1d2)

In the 8th SOW, CMS incorporated Task 1e of the 7th SOW (underserved and rural populations) into the physician practice setting task. Under Task 1d2, the QIOs work statewide as well as with two identified participant groups whose members may overlap. Statewide, QIOs work to improve performance on measures of diabetes care, mammography, and adult immunizations for one of the following populations (CMS, 2005c):

- African Americans,
- Asians-Pacific Islanders,
- American Indians-Alaska Natives, and
- Hispanics and Latinos.

Unlike the 7th SOW, rural and dual-eligible populations do not qualify for this task (see the discussion of underserved and rural populations later in this chapter). To work on this task, at least 3 percent of the state's beneficiary population must fall into one of the categories listed above. The QIOs in the U.S. Virgin Islands and Puerto Rico are automatically excluded from this task.

QIOs work with a Task 1d1 underserved identified participant group on the same activities described for Task 1d1. The practices in this group must proportionately represent the underserved population in that state or jurisdiction. With the second group, QIOs promote Culturally and Linguistically Appropriate Services (CLAS) standards and cultural competency. This group is known as the CLAS/Cultural Competency identified participant group. For this group, the QIOs promote the adoption of cultural standards and requirements at both the practice level and the practitioner level using a tool from the Office of Minority Health of the U.S. Department of Health and Human Services and self-assessments. This group must include 5 percent of the total number of primary care practices, within boundaries of between 20 and 50 participants. At the practitioner level, the group must include at least 10 percent of the practitioners from participating practices, within an accepted range of 20 to 100 practitioners (CMS, 2005c).

8th SOW: Physician Practice and Pharmacy: Medicare Part D Prescription Drug Benefit (Task 1d3)

As a result of enactment of the Medicare Prescription Drug, Improvement, and Modernization Act of 2003, CMS added Part D (the Medicare prescription drug benefit) as a new topic area for the QIOs in the 8th SOW. CMS plans to work with the QIOs on developing methods for improving the dissemination of information and the implementation of registries. The QIOs will work with identified participants (physicians' practices or pharmacies) to improve safety in prescription delivery. Their services may range from providing information to physicians to modify their practices to helping with the implementation of electronic prescribing systems. The QIOs will partner with prescription drug plans on this task, including Medicare Advantage prescription drug plans. Section 109(b) of the Medicare Prescription Drug, Improvement, and Modernization Act authorizes QIOs to offer assistance regarding improving the quality of prescription drug therapy for all Medicare providers, Medicare Advantage organizations offering prescription drug plans under Part C, and organizations offering prescription drug plans under Part D (CMS, 2005c). The Part D benefit is scheduled to start on January 1, 2006, and as of this writing, the QIOs will begin quality improvement projects the following August. These projects will include baseline assessments of performance, implementation of an intervention, identification of targets, and follow-up assessments. CMS will identify appropriate measures for this task on the basis of evidence-based guidelines and collaborations with multiple partners.

The contract for the 8th SOW outlines four preliminary options for QIO activities in this task. The QIO must select two options—either Option 1 or Option 2 and either Option 3 or Option 4 (see below)—for which the QIO will submit concept papers to CMS (CMS, 2005c). If CMS determines that the concept papers from all QIOs are varied enough, the QIOs will then submit project proposals. The QIOs will partner with prescription drug plans for all of these activities.

Option 1: Improve prescribing using Part D data   This option focuses on electronic prescribing. The measures will likely address drugs whose use by elderly populations should be avoided, drug interactions, the use of generic drugs, preferred drugs, and polypharmacy.

Option 2: Improving patient self-management through medication therapy management services   This option focuses on the delivery side of drug therapy. Measures will likely address process measures (such as the identification of appropriate patients) and outcomes measures (such as those related to patient experience and rehospitalization rates). As of this writing, the QIO will have to recruit a group of participants representing at least 5 percent of the total number of pharmacies working with a prescription drug plan.

Option 3: Improving disease-specific therapy using integrated Medicare Part A, B, and D data   This option focuses on physicians' practices that use electronic health records or electronic prescribing tools. It requires working with the identified participants for Task 1d1 who are using these technologies, as well as with others who are using the technologies but who are not working in the Task 1d1 identified participant group. Measures will likely address drug–disease interactions and therapeutic monitoring.

Option 4: QIO-directed project   This option requires approval of the Project Officer and the Task 1d3 Government Task Leader.

UNDERSERVED AND RURAL BENEFICIARIES

7th SOW

Under Task 1e of the 7th SOW, each QIO worked to reduce a health disparity in its state. Work with underserved populations began in the 6th SOW, and in the 7th SOW, the QIOs could continue the same project or start a new one (CMS, 2002, 2004). The disparity had to exist between a medically underserved population and a reference group from the general population of all Medicare beneficiaries. The following is a list of the acceptable populations for this subtask during the 7th SOW (the numbers of QIOs that chose each of the populations to work with are given in parentheses) (CMS, 2004):

- African Americans (22),
- American Indians-Alaska Natives (3),
- Asians-Pacific Islanders (1),
- Hispanics (4),

- Dually enrolled (3), and
- Rural beneficiaries (19).

The reference group for nonrural projects was white, non-dually eligible Medicare beneficiaries residing or receiving care in the same geographic area as the underserved population. The reference group for rural projects was Medicare beneficiaries residing or receiving care in all urban counties of the state. CMS granted a waiver to the QIO for the U.S. Virgin Islands because the entire population was considered "underserved" (CMS, 2002, 2004). The QIOs targeted a subset of the underserved population in their states, called the intervention group, which had to be at least 25 percent of the underserved population's entire size. The QIO addressed one quality measure used in either Task 1c or Task 1d for its underserved population. If the QIO was continuing a project from the 6th SOW, the QIO was encouraged to increase the size of its intervention group. In this subtask, the QIOs also supported state Quality Assessment and Performance Improvement projects to reduce health disparities (see the discussion of managed care later in this chapter).

The story presented in Box 8.4 demonstrates a successful intervention by Florida Medical Quality Assurance, Inc. (Florida's QIO), which used multiple techniques, including beneficiary education, the use of opinion leaders, partnering with key stakeholders, communications tools, use of QIOSC materials, and individualized assistance to providers to improve the rate of hemoglobin A1c testing in the African-American population (CMS, 2002, 2004).

Telephone Interviews: Challenges

In telephone interviews, many QIO CEOs mentioned difficulties with the design of interventions for the underserved population, including access versus quality; the resource-poor state of some providers; and the ability to track changes in populations whose providers bundled charges for tests into visits, such as the Indian Health Service. They expressed concern that access issues are not addressed by the QIOs as much because there is a tendency to look at the care of people who already have access. They also related logistical difficulties with the study of underserved populations, including sufficient sample sizes, the increased use of services by all populations, and special geographical needs. The following are comments of some of the CEOs:

- "I don't think the issue is the quality of care delivered in the area, but it is the issue of access instead. For example, people in rural areas or even midcity often do not have transportation to care."

BOX 8.4 Glycosylated Hemoglobin A1c Testing
Among African Americans in Florida

"The Florida Medical Quality Assurance, Inc. (FMQAI) sought to reduce the disparity in glycosylated hemoglobin A1c (HbA1c) use between African American Medicare beneficiaries and non-African American Medicare beneficiaries with diabetes in the state.

"FMQAI used previous statement of work (scope of work) research to identify barriers, such as beneficiary knowledge regarding the importance of healthcare screening techniques for diabetes. FMQAI also found a need for providers to learn about the healthcare disparity, existent barriers to care, and providers systemic changes that could address prescribing HbA1c for African Americans such as diabetic beneficiary identification and follow up by the provider.

"The QIO identified existing networks, used them to enhance communication, and employed African Americans from the community to lead the project team and build partnerships with community champions. Outreach tools were designed with target audience involvement and included mailings, radio public service announcements, and press releases. The QIO also worked with stakeholders to develop a culturally sensitive education program. FMQAI made presentations at public meetings with local health departments and church groups and developed an Internet website. Intervention tools included key chains inscribed with the phrase 'Dia-

---

• "In a rural area there might only be five or six Medicare admissions a month, so it is hard to break down rural facilities on an individual basis; we need 10 to 12 facilities to have adequate data."

• "Trying to meet the needs of lower-scoring rural hospitals really adds to the QIOs' costs not only because of their needs but because of the distance required to go to serve their needs."

8th SOW

In the 8th SOW, CMS integrated efforts to take a more community-based approach to improve beneficiary health by incorporating underserved populations into Tasks 1a to 1d, by requiring the adequate representation of providers to underserved populations and, in many cases, in the selection of identified participants. Underserved populations are specifically addressed in Task 1d2 (CMS, 2005b).

betes HbA1c <7,' a train-the-trainer module, and a diabetes education module for beneficiaries. Another beneficiary intervention involved face-to-face interaction and educational presentations, seminars, and involvement at trade shows. FMQAI implemented the Front Porch initiative, which involved a 'Closing the Gap' grant, the SHARE program, the Frenchtown initiative, and diabetic educators.

"The QIO provider intervention targeted physicians' offices and included an adaptation of the Oklahoma Foundation for Medical Quality, Inc. methodology. FMQAI visited 'best practice' offices and recruited those physicians to become FMQAI consultants, who conducted other provider office visits. The QIO also made direct mailings, which contained recruitment materials and a 'project-in-a-box' with tools for system changes. Other efforts involved physician-to-physician mailings, QIO partner articles, presentations, and face-to-face contact with providers by teleconferencing. Diabetic educators and pharmacists also assisted the QIO in working with physicians.

"The HbA1c-testing rate for the target population showed an absolute improvement of 14.6 percent. There was a reduction in the disparity of HbA1c use between African American Medicare beneficiaries and non-African American Medicare beneficiaries with diabetes of 3.1 percent."

SOURCE: QSource: The Center for Healthcare Quality (2005).

MANAGED CARE

By law, the QIOs must also review the services provided to beneficiaries in managed care plans. Independent of the QIO program, all Medicare managed care organizations must execute one national Quality Assessment and Performance Improvement (QAPI) project to improve health outcomes and beneficiary satisfaction. CMS chooses the clinical topic for the national project each year. Past topics included diabetes, community-acquired pneumonia, congestive heart failure, and clinical health care disparities or culturally and linguistically appropriate services (CMS, 2005a). In 2005, CMS did not assign a specific topic because of the overwhelming work that resulted from implementation of the Medicare Prescription Drug, Improvement, and Modernization Act (P.L. 108-173). Instead, organizations performed a task of their choosing based on local needs (Moreno, 2004). In years with an identified clinical topic, the organizations could initiate additional projects on topics in response to local needs.

Under Task 1f of the 7th SOW, the QIOs supported Medicare+Choice organizations' (M+COs') performance of QAPI projects. The QIOs encouraged consistent practice patterns for beneficiaries, regardless of the type of plan in which they were enrolled. CMS required the QIOs to invite all Medicare+Choice organizations in the state to participate in any projects related to Tasks 1a to 1e. If possible, a QIO was supposed to offer technical assistance to Medicare+Choice organizations for any quality improvement activities not specifically related to QAPI project requirements. This work continued collaborations initiated during the 6th SOW. No specific set of measures existed for this task, but the QIOs reported on their activities to CMS on a quarterly basis (CMS, 2002). Box 8.5 gives an example of how

---

BOX 8.5   Cultural Competency Organizational Assessment (CCOA) Pilot

"CMRI (now known as Lumetra) sponsored a pilot project utilizing the Organizational Self-Assessment tool and protocol developed by Dennis Andrulis, PhD, MPH, a research professor at the department of Preventive Medicine & Community Health at the State University of New York, Downstate Medical Center.

"In consultation with Dr. Andrulis, the original self-assessment tool was modified to meet the needs of the managed care community. Five California M+COs participated in the pilot project. The participating plans contributed to the adaptation of the tool and shared their experiences with other M+COs at a meeting in December 2002 in Oakland, California.

"The M+COs who participated in the CCOA Pilot have been given permission by CMS to use that experience as the basis for their 2003 QAPI Project. More importantly, the participants contributed to the development of an organizational self-assessment tool that can be used by all types of managed care organizations nationwide. Dr. Andrulis is consulting with each participant plan confidentially about their scoring results and 'next steps.' Although all participants note that the self-assessment took a lot of hard work, they enthusiastically acknowledge how valuable the experience has been to their organization. They report increased awareness of organizational resources and improved inter-departmental communications. The CCOA pilot results help their organizations to develop a multi-year action plan to address issues related to cultural competency."

SOURCE: Lumetra (2005).

Lumetra (California's QIO) interacted with managed care plans in that state on its national project for 2003.

In the 8th SOW, CMS did not define a separate task for the Medicare Advantage beneficiary population, but the QIOs must include Medicare Advantage organizations in all of their activities at a level that is equivalent to their representation in the state.

QIO SUPPORT CENTERS

As described in Chapter 7, a QIOSC is a QIO that acts as a central resource on a specific task or crosscutting topic. QIOSCs conduct analyses, develop materials, and share information. In interviews with four QIOs (representing seven QIOSCs), all stated that they had various levels of interaction with the QIOs. They provided information when they were asked, but they could not intervene in a QIO's activities unless they were asked to do so. They agreed that individual QIOs needed different levels of help, depending on their own skills. All QIOSCs saw their role as assistants to QIOs in their activities and as sources for the sharing of knowledge. The following sections present specific examples of QIOSC activities related to the role of QIOs in offering technical assistance to providers.

Nursing Home QIOSC

During the 7th SOW, Quality Partners of Rhode Island (Rhode Island's QIO) served as the Nursing Home QIOSC. In addition to providing general support, it provided technical information and reports, training, and implementation materials to the QIOs. The QIOSC served a convening function for QIOs to communicate among themselves through the establishment of a community of practice, a group that comprised staff working on this specific task in each QIO. Communities of practice regularly engaged in roundtables by telephone and communicated through a listserve. Additionally, the QIOSC helped develop and maintain a Nursing Home Information Clearinghouse, an Internet-based database of best practices, change concepts, interventions, and guidelines available to the QIOs and nursing homes. The data included findings from the literature, as well as the experiences of QIOs and nursing homes (CMS, 2004). Quality Partners of Rhode Island continues these activities as the Nursing Home QIOSC in the 8th SOW.

Box 8.6 represents part of a document developed by the Nursing Home QIOSC in the 7th SOW to serve as a resource guide for the QIOs when they are working on delirium.

**BOX 8.6   Delirium: Tools and Web Links
Resources for Creating Your Own
Delirium Relief Resource Manual**

"**Assessment:**
10-Point Clock Test Screens
http://www.psychiatrictimes.com/p981049.html
A method of using clock-drawing tests to identify delirium. This tool is accompanied by an article, which describes the administration of the 10-Point Clock Test, as well as the interpretation of the score for cognitive impairment.
Source: Psychiatric Times

Confusion Assessment Method
http://www.hartfordign.org/publications/trythis/issue13.pdf
The Confusion Assessment tool has two parts. Part one is an assessment instrument that screens for overall cognitive impairment. Part two includes only those four features that were found to have the greatest ability to distinguish delirium from other types of cognitive impairment.
Source: The Hartford Institute for Geriatric Nursing [adapted from Inouye, S., van Dyck, C., Alessi, C., Balkin, S., Siegal, A. & Horwitz, R. (1990). Clarifying confusion: the confusion assessment method. Annals of Internal Medicine, 113(12), 941–948.]

Mini-Mental State Examination (MMSE)
http://www.minimental.com

Home Health QIOSC

In the 7th SOW, the Maryland-based QIO of the Delmarva Foundation for Medical Care served as the Home Health QIOSC as a result of a pilot study that it led during the 6th SOW. As with the Nursing Home QIOSC, the Home Health QIOSC offered general assistance as well as technical information, reports, and implementation materials to the QIOs. Because this was a new setting for QIOs, the QIOSC worked to orient the QIOs to the home health setting in general. They also provided OBQI system train-the-trainer programs to all the QIOs. The 3-day training included lectures on the state of the home health industry and OASIS (CMS, 2004). The Home Health QIOSC operated in a fashion similar to that described above for the Nursing Home QIOSC and maintained an information clearing-

A practical method for grading the cognitive state of patients for the clinician.
Source: Marshal F. Folstein, MD; Susan E. Folstein, MD; Paul R. McHugh, MD

Guidelines:
Acute confusion and delirium
http://www.guideline.gov/VIEWS/summary.asp?guideline=000536&summary_type=brief_summary&view=brief_summary&sSearch_string=delirium
Major recommendations including the assessment and management of delirium.
Source: Research Dissemination Core. Acute confusion/delirium. Iowa City (IA): University of Iowa Gerontological Nursing Interventions Research Center; 1998. 41 p. [81 references]

Practice Guideline For the Treatment of Patients with Delirium
http://www.psych.org/clin_res/pg_delirium.cfm
This practice guideline seeks to summarize data regarding the care of patients with delirium. It begins at the point where the psychiatrist has diagnosed a patient as suffering from delirium according to the DSM-IV criteria for the disorder. The purpose of this guideline is to assist the psychiatrist in caring for a patient with delirium.
Source: American Psychiatric Association"

SOURCE: Quality Partners of Rhode Island (2005).

house. In the 8th SOW, the West Virginia Medical Institute (West Virginia's QIO) acts as the Home Health QIOSC.

Hospital QIOSCs

In the 7th SOW, the Colorado Foundation for Medical Care (Colorado's QIO) served as the Heart Failure QIOSC and focused on hospital-based measures of acute myocardial infarction and heart failure, whereas the Oklahoma Foundation for Medical Quality (Oklahoma's QIO) served as the Infectious Disease QIOSC and supported hospital tasks related to pneumonia and the prevention of surgical infections. These QIOSCs operated in the same fashion described above for the other QIOSCs. For example, the Infectious Disease QIOSC brought together representatives of the Infectious Diseases Society of America and the American Thoracic Society to develop joint guidelines for the treatment of community-acquired pneumonia. Examples of fact sheets include Antibiotic Timing and Selection (developed by the Infectious Disease QIOSC) and Successful Inpatient Intervention Factors (developed by the Heart Failure QIOSC) (CMS, 2004).

In the 8th SOW, the Iowa Foundation for Medical Care (Iowa's QIO) acts as the newly designed Hospital Reporting QIOSC. This QIOSC will provide data support for hospital reporting initiatives, help with the CMS Abstraction and Reporting Tool (see Chapter 13), and support validation for hospital-generated data and will perform overall data management (Qualis Health, 2005). The Oklahoma Foundation for Medical Quality (Oklahoma's QIO) operates the newly designed Hospital Interventions QIOSC to provide support for all Task 1c1 and Task 1c2 activities.

Physician Office QIOSC

In the 7th SOW, the Virginia Health Quality Center (Virginia's QIO) acted as the Physician Office QIOSC and thereby supported the QIOs in the same manner described above. Monthly calls included discussions of national topics, as well as topics designed to target smaller groups of QIOs with specific demographic challenges. The QIOSC also supported the Medicare Quality Improvement Community website through coordination with the Interventions QIOSC (CMS, 2004). The Virginia Health Quality Center acts as the Physician Office QIOSC in the 8th SOW. Additionally, it has three subcontractors: (1) Lumetra (California's QIO) for Medicare Advantage, (2) Lumetra (under a second subcontract) for Electronic Health Record Vendor Relations Updates, and (3) the Northeast Health Care Quality Foundation (New Hampshire's QIO) for Office System Survey (Qualis Health, 2005).

Underserved QIOSC

In the 7th SOW, the Center for Healthcare Quality (Tennessee's QIO) served as the Underserved/Rural QIOSC. This QIOSC provided support to the QIOs in a manner similar to that described above and collected a large scientific evidence base on disparities in health care quality. Specific efforts included participation in the Healthy People 2010 Partnership for Heart Disease and Stroke and the Southeast Health Disparities Collaborative. The Underserved/Rural QIOSC also conducted a needs assessment in January 2003 (5 months after the first round of the 7th SOW started) in which it surveyed the QIO community on how the QIOSC could best serve its needs. The survey found that QIOs had a strong preference to learn from other

QIOs and other experts. As a result of this and other findings, the QIOSC held conference calls on intervention strategies, convened a 1-day conference on rural health for hospitals and outpatient rural projects, led web-based training sessions, and provided written educational materials (CMS, 2004). The Center for Healthcare Quality continues its activities as the Underserved QIOSC in the 8th SOW.

Medicare Advantage QIOSC

In the 7th SOW, Lumetra (California's QIO) acted as the Medicare +Choice QIOSC. The QIOSC provided support in a way similar to that described above for other QIOSCs. In the 8th SOW, no QIOSC is dedicated solely to Medicare Advantage issues. Instead, Lumetra acts as a supporting contractor to the Physician Office QIOSC for Medicare Advantage issues.

SUMMARY

This chapter has discussed issues related to the technical assistance activities of the QIO program. The following are some of the main themes of this chapter, which are reflected in the finding and conclusions presented in Chapter 2:

• The activities involved under the broad term of technical assistance vary widely and include the implementation of interventions, the provision of support with public reporting, the provision of assistance with data collection and manipulation, and collaboration with stakeholders.

• Recruitment of voluntary identified participants is largely left to the discretion of the QIO (aside from certain specific numeric or demographic requirements). The QIOs largely favor working with those showing an eagerness and readiness for change.

• The QIOs have experience with many methods for interacting with providers, including collaboratives, one-on-one consulting, teleconferences, local or regional conferences, newsletters and other printed materials, and web-based tools.

• The QIOs favor an increased ability to tailor interventions to local needs.

• Because of the history of the QIO program, QIOs have the longest-standing relationships with hospitals. For some providers, particularly physicians in ambulatory care, their interaction with QIOs has occurred over a much shorter length of time, and so many of those relationships are not fully developed.

• The 8th SOW has many more detailed requirements for technical assistance activities than the 7th SOW did. The identified participant groups are intricately described, including how they may be chosen, and more complex evaluation criteria are used to determine the QIOs' success on these tasks. The 8th SOW also includes many new challenging areas to be addressed, such as the Part D prescription drug benefit and a program to work with physicians' offices on the adoption of information and communication technology.

 • Task-specific QIOSCs exist for each of the provider settings. These QIOSCs are very active in producing materials, disseminating information, and otherwise supporting the QIOs in their technical assistance activities.

REFERENCES

Bradley EH, Carlson MDA, Gallo WT, Scinto J, Campbell MK, Krumholz HM. 2005. From adversary to partner: Have quality improvement organizations made the transition? *Health Services Research* 40(2):459–476.

CMS (Centers for Medicare and Medicaid Services). 1999. *6th Statement of Work (SOW)*. [Online]. Available: http://www.cms.hhs.gov/qio [accessed April 9, 2005].

CMS. 2002. *7th Statement of Work (SOW)*. [Online]. Available: http://www.cms.hhs.gov/qio [accessed April 9, 2005].

CMS. 2004. *The Quality Improvement Organization Program: CMS Briefing for IOM Staff*. [Online]. Available: http://www.medqic.org/dcs/ContentServer?cid=1105558772835&pagename=Medqic percent2FMQGeneralPage percent2FGeneralPageTemplate&c=MQGeneralPage [accessed December 26, 2005].

CMS. 2005a. *Quality in Managed Care, National QAPI Project Information*. [Online]. Available: www.cms.hhs.gov/healthplans/quality [accessed May 25, 2005].

CMS. 2005b. *8th Statement of Work (SOW)*. [Online]. Available: http://www.cms.hhs.gov/qio [accessed April 9, 2005].

CMS. 2005c. *8th Statement of Work (SOW), Version 080105-1*. [Online]. Available: http://www.cms.hhs.gov/quality improvementorgs/downloads/8thsow.pdf [accessed November 4, 2005].

Davis D. 1998. Does CME Work? An analysis of the effect of educational activities on physician performance or health care outcomes. *International Journal of Psychiatry in Medicine* 28:21–39.

Eloranta S. 2005. *Brief Report: National Nursing Home Improvement Collaborative Outcomes Congress*. [Online]. Available: http://www.ihi.org/IHI/Topics/Improvement/ImprovementMethods/ImprovementStories/BriefreportNationalNursingHomeImprovementCollaborativeOutcomesCongress.htm [accessed May 11, 2005].

iHealthBeat. 2005. *CMS Expands DOQ-IT Program Nationwide*. [Online]. Available: http://www.ihealthbeat.org/index.cfm?Action=dspItem&itemID=114658 [accessed September 13, 2005].

Institute for Healthcare Improvement. 2003. *The Breakthrough Series: IHI's Collaborative Model for Achieving Breakthrough Improvement*. Cambridge, MA: Institute for Healthcare Improvement.

Institute for Healthcare Improvement. 2005. *The Spread Initiative*. [Online]. Available: http://www.ihi.org/IHI/Programs/CollaborativeLearning/TheSpreadInitiative.htm [accessed April 21, 2005].

Jencks SF, Huff ED, Cuerdon T. 2003. Change in the quality of care delivered to medicare beneficiaries, 1998–1999 to 2000–2001. *Journal of the American Medical Association* 289(3):305–312.

Jones J. 2003. *Improvement Story: Clarifying the Definition for Intractable Pain Makes the Difference.* [Online]. Available: http://www.medqic.org/dcs/ContentServer?cid=1110810401913&pagename=Medqic percent2FMQStories percent2FImprovement StoryTemplate&c=MQStories [accessed April 21, 2005].

Joshi M. 2000. Effecting and leading change in health care organizations. *Journal of Quality Improvement* 26(7):388–399.

Lumetra. 2005. *QAPI—Cultural Competency.* [Online]. Available: http://www.lumetra.com/healthplans/culturalcompetency/index.asp [accessed May 24, 2005].

Moreno C (Director, Health Plan Benefits Group). 2004, March 3. *Memo: Selection of 2005 QAPI Project Focus.* [Online]. Available: http://www.cms.hhs.gov/healthplans/quality/2005memo2.pdf [accessed May 24, 2005].

Oklahoma Foundation for Medical Quality. 2005, March 7. *Improvement Story: Mammography Scheduling Block Improves Rate.* [Online]. Available: http://www.medqic.org/dcs/ContentServer?cid=1110810342250&pagename=Medqic percent2FMQStories percent2FImprovementStoryTemplate&c=MQStories [accessed September 14, 2005].

Ovretveit J, Bate P, Cleary P, Cretin S, Gustafson D, et al. 2002. Quality collaboratives: Lessons from research. *Quality and Safety in Health Care* 11(4):345–351.

QSource: The Center for Healthcare Quality. 2005. *Diabetes: African American Population.* [Online]. Available: http://www.qsource.org/HDS/African percent20American percent20 Diabetes percent20-v1.pdf [accessed May 11, 2005].

Qualis Health. 2005. *QIO Guidebook to QIOSC Resources.* Unpublished. Seattle, WA: Qualis Health.

Quality Partners of Rhode Island. 2005. *Tools and Weblinks Related to Delirium.* [Online]. Available: http://www.medqic.org/dcs/ContentServer?cid=1110810477361&pagename=Medqicpercent2FMQTools percent2FToolTemplate&c=MQTools [accessed May 1, 2005].

Rollow WC. 2005. *The Medicare Quality Improvement (QIO) Program 7th SOW and Results.* PowerPoint Presentation to the Committee on Redesigning Health Insurance, June 13, Washington, DC.

Shortell SM, Marsteller JA, Lin M, Pearson ML, Wu SY, et al. 2004. The role of perceived team effectiveness in improving chronic illness care. *Medical Care* 42(11):1040–1048.

Soumerai S, McLaughlin TJ, Gurwitz JH, Guadagnoli E, Hauptman PJ, et al. 1998. Effect of local medical opinion leaders on quality of care for acute myocardial infarction: A randomized controlled trial. *Journal of the American Medical Association* 279:1358–1363.

Thomson O'Brien M, Oxman A, Haynes R, Davis D, Freemantle N, Harvey E. 2005. Local opinion leaders. *Cochrane Database of Systematic Reviews* 2005(2).

9

Impact of Technical Assistance for Quality Improvement and Knowledge Transfer

CHAPTER SUMMARY

This chapter reviews the literature base for quality improvement and knowledge transfer, two concepts important to the provision of technical assistance to help health care providers improve the quality of care that they provide. To understand the effectiveness of the technical assistance provided through the Quality Improvement Organization (QIO) program or the extent to which the program goals have been achieved, it is necessary to first understand how similar quality improvement efforts have fared in the larger health care environment outside of the QIO program. This chapter presents discussions on the following topics related to quality improvement: quality improvement interventions in general and in QIOs, approaches to quality improvement, and an overview of knowledge transfer and its impact within the QIO environment.

QUALITY IMPROVEMENT

The Quality Improvement Organizations (QIOs) seek to achieve quality improvement through the use of various interventions to enhance the efficiency and effectiveness of care received by Medicare beneficiaries. This section examines the impacts that QIOs' quality improvement interventions have on the delivery of health care. With specific reference to the QIOs, the Centers for Medicare and Medicaid Services (CMS) defines interventions as activities adopted by providers, beneficiaries, or the QIOs to facilitate change to improve health care delivery processes, structures, or behaviors (CMS, 2005b). To assess and explain the impacts of quality interventions by the QIOs, the impacts of these interventions throughout the health care industry must be reviewed. Thus, this discussion first examines the litera-

ture regarding quality improvement in general and then assesses the literature on QIO quality improvement interventions.

A literature review conducted for this project provides an overview of
evidence on improving health care quality. (For details on each study, see
Table A.1 in Appendix A.) The studies included in the literature review
were categorized by study design; the findings of studies with more rigorous
methodologies were considered more heavily (see Table A.2 in Appendix
A). The studies reviewed paint an inconclusive picture of the effectiveness
of quality improvement programs, whether they are conducted by QIOs or
other organizations, for both Medicare and nonMedicare services.

Although health care quality improvement interventions have been discussed for decades, the emerging evidence base supporting their effectiveness remains sparse and therefore difficult to use as a basis for making
policy decisions. Comprehensive studies of specific types of interventions
are limited in part because of the many different methods of approaching
quality improvement. Quality improvement resulting from specific interventions, however, is difficult to measure because many of the impacts of
the interventions are qualitative, it often takes more time than is allowed by
the study to demonstrate measurable improvements, and the interventions
themselves are not described at a level of detail that allow them to be
replicated.

Quality improvement interventions tend to target multiple components
of complex organizations, all of which are subject to many internal and
external influences, making evidence of effectiveness almost impossible to
detect (Ovretveit and Gustafson, 2003). If improvement has been made,
attribution of this success cannot be determined because of the wealth of
players often involved in enhancing the quality of care. Conversely, the
reason why quality improvement interventions fail also remains inconclusive, despite qualitative studies suggesting that specific organizational culture characteristics play a role (Bradley et al., 2001).

These limitations in the assessment of quality improvement overall, as
well as the assessment of specific quality improvement interventions, result in various types of study designs and different levels of reliability of
the study results. Few of the studies reviewed contained true control
groups, and even fewer were the more stringently devised randomized
control trials. The majority of the studies measured improvement as the
change from the baseline in the group receiving the intervention and were
either prospective or retrospective in design. One research method used to
temper some of the limitations and control for changes in the environment is to stagger implementation of the intervention. The intervention is
put into practice twice: once in the original study intervention group and
once again in the designated control group after the conclusion of the
original study (Chu et al., 2003). Analyses assessing time trends are espe-

cially important in evaluations of quality improvement interventions, as the desired changes often take longer to achieve than the lengths of the interventions themselves and because a potential disparity exists between short- and long-term achievements.

Impact of Health Care Quality Interventions

As mentioned above, many different approaches have been tried to achieve quality improvement in health care. Although some studies that the committee examined found no change in the quality of care delivered as a result of the selected interventions; most cited some level of improvement ranging in levels of statistical significance. Most interventions approach quality improvement by targeting three aspects of health care: structure, process, and outcome. Structure refers to the characteristics of a care setting, including material resources, human resources, and organizational structure. Process describes what and how care is actually provided and received. Outcome denotes the impact of health care services on health status and patient satisfaction. In theory, improvement in structure drives a good process, which in turn drives a good outcome (Donabedian, 1988). The following discussion assesses the literature on interventions that target processes and outcomes and then discusses the literature on other interventions that focus on structure and audit-feedback.

Process Measures

One common finding in the literature was the demonstrated improvement in process measures due to the implementation of clinical practice guidelines. This conclusion was determined from the findings of both randomized controlled trials and cohort studies (Ornstein et al., 2004; Joseph et al., 2004; Halm et al., 2004). Clinical practice guidelines are evidence-based recommendations developed to direct decision making for the provision of care. An example of a guideline for a process measure is the percentage of providers who document taking a patient's blood pressure during an office visit. The use of process guidelines generally led to increases in the documentation of care processes for a variety of conditions (cardiovascular diseases, pneumonia, and tobacco use) and a variety of care settings (physicians' offices and hospitals). However, the resulting levels of statistical significance varied, with studies citing significant improvement in only one of many measures (one study looked at 14 process measures) (see Table A.1 in Appendix A). One randomized controlled trial, however, evaluated guidelines in the context of a larger, more systemwide intervention, and found only marginal change in physician adherence (Ornstein et al., 2004). The more systemwide effects of the intervention were not separated from those of the guidelines themselves, complicating any conclusions that guidelines alone enhance quality. The provision of guidelines also does not necessarily lead to the dissemination of new knowledge regarding care practices (Centor et al., 2003).

Outcomes

Another theme detected in the literature review was a lack of demonstrated improvement in health outcomes (such as patient health status) as a result of the use of treatment guidelines for desired outcomes. For example, a desired outcome derived from the observance of diabetes care guidelines is control of hemoglobin A1c levels in diabetes patients to less than 8 percent mg/dL. The same studies that failed to demonstrate improvement in process measures were used to evaluate outcomes. These studies were designed as randomized controlled trials and cohort studies. The studies evaluated multiple conditions and care settings. Outcomes based on treatment guidelines did not change significantly during the study periods, with use of the guidelines having from no impact to only a marginal impact (Ornstein et al., 2004; Joseph et al., 2004; Halm et al., 2004) (see Table A.1 in Appendix A). The impacts of interventions on outcomes may, however, take longer to identify than the duration of the study, thereby resulting in false conclusions about an intervention. Changes in outcomes may also be influenced by patient behaviors, over which providers have limited control.

Other Interventions

Conclusions about other types of interventions cannot be drawn because of a lack of a robust evidence base and inconsistent results. For instance, research gaps exist concerning structural issues and audit-feedback (Jamtvedt et al., 2004; Coleman et al., 2004; Mark et al., 2004).

Although improved performance on the process and outcome measures presented in studies are a good starting point for obtaining improvements in quality, performance should ultimately keep getting better. Structural issues such as nurse staffing levels were addressed in a cohort study. Improvements in mortality rates were found in association with increases in the numbers of registered nurses on staff, but the improvements could not be solely ascribed to those increases. Also, a diminishing marginal effect of increased staff members was found on improvements of mortality rates. Although the evidence base for improvements in health care quality attributable to structural changes is emerging, it is sparse (Mark et al., 2004).

Provider and organizational characteristics are also important structural issues to be considered for the achievement of continuous improvements. One qualitative study used interviews to evaluate whether correlations between provider characteristics and quality improvement exist (Bradley et al., 2001). The researchers identified provider characteristics and measured quality improvement in terms of the percentage of patients who had received beta-blockers at discharge. Hospitals with greater amounts of improvement had four similar characteristics: shared goals throughout the institution, strong administrative support, high levels of physician leadership, and high-quality feedback. The levels of innovation were not, however, found to correlate with high or low levels of performance (Bradley et al., 2001).

To prepare an organization to be receptive to change, researchers identified the following dimensions of success: strategy, culture, technique, and structure. The improvement mechanism must target strategic conditions and processes within the organization. The organization must foster a culture that supports the mechanism, and it must ensure that staff are properly trained and given the necessary tools to implement the intervention technically. The last dimension is structure, which refers to the mechanisms used to adopt and spread better practices throughout the organization. All four dimensions must be present for successful change to occur (Shortell et al., 1998; Heller and Arozullah, 2001). However, it is very difficult to develop the strategic and cultural dimensions if the organization does not already have these attributes. Technique and structure are somewhat easier to develop. For example, the organization can purchase expertise, but it takes longer to develop a supportive culture.

In health care settings, audit and feedback refers to the process in which provider performance is evaluated and reported back to the provider, which allows the provider to make improvements. The committee's present review found that the audit and feedback method inconsistently provides significant improvements. The coupling of these efforts with other types of improvement interventions also did not yield better results. A major limitation to the committee's systematic review was the lack of high-quality studies, as it was noted that the participants in many studies had low levels of compliance at the baseline and the studies had small sample sizes. Improved reporting of the details about the actual intervention was also found to be needed (Jamtvedt et al., 2004).

Impact of QIO Quality Improvement Interventions with Providers

The evidence about the impact of QIO quality interventions compared with the impact of other health care quality interventions is mixed. This conclusion is most prominently derived from studies in which researchers found that the trends for hospital systems and hospitals that did and did not participate in QIO interventions were similar (Ellerbeck et al., 2000; Dellinger et al., 2005).

Process Measures

Studies using process measures to evaluate the effects of QIO efforts to improve quality used a variety of designs: randomized controlled trial designs, quasiexperimental designs, cohort study designs, and cross-sectional study designs. These studies looked at the use of practice guidelines for the care processes for multiple conditions (diabetes, cardiovascular disease, and pneumonia) and were conducted in hospitals, academic medical centers, and physicians' offices. Echoing the findings from the quality improvement intervention literature of studies assessing non-QIO-related interventions, improvements in quality were found as a result of the QIO-related interventions (Marciniak et al., 1998; Ellerbeck et al., 2000; Holman et al., 2001; Kiefe et al., 2001; Sheikh and Bullock, 2001; Sutherland et al., 2001; Luthi et al., 2002; Gould et al., 2002; Chu et al., 2003; Burwen et al., 2003; Berner et al., 2003; McClellan et al., 2003; Massing et al., 2003; Daniel et al., 2004a).

Outcomes

Many studies looked at the impact that QIO interventions have on outcomes. Those studies examined a variety of outcomes in patients with diabetes, cardiovascular disease, and pneumonia seen in the hospital and the physician's office settings and used quasiexperimental and cohort methodological designs. As has been found in the broader literature on quality improvement, interventions by QIOs to improve outcomes have not yet been demonstrated to result in significant change. Although some studies found improvements in quality, the results of many of them are inconclusive. The limitations described in the broader literature on quality improvement are the same, such as a limited ability to control patient behaviors (Marciniak et al., 1998; Ellerbeck et al., 2000; Sheikh and Bullock, 2001; Sutherland et al., 2001; Holman et al., 2001; Luthi et al., 2002; Gould et al., 2002; Chu et al., 2003; McClellan et al., 2003; Massing et al., 2003; Daniel et al., 2004a) (see Table A.1 in Appendix A).

Only one study evaluated in the committee's literature review focused on patient behaviors. That study examined patient adherence to a health maintenance organization's guidelines for the frequency of mammography upon receipt of one of three types of reminders. This QIO-related randomized control trial found that only telephone reminders coupled with the option to schedule an appointment were effective; publicity campaigns encouraging screening and mail reminders were not effective (Barr et al., 2001).

Other Interventions

Studies of other types of interventions that have been performed by QIOs or that use improvement tools developed by QIOs have yielded inconclusive results. For example, the impact of educating second-year medical students on the use of process guidelines and reminders provided by QIOs generated some significant improvement (Gould et al., 2002). A study conducted by a QIO audit and feedback in hospitals could not conclusively find methods to yield improvements for the following five conditions: acute myocardial infarction, heart failure, pneumonia, stroke, and atrial fibrillation. Consistent with the general limitations of quality intervention studies, a true causal relationship could not be drawn because of the lack of controls in that study (Schade et al., 2004).

National Evaluations of QIO Technical Assistance Efforts

Various reviews have evaluated various elements of the technical assistance provided by the QIO program, but none could ascribe the improvements directly to the efforts of the QIOs.

One study compared the national and state-level improvements in 22 QIO measures of quality in the hospital and the physician's office settings between the time periods of 1998–1999 and 2000–2001 (from the end of the 6th scope of work [SOW] to the beginning of the 7th SOW). That cross-sectional study built upon earlier efforts that found that the quality of care provided by the states was inconsistent (Jencks et al., 2000). The study found that care for fee-for-service beneficiaries on the whole improved during this time period, as the national and the state averages for 20 of the 22 measures increased. In general, states with lower baselines yielded higher rates of absolute improvement in the quality of care. The study also ranked states on the appropriate provision of care on the basis of the same 22 measures. The result was a geography-specific pattern of care, with better care being delivered in the northern states than in the southern states. The levels of improvement followed a similar pattern. The improvements cited in that study could not be attributed directly to the QIO program, however, for many of the reasons discussed above. However, that study was designed to look at quality trends and not to assess the impact of the QIO program (Jencks et al., 2003).

Another study randomly surveyed 105 hospital directors of quality of care across the nation to determine their perceptions of QIO effectiveness. That cross-sectional study found that 60 percent of quality directors believed that certain QIO interventions, such as the provision of performance data and education materials, were helpful or very helpful. However, the same survey disclosed that in the absence of QIO interventions, only 25 percent of directors thought that the quality of the care delivered would have been worse. Although the study found that QIOs were mostly viewed as partners for improving care, as opposed to their previous role as adversaries, the researchers noted the need to engage senior-level support (both physicians and hospital management) to further the QIOs' impacts. These findings were based on the opinions of those interviewed and not on quantitative measures of actual impacts (Bradley et al., 2005).

A recent study evaluated the effectiveness of QIO interventions on improving the quality of care in hospitals. That quasiexperimental study compared the differences in care in five clinical areas (atrial fibrillation, acute myocardial infarction, heart failure, pneumonia, and stroke) delivered by participating (n = 199) and nonparticipating (n = 142) hospitals in Maryland, New York, Nevada, Utah, Washington state, and Washington, D.C. The researchers collected data on 15 indicators at the baseline (1998–1999) and at the follow-up (2000–2001). The data revealed that nonparticipating hospitals were generally for profit and smaller than the participating hospitals. (The researchers defined "participating hospitals" as those that either collected measurement data or implemented changes in their procedures as a result of efforts made by their respective QIOs.) At the baseline, data for 5 of 15 indicators differed significantly, with nonparticipating hospitals performing better than participating hospitals on 2 of these 5 indicators; participating hospitals performed better on the other three indicators. At the follow-up, the data showed significant differences on four indicators, with the participating hospitals performing better on all of them. However, at the baseline, differences between participating and nonparticipating hospitals were found on only two of these four indicators. When the baseline performance and the follow-up performance were compared, researchers found significant differences (P < 0.05) between participating and nonparticipating hospitals for only 1 of the 15 indicators (the patient was screened for pneumococcal immunization or given the pneumococcal vaccine [P = 0.005]). They concluded that, overall, hospitals participating with QIOs were no more likely to improve than nonparticipating hospitals. Importantly, a general trend of improvement was found for both participating and nonparticipating hospitals (Snyder and Anderson, 2005).

The findings of that study concur with those of other studies that show that quality improvements have been made over time, but the study concludes that the improvements cannot be directly attributed to the activities of the QIOs (Jencks et al., 2003). Although that study has strength because of its use of a comparison group, it also has limitations. In particular, the distinction between participating and nonparticipating hospitals is very broad, and precise descriptions of the interventions are lacking. A lack of descriptive details also makes it difficult to discern the exact roles that the QIOs played. The effects of other quality interventions that were concurrently under way in the hospitals included in the study are unknown. Each participating hospital did not necessarily participate in QIO activities or focus on improving all 15 indicators at the same time, which biased the impacts of the interventions and thus does not allow comparisons of the improvements on specific indicators within a clinical area. Additionally, the study examined only a limited subset of the hospitals in the country and only one portion of the QIO program. Moreover, the data reflect the results from the 6th SOW; evaluated changes thus do not reflect the major strategic shifts made by the QIO program in the 7th SOW and is not indicative of the effectiveness of the current program.

Although the studies described above cannot ascribe improvements in the quality of the care delivered directly to the efforts of the QIOs, this is not to say that QIO interventions have been unsuccessful. Some studies find that the efforts of QIOs have had positive impacts. One of the building blocks for promoting quality improvement through the QIO program is the Cooperative Cardiovascular Project (see Chapter 1). The Cooperative Cardiovascular Project was part of the initial movement in 1992 to shift the strategy of CMS to providing technical assistance to providers (Jencks and Wilensky, 1992). The Cooperative Cardiovascular Project pilot lasted from 1992 to 1995 and assessed quality improvement activities for acute myocardial infarction patients in Alabama, Connecticut, Iowa, and Wisconsin. The quality of care was evaluated on the basis of improvements in 26 measures of processes and outcomes. The researchers found that not all eligible patients received treatments either at all or in a timely manner. Despite this finding, the Cooperative Cardiovascular Project successfully attained significant documented improvements in process measures (Ellerbeck et al., 1995; Marciniak et al., 1998; Holman et al., 2001; Burwen et al., 2003), thereby promoting the use of quality improvement efforts.

In addition to the Cooperative Cardiovascular Project, other studies of QIO activities support the effectiveness of QIO interventions (Sutherland et al., 2001; Gould et al., 2002; Chu et al., 2003; Daniel et al., 2004b). While these studies all targeted physicians, no other commonalities were readily identified in the articles. The positive effects were limited, and do not demonstrate the impact of the QIO program overall.

Because of the QIO program's voluntary nature, its goal of the provision of a public good, and the QIOs' method of involving many partners in each intervention program, it is difficult to attribute in a causal manner the activities of QIOs to quality improvement, as these activities cannot be easily distinguished from those of other organizations also working to improve quality (Jencks et al., 2000). This does not mean that the QIO program is ineffective; rather, it is difficult to measure its effect separately, as is the case with quality improvement efforts in general. Although other organizations work to enhance the quality of care, their efforts can work in tandem with the efforts of the QIOs. For example, a demonstration project in Texas found that the efforts of a state-sponsored program did not duplicate those of a QIO that provided technical assistance (Cortes, 2004).

Given the limited research available, it remains unknown what drives both successful and unsuccessful quality interventions by QIOs. More evidence is needed to identify these potential drivers. While the QIO program looks to further develop its quality improvement activities, some lessons can be gleaned from the rest of the industry.

APPROACHES TO QUALITY IMPROVEMENT

Many approaches to managing quality improvement focus on improving systemwide processes within provider settings; these approaches are not limited to use within health care settings, however, and are often adapted from other industries for use by health care organizations. As many health care organizations work toward improving quality and decreasing costs, these approaches have become increasingly more relevant to understand. If QIOs are to successfully work in collaboration with some of the hospitals, physicians' offices, and health care plans that have turned to these methods, the QIOs need to be informed. When these processes are implemented, it is important for all players (providers) to agree to participate as well as to keep the customers (patients) as the focus for improvement. The approaches described below represent a mixture of tools, methodologies, and goals for improving quality; they are not independent of each other, as some focus on streamlining processes within individual organizations, whereas others target large organization or multi-organization systems. In addition, process and systems are often combined to achieve higher quality:

• Baldrige criteria. Baldrige criteria are indicators of organizational performance excellence used to evaluate organizations in different industries. The seven criteria are leadership; strategic planning; customer and market focus; measurement, analysis, and knowledge management; a focus on human resources; process management; and results. Organizations that apply and exemplify these criteria are awarded the Baldrige National Quality Award, which symbolizes excellence in quality and performance. The United States Congress established the Baldrige National Quality Award in 1987, and it is presented annually by the President of the United States. Awards are given for five sectors: manufacturing, service, small business, education, and health care. In any given year, awards may be given to one or more organizations in any or all of the five sectors. Recent award recipients for the health care sector include: Saint Luke's Hospital of Kansas City, Kansas City, MO (2003); Baptist Hospital, Inc., Pensacola, FL (2003); Robert Wood Johnson University Hospital Hamilton, Hamilton, NJ (2004);

and Bronson Methodist Hospital, Kalamazoo, MI (2005) (NIST, 2005). Individual states have also created similar awards on the basis of the criteria presented above.

• Collaborative methodology. The model for improvement has been extrapolated to the collaborative methodology, which refers to a semi-structured gathering of providers from various health care organizations to improve a common process of care by sharing experiences, best practices, and lessons learned with each other (Ovretveit et al., 2002). The methods used often include meetings, web-based conferences, and teleconferences (see Chapter 8 for further discussion).

• Human factors. Human factors is a tool used to redesign processes and systems to better use the attributes controlled by both the physical and the cognitive abilities of the people involved in the delivery of care. By understanding the human aspects of why errors occur, processes and systems can become more safe, effective, efficient, and patient centered (NAE and IOM, 2005; Qualis Health, 2005c).

• International Standards Organization Standard 9000 (ISO 9000). ISO 9000 is a standard that provides process guidelines and requirements for quality management. On the basis of an external audit, an organization can be certified to ISO 9000, which signifies that it has demonstrated the ability to adhere to processes of quality improvement. The ISO 9000 family includes guidelines for quality management, quality management systems, and quality assurance.

• Lean principles. Lean principles aim to streamline processes with the goal of reducing waste and eliminating zero-value-added tasks and resources. Lean principles can also be used to simplify systems. For example, by tracking patients across the care system, services can become more effective and efficient in improving quality and minimizing costs.

• Plan, Do, Study (Change), Act (PDSA) Cycle. The PDSA Cycle is a method for continuously improving the quality of processes: plan for a change, do a trial of the planned change, study the results, and act to implement the next steps based on the results. In the PDSA Cycle, change refers to implementing change in the process.

• Six Sigma. Six Sigma is a data-driven problem-solving methodology that is used to minimize variations in processes and builds on statistical process control. Individuals can build Six Sigma competencies through training and continuous practice with application of the method in various projects. The competency levels include green belt (entry level), black belt (middle), and master black belt (expert).

• Root-cause analysis. Root-cause analysis is an approach taken to understand the reasons why an event has occurred. The recurrence of adverse events can be eliminated by looking systematically at the managerial processes behind the series of actions that lead up to an event (American Society for Quality, 2005).

By learning and implementing the skills required for the use of these approaches, organizations can streamline their own resources as well as become drivers of improvement by teaching these methods to others who possess the necessary infrastructure support. QIO Support Centers (QIOSCs) and QIOs train staff on many of these approaches and instruct both other QIOs and providers to use them within their organizations (personal communication, L. A. Baseflug, August 19, 2005) (see Chapter 7 for a discussion of the accreditations and awards held by QIOs and the organizations holding QIO contracts).

The Process Improvement QIOSC conducted the Health Care Quality Improvement Project Improvement Methodologies Survey in September 2004 (the results are presented below) to measure QIOs' familiarity with and use of six of the methodologies for quality improvement described above: Baldrige criteria, collaborative methodology, human factors, ISO 9000, lean principles, and Six Sigma (Qualis Health, 2005c). In total, 99 respondents from 41 states completed the surveys. The respondents (75 percent of whom were project managers, project coordinators, or departmental directors) were the most familiar with and used the collaborative methodology. This is expected, because the QIO program strongly promoted the collaborative methodology during the 7th SOW. The survey responses showed familiarity with all methodologies, although familiarity with ISO 9000 and lean principles scored the lowest (49 and 45 percent, respectively). Even though, on average, half of the respondents stated their familiarity with the six methodologies, an average of only 28 percent of the respondents noted that they actually used the methodologies. The respondents remarked that the methodologies that they would most like to receive training on are human factors and lean principles (76 and 74 percent, respectively) (Qualis Health, 2004). Training in human factors can be very relevant in impacting patient safety (Gosbee, 2002; Silver et al., 2004), while lean principles are useful in adding value to processes (Toussaint, 2005).

Two of the methodologies described above are particularly pertinent to the QIO program: the collaborative methodology and lean principles. In the 7th SOW, CMS heavily promoted the use of collaboratives, as described in Chapter 8. In the 8th SOW, CMS identified the use of lean principles as a strategy for promoting transformational change for case review (CMS, 2005c). Although this strategy will be most closely tied to making case review more efficient, the lessons learned from lean principles will be applied where applicable.

The use of quality improvement collaboratives is beginning to be evaluated. Like quality improvement interventions, the designs of collaboratives vary widely. A randomized controlled trial used the collaborative method to assess physician adherence to guidelines for the treatment of stroke and cardiovascular disease but found only small levels of improvement (Ornstein et al., 2004). Other prospective and retrospective studies provided mixed results for a variety of conditions (Sheikh and Bullock, 2001; Holman et al., 2001; Halm et al., 2004). Another study assessed the effect of a controlled national collaborative on the outcomes of care for human immunodeficiency virus–infected patients. That controlled pre- and postintervention study concluded that the outcomes did not improve significantly (Landon et al., 2004).

One study evaluated a QIO-run national demonstration project that used the Institute for Healthcare Improvement collaborative method and was part of the National Surgical Infection Prevention Project, a project that was integrated into the 7th SOW and that was designed to improve the safety of surgical care (Dellinger et al., 2005). From April 2002 to February 2003, researchers aggregated data on changes for three process measures and one outcome measure from 44 of 56 volunteering hospitals representing 50 QIO jurisdictions and 35,543 surgical cases; some hospitals also elected to work and report on additional process measures. The study used a preintervention-postintervention design without control groups and yielded significant improvements in performance ($P < 0.05$) for the three process measures required by the study. The researchers calculated the differences in performance on measures between the beginning and the end of the study by conducting paired differences tests to adjust for confounding variables. Changes in the outcome measures were not significant from quarter to quarter, although comparison of the results at the end of the study period with those at the beginning yielded significant differences. In their summary, the investigators questioned the sustainable effects of quality improvement on outcome measures.

That study provides evidence for the positive effects of efforts toward improving patient safety in surgical care processes and suggests that QIOs can have an effect on quality improvement (Dellinger et al., 2005). Nevertheless, a limitation to the study was that not all hospitals assessed the same surgical procedures because of different case mixes or other reasons; therefore, direct hospital-to-hospital comparisons could not be made. The sustainability of these results and their ability to be spread to other providers also remain unanswered by this study. Although the interventions of process measures were well described and these processes could have produced the given outcomes, the lack of randomization remains a barrier to attribution because all participants were interested in improving. Therefore, this study is unable to discern whether these positive effects are directly attributable to the QIO program, the collaborative methodology, a combination thereof, or other variables.

Collaborative studies that have used the chronic care model have also recently been assessed. The chronic care model focuses on a system in which the patient is the manager of his or her health care. Patient preferences, evidence-based guidelines, and persistent follow-up are emphasized (IOM, 2003).These studies evaluated the collaborative methodology, with the focus being to improve the quality of care for particular disease states, such as asthma and chronic heart failure, by using quasiexperimental study designs. The participant groups showed significant improvements in the process measures compared with the improvements for the control groups, but they did not show improvements in outcomes. These results are in concert with the findings presented in the quality improvement literature (Shortell et al., 2004; Cretin et al., 2004; Schonlau et al., 2005; Asch et al., 2005).

The difficulty of sustaining the transfer of best practices to other providers—a key component to providing continuous improvement—has also been identified (Kosseff and Niemeier, 2001). Comparison of significant results from these studies is difficult, as it is not in the nature of collaboratives to determine statistical significance (Daniel et al., 2004a). In addition, the effectiveness of the collaborative model has not been established, as not enough evidence is available to affirm or deny the effectiveness of collaboratives in general or in the QIO environment in particular (Leatherman, 2002; Mittman, 2004; Greenhalgh et al., 2004).

In telephone interviews with QIO chief executive officers (CEOs), the CEOs did not mention collaboratives until they were directly asked about them. Although the Performance Improvement QIOSC trains QIOs on how to implement the Institute for Healthcare Improvement collaborative model, many states use other collaborative designs. In addition, although the QIOs are interested in learning about various approaches to improving quality, they often do not implement other methods for a variety of reasons, such as the cost of training, the intensity of work required for their success, and acceptance by the providers themselves.

KNOWLEDGE TRANSFER

The transfer of knowledge is difficult to achieve in any field, including health care. The terminology in the literature is not yet well defined and is inconsistent. Nuances exist as a result of the use of different terms, such as "dissemination," "sharing of best practices," and "knowledge transfer." In the context of this report, the term "knowledge transfer" refers to collective exchanges of ideas on how to best promote or provide high quality. Knowledge transfer is not limited to interactions between researchers and providers or decision makers. In the QIO program, the participants in knowledge transfer include CMS, the QIOSCs, the QIOs, practitioners, administrators, and beneficiaries. By affecting the components of health care delivery, such as the care processes, organizational structures, and systems in which care are delivered, the QIOs can work toward changing behaviors to promote higher-quality health care and, ultimately, better health. Knowledge transfer is thus an important function of the QIO program and is especially relevant to the QIOSCs, because despite variations in health and health care delivery systems, common fundamental components of the provision of high-quality care may exist. The next section discusses knowledge transfer in the general health care environment through an assessment of the literature, followed by a discussion of the multiple methods in which ideas are translated within the QIO program.

Knowledge Transfer in the Literature

As is the case for the health care–related quality improvement intervention literature, the evidence base for knowledge transfer in health care is limited (Heller and Arozullah, 2001). Although no single technique for the best way to transfer knowledge has been identified, many methods have been tried, with some appearing to be more successful than others. Most of the literature tends to be descriptive and observational and, thus, is based on inference and extrapolation (Berwick, 2003). Existing studies demonstrating knowledge transfer in health care are often cited as being of poor design and as containing methodological flaws (Greenhalgh et al., 2004; Mittman, 2004; Fleuren et al., 2004).

Internal and external factors affect knowledge transfer. One important aspect is the development of new ideas internally within an organization. Rogers' diffusion of innovations theory (see Chapter 8) discusses five organizational characteristics that impact how quickly organizational behaviors change: relative advantage, compatibility, complexity, triability, and observability. In addition to these characteristics, organizational commitment and readiness for change are necessary elements for successful knowledge transfer. Support must come from the organization leadership (Greenhalgh et al., 2004; Wang et al., 2004; Mills and Weeks, 2004). The organizations contributing to the literature typically want to improve and thus already have some important organizational support in place. To operationalize the adoption of quality improvement, a clear plan of how to implement change is necessary. In health care, the value of interpersonal influence among providers should not be underestimated, as the literature suggests that the presence of clinical leaders and champions promotes knowledge transfer, despite a lack of conclusive evidence of their effectiveness (Berner et al., 2003; Shortell et al., 2004; Jamtvedt et al., 2004; Greenhalgh et al., 2004; Thomson O'Brien et al., 2005).

Knowledge transfer may also be influenced by external factors, such as financial incentives and politics. Depending on the design of the payment structure, financial incentives such as pay for performance could inhibit or expedite knowledge transfer. If competition to improve arises, providers may not want to exchange ideas about best practices and lessons learned; however, if such exchanges are rewarded, knowledge transfer may be promoted. Political factors outside of an organization can also affect an organization's readiness for change (Greenhalgh et al., 2004).

The literature discusses many barriers to successful knowledge transfer, some of which are mentioned below. Within an organization, issues such as competing priorities, resource allocation, and delayed acceptance by key stakeholders are among the numerous difficulties. Another barrier is the lack of willingness to share due to fear that competitors will fare better upon collaboration. Other issues, such as physician autonomy, make behavioral changes in the health care industry particularly complicated. Because physicians are considered experts because of their highly specialized knowledge of the complex field of medicine, it can be difficult for non-physicians to evaluate the work of physicians and be heeded. The presence of many small group practices adds to the insularity of health care providers, making the widespread transfer of knowledge challenging. Transfers of knowledge between different health care settings are often of inconsistent quality and thus an additional barrier to knowledge transfer. The largely decentralized nature of health care research is another barrier.

With the copious amounts of new ideas and technologies that are constantly being introduced, researchers need to develop a filter for use among providers that will allow providers to differentiate good and bad ideas. Guidelines for good ideas are difficult to develop, however, because of issues such as a provider's need to alter interventions to fit local needs, as well as the time required to elicit measurable changes in outcomes. Widespread knowledge transfer of health care practices is challenging and is an area requiring increased attention and research.

Knowledge Transfer Within the QIO Program

With the multitude of players in the health care delivery system, knowledge is gained on many fronts and can be transferred in many directions, as displayed in Figure 9.1. In the QIO program, sharing occurs mainly between CMS and the QIOs through the QIOSCs and between the QIOs and the providers. However, ideas are also exchanged between QIOs, among providers, from providers to QIOs, from QIO to QIOSCs, and from QIOSCs to CMS. Beneficiaries also play an integral role in this process through beneficiary education (the transfer of knowledge from QIOs and providers to beneficiaries) and through assessments of beneficiaries' perspectives of care (from beneficiaries to QIOs and providers). In combination, these multiple paths of knowledge transfer can help strengthen the communication and effectiveness of the QIO program.

QIO Support Centers

QIOSCs provide technical assistance to QIOs, just as the QIOs offer technical assistance to providers, to achieve improvements in care, as discussed in Chapters 7 and 8. QIOSCs are critical to the sharing of information among QIOs. Unlike the core QIO contracts, which are based on a point scale (see Chapter 10), CMS assesses QIOSCs on how satisfactorily their deliverables are met on the basis of the judgment of the Government Task Leader in charge of each QIOSC (see Chapter 13). CMS's evaluations of the QIOSCs in the 7th SOW led to a redesign of the QIOSC system for the 8th SOW (see Chapter 8) (personal communication, J. Taylor, April 29, 2005). With recognition of the unique feedback that QIOs can provide to the QIOSC system as the customers of the QIOSCs, a survey that assessed QIO satisfaction with the QIOSCs was added to the 8th SOW as part of the redesign of the SOW. Evaluation of QIOSC effectiveness by CMS will therefore be a function of satisfaction from both the Government Task Leaders and the QIOs.

One approach used to transfer knowledge in the QIO program is the Process Improvement QIOSC, which was created in the 7th SOW and which has been renamed the Performance Improvement QIOSC in the 8th SOW. Qualis Health led this QIOSC in both the 7th and the 8th SOWs. The goal of this QIOSC is to ensure the efficiency and effectiveness of QIO processes by creating a "culture of shameless stealing" to exchange best practices (Qualis Health, 2005b). To achieve this goal, this QIOSC trains both QIOs and providers on running and facilitating collaboratives following the design of the Institute for Healthcare Improvement Breakthrough Series Col-

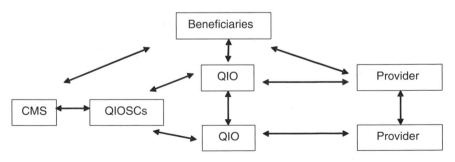

FIGURE 9.1   Knowledge transfer in the QIO program.

laborative (see Chapter 8). Although the evidence base for collaborative initiatives remains inconclusive, as discussed earlier in this chapter, in the 7th SOW, Qualis Health assisted with the implementation of more than seven collaboratives, each of which focused on different aspects of technical assistance tasks. Many of the providers involved in collaboratives made improvements, such as increasing the rate of antibiotic use from 78 to 91 percent among patients with pneumonia in 14 critical access hospitals in an 8-month collaborative in Idaho (Qualis Health, 2005a). However, because of the limitations of measuring and attributing improvement, the impact of the QIO intervention cannot be separated from those of other possible interventions or factors. Beyond instilling a culture of quality improvement through collaboration, the leaders of these initiatives hope that the providers involved transfer the knowledge that they have gained to others in their communities.

On the basis of the interviews with QIOSC CEOs and staff, the QIOSCs mentioned the following as barriers to their missions: imprecise evaluation methods, the rigidity of CMS oversight, a lack of contract flexibility, the timing of the QIOSC contract (which is aligned with the start of the SOW, and thus does not allow the QIOSCs time to develop materials before the beginning of the SOW), and the timing of the approval and distribution of the tools developed by the QIOSCs.

In telephone interviews with 20 QIO CEOs, the QIOSCs received mixed reviews in terms of both expertise and timeliness. The following are some of the criticisms of the QIOSCs from the overall assessments of the QIOSCs by the QIO CEOs:

• QIO task-related materials were not made available in a timely enough manner, at times forcing QIOs to produce their own.
• The focus or the target of the materials was not always applicable to all states because of differences in state sizes, regional influences, and population demographics.
• The innovativeness of the interventions and the materials did not necessarily lead to significant changes in areas where the QIOs needed support.
• The flow of information was backwards, in that the QIOs offered more support to the QIOSCs than the other way around.

QIO-to-QIO Knowledge Transfer

The development and alteration of interventions at the state level but with maintenance of the core attributes of the interventions that can result in improvement are key to successful quality improvement within each state because of differences in local environments. The QIOs can develop and alter interventions independently or partner with other public or private organizations. Interventions often develop in the QIO program as part of pilot tests or special studies. An example of a successful pilot program was the Cooperative Cardiovascular Project, which began as a four-state pilot project in 1995 that was eventually implemented on a national scale. An 11-state pilot project that was under way at the time of this writing and that was expected to conclude in July 2005 is testing the ability of providers to assess specific process and outcome measures to reduce preventable hospitalizations in the home health setting (AHQA, 2005). If the pilot is successful, the 11 states in the pilot will be able to pass on the lessons learned and help other QIOs implement the intervention. In telephone interviews with the QIO CEOs, 8 of 20 CEOs commented that pilot testing is beneficial because it allows experience with the task at hand to be obtained before all QIOs are required to do the task.

In the telephone interviews, the CEOs also identified non-QIOSC QIOs as sources of information and assistance. This is echoed by responses to a question in the web-based data collection tool that asked the respondents to name the top three QIOs that they would turn to for help with technical assistance tasks. Fifty-seven percent of all the responders (88 of 155) said that they would approach a non-QIOSC QIO for support.

Best Practice Methods Special Study

Innovations created at the state level may not, however, be applicable to all QIOs because of variations among the states. A special study entitled the Best Practice Methods Special Study, run by the Process Improvement QIOSC, was a two-part study of the 7th SOW for determination of how successful interventions and lessons learned can best be transferred among the QIOs. The first part of this special study distinguished high-performing QIOs from low-performing QIOs on the basis of statistically significant comparisons of statewide performance with national performance on the 12 hospital measures used in both the 6th and the 7th SOWs. Using this categorization of QIOs as a platform, the QIOSC administered surveys to the QIOs in the high-performing group (eight QIOs) and low-performing group (nine QIOs). With the recognition of limitations because of recall bias and the relatively small sample size, the study identified the organizational characteristics of high-performing QIOs that resulted in the high-quality performance: staff empowerment, low staff turnover, flexibility, and staff in place at the beginning of the SOW. The QIOs with good reputations among providers scored higher. Greater CEO and board involvement were also associated with higher-performing QIOs. Standardized ("one-size-fits-all") interventions were associated with lower-performing QIOs; the higher-performing QIOs were able to customize interventions to meet their local needs. Differences in patient age, population education, and the frequency of provider interactions were not found to be associated with either high- or low-performing QIOs.

The second part of the Best Practice Methods Special Study examined the portability of the best practices identified in the first part of the study. Fifty hospitals participated in the second part of the study, 10 hospitals from each of the five participating QIOs from the states of Arizona, Colorado, Maryland, South Carolina, and Washington. Upon the implementation of similar processes of care for smoking cessation counseling and discharge planning, the special study attempted to determine whether certain QIO characteristics or interventions are transferable to other states, which would delineate the ability to transfer knowledge of best practices among QIOs in various environments (CMS, 2005a).

The Medicare Quality Improvement Community (MedQIC) is a publicly available web-based resource that primarily serves as an interface among CMS, QIOs, and Medicare providers. Support is available in the forms of tools such as fact sheets, templates, slides, presentations, specific information on process measures and guidelines for their collection, literature, and success stories for both clinical and consumer education. The QIOs and providers may also find contact information on the website for staff at the appropriate QIOSC. Providers can rank the tools available, as well as suggest new tools. A forum within MedQIC called QNet Quest is a database of answers to frequently asked questions. Through this database, providers can directly ask the QIOs for support (see Chapter 13 for a further discussion of MedQIC).

CMS-to-QIO Knowledge Transfer

CMS uses a variety of methods to communicate with QIOs, including memos, e-mails, face-to-face meetings, and various information and communications technology tools (see Chapter 13). In the telephone interviews, the QIO CEOs also cited CMS working groups and meetings with CMS Regional Offices as methods of knowledge transfer. CMS uses QIONet, an intranet site provided under the auspices of CMS's Standard Data Processing System available only to QIOs and CMS groups, to share information and tools for the purpose of improving program management and achieving program goals (see Chapter 13).

QIO-to-Provider Knowledge Transfer

The transfer of knowledge from QIOs to providers stemmed from the widespread sharing of materials beyond the identified groups of participants through the inclusion of a broader group of providers in meetings and through the inclusion of stakeholder groups that could then communicate with their memberships. Participants are provided with materials so that they can try to make changes on their own without receiving additional technical assistance from the QIO. In the telephone interviews with the QIO CEOs, the CEOs stressed the importance of champions and the use of stakeholder organizations. Additionally, the CEOs often mentioned how the electronic age aids with the transfer of knowledge within their states, particularly when providers are dispersed geographically or have limited time to spend away from their offices. QIOs use on-site meetings and technology like webex and other video teleconferencing methods. Some QIOs develop and send out compact discs containing quality improvement–related presentations to those providers who do not attend their meetings. Many QIOs hold statewide quality forums for the presentation of best practices for providers within their states and give out awards for achievement. Other QIOs publish articles in their state medical journals as well as in national medical journals. In telephone interviews, one QIO CEO mentioned the possibility of tying some quality improvement efforts to continuing medical education credits for physicians as a way to increase their participation.

Knowledge Transfer with Beneficiaries

Beneficiaries are an integral part of knowledge transfer. Input on how care is received is important in CMS's and QIOs' evaluations of the QIO program and the performance of individual QIOs. Beneficiaries also relate their perceptions of care to providers, who can then provide feedback to the QIOs. Knowledge is indirectly transferred from beneficiaries to CMS through the QIOs. Examples of the means of knowledge transfer from beneficiaries to QIOs include consumer advisory councils, representation of consumers on QIO boards, and beneficiary surveys on their satisfaction with the mediation of beneficiary complaints (see Chapters 11 and 12).

It is also important for beneficiaries to receive information from CMS, QIOs, and providers on the quality of care being delivered and what beneficiaries themselves can do to promote better health. CMS publicly reports data on the quality of care for individual nursing homes, home health agencies, and hospitals through its Compare websites (see Chapter 11). For example, CMS requires QIOs to maintain help lines to assist beneficiaries. QIOs sometimes also supply providers with fact sheets to distribute to patients.

How well knowledge has been transferred between beneficiaries and CMS, QIOs, and providers is not well documented. In the 7th SOW, beneficiary satisfaction surveys covered only mediation activities; in the 8th SOW, however, beneficiaries will be surveyed on all the care that they receive.

The telephone interviews disclosed that many QIO CEOs found beneficiary education to be valuable for quality improvement. For example, these activities may help QIOs build rapport with providers. It is also unknown whether consumers effectively use the data presented on the CMS Compare websites or call in to the QIO help lines (see Chapter 11). The actual impacts that these efforts have on beneficiaries and the quality of care that they receive remain unclear.

Other Knowledge Transfer Mechanisms

Other mechanisms of spreading knowledge among the QIOs have developed, such as those carried out through the American Health Quality Association (AHQA), which is the trade organization for the QIOs. Informal, unofficial groups of CEOs often come together on the basis of their geographic region or state size, such as the Coral Initiative, which started among five QIOs in the Midwest. Through AHQA and these other coalitions, QIOs meet periodically; learn about the latest program changes; and share successes and failures via telephone conference calls, listserves, e-mail, newsletters, etc. These groups foster a culture of sharing among the QIOs. As described by the QIO CEOs in the telephone interviews, "The problem is not the sharing but sifting out the scientifically based from the noise and self-promotion," and "Already we have free flow of information. Perhaps we have too much free flow because the focus is not on rigor in documentation. Lots of assertions are made about what works." The CEOs praised the specialized groupings of QIOs for their effectiveness in sharing and solving problems as well as the sharing that they perform through AHQA committees and conferences.

Many QIOs have been innovators of quality improvement, as interventions are often adapted to best fit the needs of each state or jurisdiction. However, if the development processes and successes of these variations are not shared with other QIOs, opportunities for improvement may be lost. Although some QIOs share their stories of innovation with others, an "owner" of this function who can make the information widely available is lacking. Although the QIOs are encouraged to publish articles regarding their work, QIO evaluation formulas did not emphasize those efforts in the 7th SOW. In the 8th SOW, CMS added acceptance for publication in peer-reviewed journals as an extra-credit point to the Hospital Payment Monitoring Program but not for other aspects of the SOW. Therefore, as QIOs are under performance-based contracts with limited time and resources, CMS provides little incentive to contribute to the literature.

SUMMARY

This chapter has discussed issues related to the impact of technical assistance for quality improvement and knowledge transfer both in the health care environment in general and in the QIO program in particular. The following are some of the main themes of this chapter, which are reflected in the findings and conclusions presented in Chapter 2:

- Quality improvement is difficult to achieve.
- The evidence for the impact of quality improvement interventions is mixed. Conclusions drawn from the literature base for quality improvement show that the quality improvements resulting from interventions in health care in general and the QIO program in the particular are similar.
- Quality improvement interventions were able to consistently produce significant improvements in process measures; other interventions, such as those focusing on outcomes and structure, were not found to yield improvements. There are, however, many limitations to the methods by which quality improvement interventions are documented and evaluated.
- Although the quality of care received by Medicare beneficiaries has improved somewhat, researchers have been unable to attribute these changes to the QIO program. This can be the result of various limitations, such as how QIO interventions are currently evaluated or the fact that QIO interventions do not improve quality.
- A variety of approaches to quality improvement are being tried in many industries, and QIOs are learning from these approaches.
- Collaboratives were often used to incite quality improvement in the 7th SOW. However, evaluations of collaboratives in the literature—both in the general health care environment and in the QIO program—have provided inconclusive results on their impact on improving quality.
- On the basis of the information in the literature, it cannot be determined what drives knowledge transfer in the general health care environment.
- Knowledge transfer in the QIO program is not well documented, making it difficult for the committee to find evidence for how effectively the QIOs achieve it. There are many paths for the transfer of knowledge in the QIO program; these could all be leveraged to achieve increased quality.

REFERENCES

AHQA (American Health Quality Association). 2005. Home health pilot project to provide model for SOW8 work. *AHQA Matters* 6(8):12–13.
American Society for Quality. 2005. *American Society for Quality.* [Online]. Available: www.asq.org [accessed September 7, 2005].

Asch SM, Baker DW, Keesey JW, Broder M, Schonlau MP, et al. 2005. Does the collaborative model improve care for chronic heart failure? *Medical Care* 43(7):667–675.

Barr JK, Franks AL, Lee NC, Antonucci DM, Rifkind S, Schachter M. 2001. A randomized intervention to improve ongoing participation in mammography. *American Journal of Managed Care* 7(9):887–894. (Erratum, 7(12):1116.)

Berner ES, Baker SC, Funkhouser E, Heudebert GR, Allison JJ, et al. 2003. Do local opinion leaders augment hospital quality improvement efforts?: A randomized trial to promote adherence to unstable angina guidelines. *Medical Care* 41(3):420–431.

Berwick DM. 2003. Disseminating innovations in health care. *Journal of the American Medical Association* 289(15):1969–1975.

Bradley EH, Holmboe ES, Mattera JA, Roumanis SA, Radford MJ, Krumholz HM. 2001. A qualitative study of increasing beta-blocker use after myocardial infarction: Why do some hospitals succeed? *Journal of the American Medical Association* 285(20):2604–2611.

Bradley EH, Carlson MDA, Gallo WT, Scinto J, Campbell MK, Krumholz HM. 2005. From adversary to partner: Have quality improvement organizations made the transition? *Health Services Research* 40(2):459–476.

Burwen DR, Galusha DH, Lewis JM, Bedinger MR, Radford MJ, et al. 2003. National and state trends in quality of care for acute myocardial infarction between 1994–1995 and 1998–1999: The Medicare Health Care Quality Improvement Program. *Archives of Internal Medicine* 163(12):1430–1439.

Centor RM, Allison JJ, Weissman NW, Canto J, Heudebert G, et al. 2003. Diffusion of troponin testing in unstable angina patients: Adoption prior to guideline release. *Journal of Clinical Epidemiology* 56(12):1236–1243.

Chu LA, Bratzler DW, Lewis RJ, Murray C, Moore L, et al. 2003. Improving the quality of care for patients with pneumonia in very small hospitals. *Archives of Internal Medicine* 163(3):326–332.

CMS (Centers for Medicare and Medicaid Services). 2005a. *Best Practice Methods Special Study: Report of First Year Scan of QIO Inpatient Practice.* Unpublished. Baltimore, MD: Centers for Medicare and Medicaid Services.

CMS. 2005b. *MedQIC Glossary.* [Online]. Available: http://medqic.org/content/Common Items/Article/glossary.jsp?g11n.enc=ISO-8859-1&topicID=&search=yes [accessed January 5, 2005].

CMS. 2005c. *8th Statement of Work (SOW).* [Online]. Available: http://www.cms.hhs.gov/qio [accessed April 9, 2005].

Coleman EA, Smith JD, Frank JC, Parry CP, Kramer AM. 2004. Preparing patients and caregivers to participate in care delivered across settings: The care transitions intervention. *Journal of the American Geriatrics Society* 52(11):1817–1825.

Cortes LL. 2004. *The Impact of Quality Improvement Programs in Long Term Care: Are State and Federal Quality Improvement Initiatives for Nursing Homes Redundant?* Austin: Texas Department of Human Services Division of Long Term Care.

Cretin S, Shortell SM, Keeler EB. 2004. An evaluation of collaborative interventions to improve chronic illness care framework and study design. *Evaluation Review* 28(1):28–51.

Daniel DM, Norman J, Davis C, Lee H, Hindmarsh MF, et al. 2004a. Case studies from two collaboratives on diabetes in Washington state. *Joint Commission Journal on Quality and Safety* 30(2):103–108.

Daniel DM, Norman J, Davis C, Lee H, Hindmarsh MF, et al. 2004b. A state-level application of the chronic illness breakthrough series: Results from two collaboratives on diabetes in Washington state. *Joint Commission Journal on Quality and Safety* 30(2):69–79.

Dellinger EP, Hausmann SM, Bratzler DW, Johnson RM, Daniel DM, et al. 2005. Hospitals collaborate to decrease surgical site infections. *American Journal of Surgery* 190(1):9–15.

Donabedian A. 1988. The quality of care. How can it be assessed? *Journal of the American Medical Association* 260(12):1743–1748.

Ellerbeck EF, Jencks SF, Radford MJ, Kresowik TF, Craig AS, et al. 1995. Quality of care for medicare patients with acute myocardial infarction: A four-state pilot study from the cooperative cardiovascular. *Journal of the American Medical Association* 273(19):1509–1514.

Ellerbeck EF, Kresowik TF, Hemann RA, Mason P, Wilblin RT, Marciniak TA. 2000. Impact of quality improvement activities on care for acute myocardial infarction. *International Journal for Quality in Health Care* 12(4):305–310.

Fleuren M, Wiefferink K, Paulussen T. 2004. Determinants of innovation within health care organizations. Literature Review and Delphi Study. *International Journal for Quality in Health Care* 16(2):107–123.

Gosbee J. 2002. Human factors engineering and patient safety. *Quality and Safety in Health Care* 11(4):352–354.

Gould BE, Grey MR, Huntington CG, Gruman C, Rosen JH, et al. 2002. Improving patient care outcomes by teaching quality improvement to medical students in community-based practices. *Academic Medicine* 77(10):1011–1018.

Greenhalgh T, Robert G, Macfarlane F, Bate P, Kyriakidou O. 2004. Diffusion of innovations in service organizations: Systematic review and recommendations. *Milbank Quarterly* 82(4):581–629.

Halm EA, Horowitz C, Silver A, Fein A, Dlugacz YD, et al. 2004. Limited impact of a multicenter intervention to improve the quality and efficiency of pneumonia care. *Chest* 126(1):100–108.

Heller C, Arozullah A. 2001. Implementing change: It's as hard as it looks. *Disease Management and Health Outcomes* 9(10):551–563.

Holman WL, Allman RM, Sansom M, Kiefe CI, Peterson ED, et al., for the Alabama CABG Study Group. 2001. Alabama coronary artery bypass grafting project: Results of a state-wide quality improvement initiative. *Journal of the American Medical Association* 285(23):3003–3010.

IOM (Institute of Medicine). 2003. *Priority Areas for National Action: Transforming Health Care Quality.* Washington, DC: The National Academies Press.

Jamtvedt G, Young J, Kristoffersen D, Thomson O'Brien M, Oxman A. 2004. Audit and feedback: Effects on professional practice and health care outcomes. *Cochrane Database of Systematic Reviews* (4).

Jencks SF, Wilensky GR. 1992. The health care quality improvement initiative. A new approach to quality assurance in Medicare. *Journal of the American Medical Association* 268(7):900–903.

Jencks SF, Cuerdon T, Burwen DR, Fleming B, Houck PM, et al. 2000. Quality of medical care delivered to Medicare beneficiaries: A profile at state and national levels. *Journal of the American Medical Association* 284(13):1670–1676.

Jencks SF, Huff ED, Cuerdon T. 2003. Change in the quality of care delivered to Medicare beneficiaries, 1998–1999 to 2000–2001. *Journal of the American Medical Association* 289(3):305–312.

Joseph AM, Arikian MJ, An LC, Nugent SM, Sloan RJ, Pieper CF. 2004. Results of a randomized controlled trial of intervention to implement smoking guidelines in veterans affairs medical centers: Increased use of medications without cessation benefit. *Medical Care* 42(11):1100–1110.

Kiefe CI, Allison JJ, Williams OD, Person SD, Weaver MT, Weissman NW. 2001. Improving quality improvement using achievable benchmarks for physician feedback: A randomized controlled trial. *Journal of the American Medical Association* 285(22):2871–2879.

Kosseff AL, Niemeier S. 2001. SSM health care clinical collaboratives: Improving the value of patient care in a health care system. *Joint Commission Journal on Quality Improvement* 27(1):5–19.

Landon BE, Wilson IB, McInnes K, Landrum MB, Hirschhorn L, et al. 2004. Effects of a quality improvement collaborative on the outcome of care of patients with HIV infection: The EQHIV study. *Annals of Internal Medicine* 140(11):887–896.

Leatherman S. 2002. Optimizing quality collaboratives. *Quality and Safety in Health Care* 11(4):307.

Luthi JC, McClellan WM, Fitzgerald D, Krumholz HM, Delaney RJ, et al. 2002. Mortality associated with the quality of care of patients hospitalized with congestive heart failure. *International Journal for Quality in Health Care* 14(1):15–24.

Marciniak TA, Ellerbeck EF, Radford MJ, Kresowik TF, Gold JA, et al. 1998. Improving the quality of care for medicare patients with acute myocardial infarction: Results from the cooperative cardiovascular project. *Journal of the American Medical Association* 279(17): 1351–1357.

Mark BA, Harless DW, McCue M, Xu Y. 2004. A longitudinal examination of hospital registered nurse staffing and quality of care. *Health Services Research* 39(2):279–300.

Massing MW, Henley N, Biggs D, Schenck A, Simpson RJ Jr. 2003. Prevalence and care of diabetes mellitus in the Medicare population of North Carolina. Baseline findings from the Medicare Healthcare Quality Improvement Program. *North Carolina Medical Journal* 64(2):51–57.

McClellan WM, Millman L, Presley R, Couzins J, Flanders WD. 2003. Improved diabetes care by primary care physicians: Results of a group-randomized evaluation of the Medicare Health Care Quality Improvement Program (HCQIP). *Journal of Clinical Epidemiology* 56(12):1210–1217.

Mills PD, Weeks WB. 2004. Characteristics of successful quality improvement teams: Lessons from five collaborative projects in the VHA. *Joint Commission Journal on Quality and Safety* 30(3):152–162.

Mittman BS. 2004. Creating the evidence base for quality improvement collaboratives. *Annals of Internal Medicine* 140(11):897–901.

NAE and IOM (National Academy of Engineering and Institute of Medicine). 2005. *Building a Better Delivery System: A New Engineering/Health Care Partnership*. Washington, DC: The National Academies Press.

NIST (National Institute of Standards and Technology). 2005, July 13. *Malcolm Baldrige National Quality Award*. [Online]. Available: http://www.nist.gov/public_affairs/factsheet/mbnqa.htm [accessed December 30, 2005].

Ornstein S, Jenkins RG, Nietert PJ, Feifer C, Roylance LF, Nemeth L, Corley S, Dickerson L, Bradford WD, Litvin C. 2004. A multimethod quality improvement intervention to improve preventive cardiovascular care: A cluster randomized trial. *Annals of Internal Medicine* 141(7):523–532.

Ovretveit J, Gustafson D. 2003. Using research to inform quality programmes. *British Medical Journal* 326(7392):759–761.

Ovretveit J, Bate P, Cleary P, Cretin S, Gustafson D, McInnes K, McLeod H, Molfenter T, Plsek P, Robert G, Shortell S, Wilson T. 2002. Quality collaboratives: Lessons from research. *Quality and Safety in Health Care* 11(4):345–351.

Qualis Health. 2004. *HCQIP Improvement Methodologies Survey Results*. Seattle, WA: Qualis Health.

Qualis Health. 2005a. *Case Study: Collaborative Experience Project, Surgical Infection Prevention*. [Online]. Available: http://www.qualishealth.org/qi/collaboratives/case-study-sipc.cfm [accessed September 13, 2005].

Qualis Health. 2005b. *Performance Improvement QIO Support Center (PI QIOSC)*. [Online]. Available: http://www.qualishealth.org/piqiosc/index.cfm [accessed November 15, 2005].

Qualis Health. 2005c. *Improvement Methodologies*. Seattle, WA: Qualis Health.

Schade C, Cochran B, Stephens M. 2004. Using statewide audit and feedback to improve hospital care in West Virginia. *Joint Commission Journal on Quality and Safety* 30(3): 143–151.

Schonlau M, Mangione-Smith R, Chan KS, Keesey J, Rosen M, et al. 2005. Evaluation of a quality improvement collaborative in asthma care: Does it improve processes and outcomes of care? *Annals of Family Medicine* 3(3):200–208.

Sheikh K, Bullock C. 2001. Urban-rural differences in the quality of care for Medicare patients with acute myocardial infarction. *Archives of Internal Medicine* 161(5):737–743.

Shortell SM, Bennett CL, Byck GR. 1998. Assessing the impact of continuous quality improvement on clinical practice: What it will take to accelerate progress. *Milbank Quarterly* 76(4):510, 593–624.

Shortell SM, Marsteller JA, Lin M, Pearson ML, Wu SY, et al. 2004. The role of perceived team effectiveness in improving chronic illness care. *Medical Care* 42(11):1040–1048.

Silver MP, Geis MS, Bateman KA. 2004. Improving health care systems performance: A human factors approach. *American Journal of Medical Quality* 19(3):93–102.

Snyder C, Anderson G. 2005. Do quality improvement organizations improve the quality of hospital care for Medicare beneficiaries? *Journal of the American Medical Association* 293(23):2900–2907.

Sutherland JE, Hoehns JD, O'Donnell B, Wiblin RT. 2001. Diabetes management quality improvement in a family practice residency program. *Journal of the American Board of Family Practice* 14(4):243–251.

Thomson O'Brien M, Oxman A, Haynes R, Davis D, Freemantle N, Harvey E. 2005. Local opinion leaders. *Cochrane Database of Systematic Reviews* (2)

Toussaint J. 2005, May 5. *Presentation at Pay for Performance Subcommittee Meeting*. Unpublished. Washington, DC.

Wang A, Wolf M, Carlyle R, Wilkerson J, Porterfield D, Reaves J. 2004. The North Carolina experience with the diabetes health disparities collaboratives. *Joint Commission Journal on Quality and Safety* 30(7):396–404.

10

Evaluation of Quality Improvement Achieved by the QIO Program

CHAPTER SUMMARY

This chapter addresses how the Quality Improvement Organizations (QIOs) performed on each subtask in the 7th scope of work (SOW) and how the Centers for Medicare and Medicaid Services (CMS) evaluated them, how CMS plans to evaluate the QIOs in the 8th SOW, the impact on quality improvement of a QIO working more intensely with an identified group of participants in a state as compared to the improvement among all providers statewide, and an assessment of provider satisfaction with QIOs.

At the end of the 3-year Quality Improvement Organization (QIO) program contracts, the Centers for Medicare and Medicaid Services (CMS) evaluates the performance of the QIOs on the basis of demonstrated improvements in the quality of care provided in their respective states or jurisdictions. The assessment of a QIO's provision of technical assistance, Task 1 of the contract for the 7th scope of work (SOW), is based on, among other things, its ability to improve clinical quality performance measures for activities in four provider settings: the nursing home, home health, hospital, and physician's office settings. CMS calculates the scores for each care setting. These scores lead to several questions: Is a QIO that successfully shows improvement in one setting likely to have high improvement scores in other settings? Does improvement in one setting lead to improvement in other settings? What patterns of improvement exist?

CMS EVALUATION OF QIO PERFORMANCE ON TECHNICAL ASSISTANCE TASKS

Evaluation of QIOs in 7th SOW

A section of the contract for the 7th SOW (Section J-7) defines CMS's plan for the evaluation of QIO performance and involves intricate formu-

TABLE 10.1   Measures of Clinical Quality

Care Setting	Clinical Quality Score Measure	Calculation
Nursing home	Relative change	1 – (follow-up/baseline)
Home health	Significant improvement (SI) rate	(Number of identified participants with SI)/(total number of providers in state eligible for SI)
Hospital	Reduction in failure rate	(Follow-up – baseline)/(1 – baseline)
Physician's office	Reduction in failure rate	(Follow-up – baseline)/(1 – baseline)

SOURCE: CMS (2005b).

las. The evaluation formulas separately consider each subtask of Task 1, technical assistance, which correlates with activities related to each care setting (see Table A.5 in Appendix A). Improvement scores are a function of clinical quality measures and provider satisfaction. CMS weights improvements in clinical quality more heavily than it does those in provider satisfaction in the calculation of overall quality improvement scores for each subtask, as depicted in the following formula[1]:

$$\text{overall subtask improvement score} =$$
$$0.8 \text{ (clinical quality score)} + 0.2 \text{ (satisfaction score)}$$

Section J-7 delineates different equations for the calculation of improvement in clinical quality measures for each care setting (Table 10.1). These clinical quality measures are then individually divided by the target levels of improvement to create a clinical quality score for each setting. Provider satisfaction scores reflect the actual satisfaction improvement rates divided by the target satisfaction improvement rates. Overall subtask improvement scores produce numerical values, which represent the quality improvement achieved by the provider. (See Box 10.1 for an example of scoring.) The scores are a function of change, so minimum and maximum scores did not exist in the 7th SOW (see Chapter 2 for further discussion).

Adding to the complexity of scoring, the clinical quality score for the nursing home, home health, and physician's office settings includes additional components: identified participant scores and statewide scores. QIOs must work more intensely with a group of providers within the state, called "identified participants." In the 7th SOW, the hospital subtask (Task 1c)

---

[1]Evaluation of the hospital subtask of Task 1 (Task 1c) differs by weighting clinical quality 0.75 and satisfaction 0.25.

did not require identified participants. Because QIOs work more closely with identified participants, improvements made by identified participants are weighted more heavily than statewide improvements in the calculation of clinical quality scores. However, QIOs spend only approximately one-third of the appropriated funds on Task 1 subtasks with identified participants; the remaining two-thirds of the funds are devoted to making improvements statewide (CMS, 2004b). CMS evaluated QIO work with underserved populations (Task 1f) on the basis of the judgment of the Project Officer; QIOs either pass or fail this subtask without an official numerical score. A hypothetical example of the scoring system is provided in Box 10.1.

Contract Renewal in the 7th SOW

To merit noncompetitive renewal of contracts for the 8th SOW, CMS required the QIOs to meet the performance criteria on 10 of the 12 subtasks in Tasks 1 to 3 of the contract for the 7th SOW. For Tasks 1a to 1e and Task 2b, the quantifiable subtasks, the QIOs had to score 1.0 or higher to meet the performance criteria. For the subtasks for which a QIO did not meet the performance criteria, the QIO had to meet the following minimums: (1) a score of 0.6 or higher on quantifiable subtasks (Tasks 1a through 1e and Task 2b) and (2) approval of the Project Officer on all nonquantitative tasks (Tasks 1f, Task 2a and 2c, and Tasks 3a through 3c). If these standards were not met, a QIO had to compete for the contract for the 8th SOW (CMS, 2002).

Evaluations in 8th SOW

For the 8th SOW, CMS developed evaluation formulas similar to those used in the 7th SOW. However, as discussed in Chapter 8, the focus of the 8th SOW broadened to include the areas of (1) clinical performance measure results, (2) clinical performance measurement and reporting, (3) systems improvement, (4) process improvement, and (5) organization culture change. CMS weights each of these areas differently, depending on the subtask (see Table A.6 in Appendix A). As in the 7th SOW, the improvements made by identified participants tend to carry greater weight than the improvements made statewide, although this does not hold true for all subtasks. The passing scores vary by subtask. Evaluation of provider satisfaction differs in the 8th SOW, with the addition of a stakeholder and a knowledge and perception survey (see the discussion below). All Task 1 subtasks require an 80 percent overall satisfaction and knowledge-perception score to pass. For all subtasks (for Tasks 1 and 3), CMS rates QIO performance as either excellent pass, full pass, conditional pass, or

---

BOX 10.1 Hypothetical Scoring Example

Charles Hill Nursing Home has volunteered to work with Quality-Quest QIO as part of QualityQuest's identified participant group. QualityQuest would like to work on reducing the incidences of the following selected four quality measures: (1) chronic care residents with pain; (2) chronic care residents with pressure sores; (3) acute care residents with pain; and (4) acute care residents with delirium.

In 2002, the baseline, Charles Hill reported that 22 percent of its chronic care residents reported having pain. In 2005, the follow-up, the nursing home reported that only 11 percent of its chronic care residents reported having pain. For the chronic pain measure, the relative change for Charles Hill is as follows:

Relative change = 1 − (performance at follow-up/performance at the baseline)
= 1 − (11 percent/22 percent) = 0.50
(50 percent relative change)

This calculation is repeated for all four measures. The worst score on a performance measure is dropped, and the scores for the remaining three measures are summed and averaged. This average score is then averaged with (1) those of the other identified participants in the state to create the QIO's identified participant score and (2) all the nursing homes in the state for the QIO's statewide score.

QualityQuest Identified Participant Clinical Quality Score

Calculation of Identified Participant Weight
Identified participant nursing homes as a percentage of all nursing homes in the state = 13.8 percent
Target percent participating = 10 percent
Identified participant weight = 0.44 × (percent participating identified participants/target percent participating)
Identified participant weight = 0.44 × (13.8 percent/10 percent) = 0.6

Calculation of Identified Participant Score
Baseline average of four measures: 9 percent
Follow-up average of four measures: 6.9 percent

---

not pass. CMS deems scores (see the discussions below for the derivation of the scores) greater than 0.95 as excellent pass, scores between 0.75 and 0.94 as full pass, scores between 0.65 and 0.74 as conditional pass, and any score below 0.65 as not pass. All QIOs must complete the core activities of each subtask to be considered for noncompetitive contract renewal.

Identified participant relative change = 23 percent improvement on the four measures

Target level of improvement for identified participants (set by CMS): 8 percent

Identified participant score = weight × (relative change in improvement/target improvement)

Identified participant score = 0.6 × (23 percent/8 percent) = 1.72

QualityQuest Statewide Clinical Quality Score

Calculation of Statewide Weight
Statewide weight = 0.8 − identified participant weight
Statewide weight = 0.8 − 0.6 = 0.2

Calculation of Statewide Score
Baseline average of four measures: 12 percent
Follow-up of four measures: 11.1 percent
Relative change statewide: 7.5 percent average improvement on the four measures
Target level of improvement statewide (set by CMS): 8 percent
Statewide score = weight × (relative change in improvement/target improvement)
Statewide score = 0.2 × (7.5 percent/8 percent) = 0.19

QualityQuest Satisfaction Score (surveys completed only by identified participants)

Identified participants: 89 percent
More than 80 percent of QualityQuest's identified participants were satisfied with the assistance that they received. Therefore, QualityQuest has passed the satisfaction component and will receive a score of 0.2.

Overall Nursing Home Improvement Score

Overall score = 0.8 (clinical quality score) + 0.2 (satisfaction score)
= 1.72 + 0.19 + 0.2 = 2.11

QualityQuest has scored above 1 and therefore has passed the nursing home subtask.

In addition, eligibility for noncompetitive renewal is generally contingent on the QIO achieving at least one conditional pass; noncompetitive renewal is rewarded if the QIO receives a full pass or an excellent pass on seven of the nine subtasks. Upon reception of a not pass on any subtask, CMS may invite the QIO to the evaluation panel (CMS, 2005c).

TABLE 10.2   QIO Results for Task 1 of the 7th SOW

Task 1 Subtask	Range of Scores[a]	Percentage of QIOs Passing	Other Subtasks
Nursing home (Task 1a)	1.71–7.37	100	No
Home health care (Task 1b)	0.22–2.2	35	No
Hospital (Task 1c)	0.77–3.2	94	No
Physician's office (Task 1d)	−0.13–2.4	56	No
Underserved/rural (Task 1e)	0.6–1.6	94	No
Managed care (Task 1f)	NA	100	No

NOTE: NA = not applicable.

[a]The range of scores indicates the lowest and the highest scores achieved among all QIOs in the 7th SOW, based on the above overall subtask improvement scoring formula.

SOURCE: Derived from data collected from CMS's Dashboard section on its internal website.

IOM ANALYSIS OF TASK 1 PERFORMANCE BY QIOs

The Institute of Medicine (IOM) committee performed the analyses described in this section on the basis of CMS's evaluation scores for the QIOs in Task 1 of the contract for the 7th SOW. The IOM committee collected data from CMS's Dashboard section, located on its internal website, QIONet (see the discussion below and in Chapter 13), as well as other data from CMS, as requested. In the interest of understanding why some states and provider settings showed more improvement on QIO quality measures than others, the committee conducted correlations between how the QIOs scored per clinical quality improvement task and the potential presence of confounding variables, such as performance on other Task 1 subtasks, the spending per beneficiary on that subtask, the QIO contract round, the QIO region, and provider satisfaction.[2] The data used to determine correlations for all tasks were current through December 2004 and were obtained from the Dashboard section of CMS's internal website, unless noted otherwise. Table 10.2 summarizes the results.

---

[2]These correlations used QIO scores determined by CMS evaluations described in Section J-7 of the 7th SOW and discussed earlier in this chapter. Correlations between improvement scores, spending per beneficiary, provider satisfaction, QIO contract round, and region were determined by calculation of the correlation coefficient, r. On a scale from −1 to 1 (with −1 indicating a direct negative correlation, 0 indicating no correlation, and 1 indicating a direct

Correlation of Overall Subtask Score with:

Spending per Beneficiary	QIO Round	QIO Region	Provider Satisfaction
No	No	No	No
No	Some	No	No
No	No	Some	No
No	No	Some	No
No	No	No	NA
No	No	No	NA

,

For all clinical quality improvement tasks, the overall improvement scores for each Task 1 subtask were not found to correlate with improvement scores in any of the other Task 1 subtasks. For example, a QIO's success in improving the quality of care provided by nursing homes did not indicate that the QIO would necessarily have success in improving the quality of care provided by hospitals. Also, the IOM committee did not detect any correlations between subtask improvement scores and QIO spending per beneficiary or provider satisfaction. Some association between the overall subtask score and the QIO contract round was shown only for the home health setting, suggesting that QIOs beginning in later contract rounds achieved greater improvements. The scores for hospitals and physicians' offices showed some association with QIO region.

As noted above, CMS calculated the scores of QIO performance in the 7th SOW for each subtask. However, no overall score for all technical assistance subtasks in Task 1 combined was calculated. During the IOM com-

positive correlation), all *r* values were less than 0.3. QIO round refers to the CMS contract cycle, which is implemented in a three-stage approach separated by 3 months for each stage. QIOs are split into four geographic regions: Boston, Dallas, Kansas City, and Seattle. Differences between QIO improvement scores per task and QIO region were calculated by using a one-way analysis of variance (ANOVA) test, followed by the Scheffe test; significance was considered if the P value was <0.05.

mittee's study, the question of being able to identify the overall high- and low-performing QIOs thus arose. Such an identification would, however, necessitate the derivation of a single composite score that could be used to rate the progress in quality improvement that each QIO had made in all four health care settings. Although the identification of high and low performers in a single care setting was possible (this was done by the Best Practices Special Study for the hospital setting) (CMS, 2005a), this was not the case when an attempt was made to include the scores for all care settings.

The IOM committee used multiple methods in its attempt to identify the overall high and low performers, but no clear method for the categorization of the QIOs on the basis of CMS scores could be devised. For instance, the scores for all four settings could be added together; however, if a QIO scored a 5.4 in the nursing home setting but scored −0.1 in the physician's office setting, there would be no way to tell that the QIO's technical assistance might have worsened in physicians' offices during the 7th SOW. The IOM committee encountered other challenges, such as how to ensure that all subtasks received equal weight and how to set the cutoff between high and low performance. The lack of a correlation among tasks and wide variations in performance, complemented by the complexity of the QIO program, thus made the committee unable to identify the high- and low-performing QIOs for Task 1 as a whole in a valid manner.

Although QIOs in general achieved improvements in measures that were calculated at the baseline (usually at the beginning of the 7th SOW) and that were then remeasured at the end of the 7th SOW, many of these improvements were not statistically significant. Many other factors may have affected provider performance, such as quality interventions from other organizations, but CMS did not document these factors. The evaluation in the 7th SOW focused on specific measures, subtasks, and individual QIO performance and does not demonstrate the actual impact of the QIO program or attribute improvements to QIO interventions; however, they do show changes in specific quality measures in each state.

Nursing Homes

7th SOW

Under Task 1a of the 7th SOW, each QIO worked to improve quality-of-care measures for identified participants as well as for all nursing homes statewide and developed a plan for this work as one of its four deliverables (see Table A.7 in Appendix A). For evaluation purposes, CMS used the reduction in failure rate to define "improvement." CMS based the evaluation of success on three components. First, the QIO had to demonstrate at least an 8 percent improvement statewide on three to five QIO-selected clinical measures (see Table A.3a in Appendix A). Second, the QIO had to demonstrate an 8 percent improvement on these measures for the identified participants. Finally, according to provider surveys conducted by CMS, at least 80 percent of nursing homes, whether they were identified participants or not, had to report an adequate level of satisfaction with the work of the QIOs. CMS rolled these three components into an overall score for Task 1a, weighting statewide improvement less heavily than improvement among the identified participants. Clinical improvement constituted 80 percent of the score, with provider satisfaction levels counting for 20 percent. QIOs that scored a value of 1 or greater passed the task; a score of less than 1 was considered failing (CMS, 2002).

For Task 1a, the IOM committee found no correlations between overall improvement scores and QIO spending per beneficiary, nursing home satisfaction rates, the QIO contract round, or the QIO region. In the 7th SOW, all QIOs achieved a passing score on this subtask (for the scoring formula, see Table A.5 in Appendix A), with improvement scores ranging from a low of 1.71 to a high of 7.37. Data from CMS's Dashboard shows that the identified participants had greater levels of improvement across all nursing home measures, with an average relative change of 46.5 percent, in comparison with the statewide average relative change of 16.7 percent. As of December 2004, all QIOs recruited more than the required 10 percent of identified participants, with one QIO involving up to 100 percent of all nursing home providers in the state (CMS, 2004a). Nationwide, during the 7th SOW half of all nursing homes participated with their QIOs with various levels of involvement in multiple interventions (personal communication, Y. Harris, December 28, 2004).

8th SOW

In the 8th SOW, the QIOs must provide 10 deliverables (see Table A.7 in Appendix A) for the nursing home task. A notable deliverable for evaluation is that QIOs set their own statewide targets for clinical improvement for all measures in this task. The identified participants must set their own personal targets for clinical improvement (CMS, 2005c).

As described earlier in this chapter, evaluation of QIO performance in the 8th SOW will build upon the components of the evaluation of performance in the 7th SOW (clinical quality and provider satisfaction) to include the following, where applicable: clinical performance measure results, process improvement, and organization culture change (see Table A.6 of Appendix A). As in the 7th SOW, CMS will weight the identified participant scores more heavily than the statewide scores, and the most emphasis will be placed on improvements in the clinical performance measure results. The total score for this subtask is 1.1 points, but the total possible score is 1.3 points, as the process improvement activities are worth 0.2 point of extra credit. However, the QIOs must meet the following core standards in the following areas: clinical performance measure results and organization culture change, as well as the satisfaction and knowledge-perception criteria. A score of 80 percent or higher on the satisfaction and knowledge-perception activities adds 0.1 point to the overall subtask score (this is discussed later in this chapter) (CMS, 2005c).

Home Health

7th SOW

The three QIO deliverables for Task 1b in the 7th SOW included the QIO training of home health agencies on the Outcome-Based Quality Improvement System (OBQI) (see Table A.7 in Appendix A). The QIOs had to demonstrate improvement in OBQI measures for the set of identified participants. The evaluation did not include a measure of statewide improvement. CMS based the evaluation of success on two components: (1) a statistically significant improvement in at least one indicator by 30 percent of the identified participants and (2) satisfaction with QIO performance by at least 80 percent of the participating home health agencies. Completion of the home health task required a score of 1 point or higher to pass (see Table A.5 in Appendix A) (CMS, 2002).

As in Task 1a, the IOM committee found no correlation between home health improvement scores and spending on that task per beneficiary, provider satisfaction, or QIO region. The QIOs in the first contract round, however, appeared to have higher evaluation scores than the QIOs in the second and third contract rounds, suggesting that the length of time invested in change may influence improvement in this subtask. Work in this provider setting was new in the 7th SOW, and 35 percent of the QIOs achieved a passing score. However, the contracts for the 65 percent of the QIOs that failed (scoring below 1.0) were not put up for bid on the basis of this failure, as most scored between 0.6 and 1.0. As of December 2004, the scores for the home health subtask ranged from 0.22 to 2.2 points (CMS, 2004a). These are not final scores for the 7th SOW, as the results for the second and the third rounds were not available as of this writing. An average of 22 percent of the identified participants in all QIOs attained significant improvement, which was less than the target of 30 percent. Only 17 QIOs reported that more than the required number of identified participants had significant improvement; one state reported that 73 percent of all home health providers in the state had significant improvements.

8th SOW

In the 8th SOW, the QIOs are responsible for providing nine deliverables (see Table A.7 in Appendix A), including lists of identified participants, the selection of one Outcome and Assessment Information Set (OASIS) measure (see Chapter 8 for a description of OASIS measures) for statewide improvement, and the home health agencies' plans to reduce acute care hospitalizations. Unlike under the 7th SOW, the QIOs will be evaluated on the basis of the improvements both statewide and among the identified participants. The target reduction in failure rates varies by measure and is prescribed by CMS for this task, unlike in the nursing home setting, in which each QIO is allowed to define its own targets. The targets for statewide reductions in failure rates for home health settings are lower than the targets for identified participant reductions (Table 10.3). The targets for identified participants were derived in order to match the 75th percentile of the 7th SOW. Selection of statewide targets included consideration of the rates for identified participants as well as the complexity of the measures.

TABLE 10.3 Task 1b Target Reduction Rates in the 8th SOW

OASIS Publicly Reported Measures	Target Statewide RFR[a] (percent)	Target Identified Participant RFR (percent)
Improvement in bathing	14	34
Improvement in transferring	8	31
Improvement in ambulation and locomotion	9	20
Improvement in management of oral medications	8	18
Improvement in pain interfering with activity	11	41
Improvement in status of surgical wounds	6	38
Improvement in dyspnea	17	41
Improvement in urinary incontinence	9	34
Provision of any emergent care[b]		
Acute care hospitalization	30	50
Discharge to community	10	35

[a]RFR = reduction in failure rate. Identified participants are excluded from calculation of the statewide reduction in failure rate.

[b]This measure will not be used in the 8th SOW.

SOURCE: CMS (2005c).

The evaluation plan for the 8th SOW weights clinical performance measures more heavily than the other components of evaluation for this task, with particular emphasis on acute care hospitalization. In addition to improving clinical performance measures statewide, the QIOs must improve immunization assessment processes statewide. As in Task 1a, the QIOs must achieve the targets set for the following core activities: improvements by identified participants in one selected OASIS measure, acute care hospitalization, and telehealth. Statewide improvements must be met for clinical performance for acute care hospitalization, immunization surveys, and the satisfaction and knowledge-perception standards. The total score for this subtask is 1.0 point; 0.27 point of partial credit and extra credit is available, making the total possible score 1.27 points. QIOs that achieve the satisfaction and knowledge-perception standards receive 0.1 point (CMS, 2005c).

Hospitals

7th SOW

The evaluation plan for Task 1c of the 7th SOW based success on statewide improvements in quality-of-care measures and hospital satisfaction with QIO performance. The only deliverable for Task 1c was a list of contact information for every hospital in the state (see Table A.7 in Appendix A). CMS calculated a combined topic average based on improvements on the quality indicators in each of the four topic areas. The QIO had to demonstrate at least an 8 percent reduction in failure rate for a combined topic average statewide. Additionally, a provider satisfaction survey had to indicate that at least 80 percent of the hospitals in the state or jurisdiction were satisfied with the activities of the QIO. CMS determined scores above 1.0 for this task to be passing (CMS, 2002).

The IOM committee found that the hospital measure improvement rates did not correlate with spending on this task per beneficiary, the QIO contract round, or provider satisfaction. An evaluation of hospital scores by QIO region did detect differences among regions ($P < 0.05$). This difference was driven by higher scores in the Kansas City region compared with those in both the Seattle and the Boston regions; the score for the Dallas region was not significantly different from that for any other region. On the basis of data from Dashboard, 94 percent of the QIOs appear to have achieved a passing score on the hospital subtask in the 7th SOW as of the end of 2004 (CMS, 2004a). At that time, the scores on this subtask ranged from 0.77 to 3.2 points.

8th SOW

For the 8th SOW, CMS subdivided hospital work into two subtasks: Task 1c1 focuses on hospitals in general, whereas Task 1c2 focuses on critical access hospitals. Successful performance on Task 1c1 requires the provision of six deliverables (see Table A.7 in Appendix A), including the implementation of systems improvement interventions, such as computerized provider order entry, bar coding, or telehealth. The eight deliverables for Task 1c2 include the submission of quality improvement measures, interventions, and change models as well as a safety culture survey (CMS, 2005c).

CMS bases its evaluations of these subtasks on both statewide and identified participant improvements. Statewide improvement carries more weight than identified participant improvement in the evaluation of Task 1c1; in Task 1c2, identified participant improvement weights more heavily than statewide improvement. Statewide, the core activities focus on the reporting of Hospital Quality Alliance measures (see Table A.3a in Appendix A) for both Tasks 1c1 and 1c2. For Task 1c1, identified participant work focuses on improving clinical performance measure results, processes for surgical care, and the use of electronic clinical information systems. For Task 1c2, identified participants must address the culture of safety in the critical access hospital, as well as the implementation of electronic systems. Task 1c1 is evaluated out of a total score of 1.1 points, with 0.2 point of extra credit and partial credit available, for a possible score of 1.3 points. The total possible score for Task 1c2 is 1.35 points. The meeting of satisfaction and knowledge-perception standards adds 0.1 point to the overall subtask score (CMS, 2005c).

Physician Office and Physician Practice

7th SOW

Task 1d had two deliverables, including a listing of all identified participants along with the participant's Unique Physician Identification Number[3] via PARTner (see Chapter 13 for a description of PARTner). CMS used three criteria to judge a QIO's success in Task 1d. First, the QIO had to demonstrate an 8 percent overall improvement statewide on quality-of-care measures for diabetes, cancer, and immunizations using a combined topic average. The score included weighting of the Health Plan Employer

---

[3]Medicare assigns a Unique Physician Identification Number to each provider or practitioner who participates in the Medicare program.

Data and Information Set (HEDIS) data so that Medicare+Choice beneficiaries and fee-for-service beneficiaries could be considered equally. The second criterion for the successful completion of Task 1d was achieving at least an 8 percent improvement on measures related to diabetes and cancer screening for the identified participant group. Finally, provider surveys had to yield at least an 80 percent satisfaction rate among the identified participants. QIOs scoring 1.0 point and above passed the physician's office task (CMS, 2002)

For this task, the IOM committee found no correlations between evaluation scores and QIO spending per beneficiary, the QIO contract round, or physician's office satisfaction. In testing for variations among QIO regions, the committee detected significant differences ($P < 0.05$) in physician's office scores, driven by the higher average scores in the Boston region compared with those in the Seattle region. Differences in performance among other regions were not significant. As of this writing, 56 percent of the QIOs appear to have achieved a passing score on this subtask. As with the home health care analysis, this does not insinuate that 44 percent of the QIO contracts were not automatically renewed, as many could have scored above 0.6 point. The scores ranged from –0.13 to 2.4 points. Physicians' offices volunteering to be an identified participant tended to have higher reductions in failure rates than physicians' offices statewide (with average reductions of 12.1 and 6.1 percent, respectively). As of December 2004, only two QIOs did not include the required 5 percent of active primary care physicians, and one QIO included up to 16 percent of all physicians' offices in the state (CMS, 2004a).

8th SOW

In the 8th SOW, CMS separated work with physicians' practices into three groups: physician practice (Task 1d1), physician practice for underserved populations (Task 1d2), and physician practice and pharmacy: Part D prescription drug benefit (Task 1d3). Task 1d1 calls for 12 deliverables, including documentation that assistance was provided to Medicare Advantage plans, documentation of support for the Physician Voluntary Reporting Program, implementation of electronic health records, and lists of identified participant groups. The core activities for this subtask are systems improvement by the identified participant groups and satisfaction and knowledge-perception surveys. Clinical performance measures are evaluated by the Project Officer and have been broadened to include the provision of statewide support for the Physician Voluntary Reporting Program, prevention and disease-based care processes, Medicare Advantage plans, End-Stage Renal Disease Networks, and offices participating in the Medicare Management Demonstration Project. The areas of focus for the identified participant groups are clinical performance measurement and reporting, process improvement, and systems improvement. The total score is 1.2 points; partial credit is offered for the systems improvement dimension of the subtask. The QIOs must achieve an 80 percent rate on the satisfaction and knowledge-participation surveys for 0.1 point (CMS, 2005c).

The four deliverables for Task 1d2 mainly consist of cultural and linguistic competencies, addressed primarily by the identified participant group. The identified participant activities for systems improvement and process improvement are the core activities for this subtask. Clinical measures focus on statewide improvements in immunization rates, mammography rates, and diabetes measures for underserved populations. CMS weights statewide improvements less heavily than improvements among the identified participants. The total score is 1.0 point; the satisfaction and knowledge-perception surveys are core activities that can add 0.1 point to the overall subtask score (CMS, 2005c).

Task 1d3—physician practice and pharmacy: Part D prescription drug benefit—has nine deliverables, including assessments of electronic prescribing feasibility, the baseline performance of Task 1d3 measures, and comprehensive responses to beneficiary complaints about prescription medications. Evaluation of performance on this subtask will be determined solely on the basis of the identified participants' activities and will be performed by the Project Officer and the Task 1d3 Government Task Leader. Achievement of the satisfaction and knowledge-perception surveys requirement is required to pass this subtask (discussed further in this chapter) (CMS, 2005c).

Underserved and Rural Beneficiaries

7th SOW

For Task 1e of the 7th SOW, CMS required the QIOs to demonstrate a reduction in a chosen disparity in a defined population from the baseline to remeasurement by the completion of three deliverables. CMS compared the improvements made by an identified group with those made by a reference group of beneficiaries; the difference in these improvements between the two groups had to be smaller at the remeasurement than at the baseline. (This is a significant distinction, because a concomitant improvement in the reference group can affect the difference in improvement between the two groups.) QIOs could earn extra points by fully documenting the description of the intervention group, the relationship between the disparity and the chosen intervention, and the effectiveness of the intervention (CMS, 2002). CMS considered a score of 1.0 point to be passing, whereas the maximum obtainable score was 1.6 points.

The IOM committee found no correlations between overall Task 1e scores and spending on this subtask per beneficiary per QIO or QIO round. In total, 94 percent of the QIOs passed this subtask; the scores ranged from 0.6 to 1.6 points (personal communication, J. Kelly, July 5, 2005).

8th SOW

In the 8th SOW, CMS has incorporated the underserved and rural beneficiary focus of the 7th SOW into selected subtasks of Task 1 (CMS, 2005c).

Managed Care Organizations

7th SOW

Successful performance of Task 1f required two deliverables, including submission of a plan of action to incorporate Medicare+Choice organizations into all other quality improvement tasks. Under Task 1f, the Project Officer considered whether the QIO demonstrated adequate initiative to include Medicare+Choice organizations in Tasks 1a to 1e. CMS also considered the Medicare+Choice organizations' satisfaction with their interactions with QIOs, with an expected minimum satisfaction level of 80 percent. Additionally, CMS looked to Medicare+Choice Quality Review organizations or other accreditation organizations to determine whether the Medicare+Choice organizations achieved demonstrable success in their Quality Assessment Performance Improvement projects. For overall evaluation of a QIO's success on Task 1f, the Project Officer gave equal weight to Quality Assessment and Performance Improvement projects (see Chapter 8) in conjunction with QIO technical assistance and achievement of an 80 percent satisfaction level (CMS, 2002). All QIOs with Medicare+Choice organizations in their states passed Task 1f.

8th SOW

QIO work with Medicare Advantage plans (formerly Medicare+Choice organizations) is incorporated into the appropriate settings during the 8th SOW. CMS did not separate out this work as a distinct task (CMS, 2005c).

IMPACT OF INTENSE QIO ASSISTANCE

In the 7th SOW, subsets of providers in the nursing home, home health care, and physician's office settings volunteered to work more closely with the QIO than other providers in the state; the QIO program recognizes

these providers as "identified participants." CMS's analyses of QIO interventions in the 7th SOW attempted to determine whether the identified
participants achieved greater improvements than the nonidentified participants; one goal of such determinations is to show whether more intense
QIO interactions yield a better quality of care. CMS shared preliminary
results in public forums, such as the American Health Quality Association
Technical Meeting in February 2005. The results suggested that the identified participants scored higher than the nonidentified participants (Rollow,
2004).

Upon initial analysis of these data, the IOM committee noted that the
results are limited by many confounders, including the following: potential
biases between identified participants and other providers, ignorance of
other quality improvement interventions in which the providers participate,
limited knowledge of the QIOs' statewide quality improvement efforts, and
the impacts of these other interventions. In addition, the methods and time
frames for determining the impacts of the intensity of work with the QIOs
are not consistent across care settings (i.e., inconsistent remeasurement periods) (personal communication, W. C. Rollow, July 8, 2005).

CMS plans to publish a study with more complete data that support
these findings; an advance summary of that study was provided to the committee. The study assesses the level of intensity of provider work with the
QIOs by separating the providers into groups (Table 10.4). Providers working more intensely with QIOs appear to have achieved greater improvements on measures than those that did not. However, the statistical significance of these improvements could not be determined from this summary.
CMS concluded that QIO assistance is, in general, valuable for improving
quality (CMS, 2005b).

PROVIDER SATISFACTION

7th SOW

In the 7th SOW, the scores on which QIO performance was based included dimensions of provider satisfaction with their interactions with QIOs
as well as the relative improvement on various performance measures.
QIOs needed to attain an 80 percent rate of provider satisfaction for Tasks
1a, 1b, 1c, 1d, and 1f, which contributed to 20 percent of the QIO's overall
score on each subtask (see Table A.5 in Appendix A). CMS contracted with
Westat to survey all the identified participants; CMS also included a selection of nonidentified participants from the nursing home and home health
settings for these surveys. The surveys yielded a response rate of 90 percent
from 21,710 providers nationwide. Westat sent the surveys by mail, the
Internet, and telephone; and the provider representative who served as the

TABLE 10.4   Summary of CMS Evaluation of 7th SOW

| Evaluation Parameter | Care Setting | | | |
	Nursing Home	Home Health	Hospital	Physician's Office
Levels of intensity	Nonidentified participants, identified participants, and select identified participants[a]	Nonidentified participants, identified participants, and select identified participants	NA[b]	Nonidentified participants and identified participants
Number of measures improved	4/6 measures improved	10/11 measures improved	17/18 measures improved	2/4 measures improved
Number of providers or beneficiaries (approximate)	13,000 providers	6,000 providers	3,700 providers	1.7 million beneficiaries
Measurement period[c]	Q2[c] 2002–Q2 2004	April 2002–January 2005	2000–Q4[c] 2004	2001–2004

[a]Select identified participants are identified participants focusing on improving a specific quality measure.
[b]NA = hospital data were unavailable for this summary.
[c]Q2 = second quarter; Q4 = fourth quarter.

SOURCE: CMS (2005b).

main point of contact with the QIO completed the survey. Questions ranged from asking about QIO-to-provider communications processes (i.e., "How satisfied or dissatisfied were you with the one-to-one e-mail communication?" and "How satisfied or dissatisfied were you with the timeliness of the QIO's response to your question or request for assistance?") to the content and outcome of QIO technical assistance (i.e., "When implementing our quality improvement projects, we used the information received from this QIO" and "Medicare beneficiaries are now better served by our organization thanks to the assistance we received from this QIO") (Westat, 2005:58–59).

The surveys covered the following six topic areas: access to health care, timeliness of response, information dissemination, technical support, professionalism and courtesy, and overall responsiveness to needs. The scores incorporated the aggregated survey responses, with each topic area weighted equally.

Westat determined satisfaction on the basis of a range of choices: very satisfied, somewhat satisfied, neither satisfied nor dissatisfied, somewhat dissatisfied, and very dissatisfied. When applicable, Westat used compa-

TABLE 10.5 Provider Satisfaction with QIOs

Task and Survey Respondent		Provider Satisfaction (percent)
Task 1a	Nursing home identified participants	91
	Nursing home nonidentified participants	75
Task 1b	Home health identified participants	94
	Home health nonidentified participants	81
Task 1c	Hospital	90
Task 1d	Physician's office	85
Task 1e	Underserved and rural	NA[a]
Task 1f	Medicare+Choice	93

[a]NA = not applicable.

SOURCE: Westat (2005).

rable choices of strongly agree, somewhat agree, neither agree nor disagree, somewhat disagree, and strongly disagree. Westat included responses of very satisfied and somewhat satisfied in the calculation of the satisfaction rate. Table 10.5 shows the providers' overall satisfaction with QIOs, listed by subtask.

Westat also performed an analysis of "key drivers" for satisfaction. That analysis determined that 93 percent of all providers responded that they were satisfied with both the ease of access of contacting QIOs and the timeliness of the response. Satisfaction with the provision of technical support varied depending on the type of assistance and ranged from a low of 84 percent (telephone conference calls) to 93 percent (training workshops, one-on-one telephone calls, and one-to-one e-mails). The overall value of QIO assistance was not equal across all types of providers and differed by participant status, as depicted in Table 10.6. The report suggests that the perceived usefulness may predict higher overall satisfaction with the QIOs (Westat, 2005).

8th SOW

In the 8th SOW, the QIO program will continue to evaluate the satisfaction of providers as a component of Task 1 subtasks. However, a new topic will be added to the survey and will ask providers about their knowledge and perception of both CMS and the QIO with which they work. Under the umbrella of satisfaction surveys, an independent contractor will also survey the beneficiaries about their interactions with the QIO program. Previously, the only beneficiary satisfaction surveys administered were by the QIOs themselves as part of their case review activities (see Chapter 12). In the 8th SOW, QIOs achieving at least an 80 percent score

TABLE 10.6   Value of QIO Assistance

Task and Survey Respondent		Overall Value (percent)
Task 1a	Nursing home identified participants	81
	Nursing home nonidentified participants	60
Task 1b	Home health identified participants	88
	Home health nonidentified participants	70
Task 1c	Hospital	77
Task 1d	Physician's office	72
Task 1e	Underserved and rural	NA[a]
Task 1f	Medicare+Choice	74

[a]NA = not applicable.

SOURCE: Westat (2005).

on the satisfaction and knowledge-perception surveys—core activities for all parts of Task 1—will add 0.1 point to their subtask scores. Task 1d3 is the only exception, for which 80 percent satisfaction is required to pass (CMS, 2005c).

A stakeholder survey and a QIO survey will also be introduced in the 8th SOW. The stakeholder survey will be conducted twice during the 3-year contract period and will measure how key health care system stakeholders view the QIOs and CMS. The QIO survey will allow the QIOs to voice their satisfaction or dissatisfaction about CMS's operation and management of the overall QIO program (personal communication, M. G. Wang, July 6, 2005). The QIOs will also be surveyed on their views toward the QIO Support Centers (QIOSCs), which will contribute to the formal performance evaluation of each QIOSC (personal communication, J. Taylor, April 29, 2005).

Although the IOM committee believes that surveys can be valuable sources of information for determination of the impact of the QIO program, as discussed in Chapter 5, the surveys must be designed and administered in a fair and clear manner with specific, actionable questions. In addition, analyses should be conducted to discern the characteristics of QIOs receiving high and low satisfaction ratings. Also, in keeping with the transparency of public reporting expected of providers, it would be appropriate to make public the various satisfaction scores of each QIO.

PROGRAMWIDE EVALUATION OF IMPACT

As shown throughout this chapter, evaluations of quality impacts have focused on specific measures, subtasks, and individual QIOs. Some data are presented for the nation as a whole but are based on summaries of changes in individual states. The program has not assessed the impact of the entire 7th SOW (including the combination of technical assistance activities with other requirements related to the protection of beneficiaries and program integrity). Although some QIOs have mentioned that the performance of case reviews sometimes brings quality improvement issues to light, these have not been documented in a method available for evaluation, nor has CMS assessed the impacts of program spending outside the core contracts, which is almost one-third of the funds apportioned.

SUMMARY

This chapter has discussed issues related to evaluation of the impact of quality improvement in the QIO program. The following are some of the main themes of this chapter, which are reflected in the findings and conclusions presented in Chapter 2:

• CMS evaluates QIO performance on the basis of a number of provider quality measures and deliverables provided for each task. Objective data that measure quality improvements are limited to what is in the evaluation scores.

• The method by which QIOs are evaluated is detailed and complicated, does not reflect any program priorities, and thus, neither reflects patterns of effective technical assistance nor helps the QIOs prioritize how best to approach the provision of technical assistance. This complicated method of evaluation is made even more complex in the 8th SOW. The levels of expectation for the various measures have implications for answering the question of whether QIOs improve quality; but because of the intricacies of CMS's evaluation formulas, the IOM committee was not able to determine whether the levels of expected improvement for each setting were adequate.

• The data used for evaluation may have selection bias. For example, QIOs may not recruit identified participants randomly; instead, identified participants may be selected on the basis of their ability to achieve the greatest improvement, thus yielding higher scores.

• Evaluation formulas do not reflect the differences between the monies spent on a particular subtask and the weight given to calculation of identified participant and statewide scores.

• Because identified participants volunteer to work with the QIO, they may be biased toward improving quality. This is important, as CMS weights identified participant improvements more heavily than statewide improvements.

On the basis of the QIO contract performance evaluations:

- In general, providers in all settings seem to be improving quality on most of the performance measures on which they are evaluated.
- The IOM committee was not able to identify correlations with substantial implications between subtasks, QIO spending per beneficiary, contract round, region, or level of provider satisfaction.
- However, a small but growing amount of evidence indicates that providers who work intensely with their QIOs achieve higher levels of improvement, are more satisfied with QIO assistance, and value QIO assistance more than those who do not.
- The lack of an overall program evaluation limits the IOM committee's ability to draw conclusions about the overall impact that the QIOs have had on quality.

REFERENCES

CMS (Centers for Medicare and Medicaid Services). 2002. *7th Statement of Work (SOW).* [Online]. Available: http://www.cms.hhs.gov/qio [accessed April 9, 2005].

CMS. 2004a. *QualityNet Dashboard.* [Online]. [accessed January 2005].

CMS. 2004b. *QualityNet Dashboard.* [Online]. [accessed August 26, 2004].

CMS. 2005a. *Best Practice Methods Special Study: Report of First Year Scan of QIO Inpatient Practice.* Baltimore, MD: Centers for Medicare and Medicaid Services.

CMS. 2005b. *Evaluation of the 7th Scope of Work: Special Advance Summary Report Submitted to the Institute of Medicine.* September. Unpublished. Baltimore, MD: Centers for Medicare and Medicaid Services.

CMS. 2005c. *8th Statement of Work (SOW), Version #080105-1.* [Online]. Available: http://www.cms.hhs.gov/qio [accessed November 4, 2005].

Rollow WC. 2004. *Presentation to IOM Committee: Evaluating the HCQIP Program.* Unpublished. October 4. Washington, DC: Institute of Medicine.

Westat. 2005. *Survey for Provider Satisfaction with Quality Improvement Organizations.* Unpublished. July 1. Rockville, MD: Westat.

11

Beneficiary Education
and Communications

CHAPTER SUMMARY

This chapter describes the activities of the Quality Improvement Organizations (QIOs) under Task 2 of the 7th scope of work (SOW), Improving Beneficiary Safety and Health Through Information and Communications. Under this task, the Centers for Medicare and Medicaid Services (CMS) charged the QIOs to inform beneficiaries about the purpose of the QIO program, their rights under the program, and how to exercise those rights (CMS, 2002, 2004b). The QIOs worked with other stakeholders in their geographic regions to coordinate beneficiary-related activities. Specific communications activities included the promotion of public reports of quality. The QIOs also assisted hospitals with preparation for self-reporting on the quality-of-care measures for these reporting efforts. Additionally, the QIOs maintained toll-free help lines; ensured consumer representation in their own organizations; and produced annual reports on their case review activities, which were available to the public. In the contract for the 8th SOW, CMS defined beneficiary education and communications activities only on a limited basis.

TASK 2A: PROMOTING THE USE OF PERFORMANCE DATA

Background

During the 7th SOW, the Quality Improvement Organizations (QIOs) assisted the Centers for Medicare and Medicaid Services's (CMS's) efforts to measure quality and disseminate quality information on Medicare providers in the nursing home, home health agency, and hospital settings through public reporting (CMS, 2002). CMS launched the Nursing Home

Quality Initiative in November 2002. That initiative sought to help beneficiaries, their families, hospital discharge planners, and others make decisions regarding long-term care as well as to encourage and help nursing homes improve the quality of care that they provide. The initiative worked in conjunction with Medicare's release of Nursing Home Compare (www.medicare.gov/NHCompare/home.asp), a website that allows consumers to compare nursing homes on the basis of certain quality measures and other information, such as staffing levels and type of ownership. In 2003, CMS began the Home Health Quality Initiative, which involved the public reporting of quality measures for home health agencies on the Home Health Compare website (http://www.medicare.gov/HHCompare/home.asp.) In March 2005, CMS launched the Hospital Compare website (http://www.hospitalcompare.hhs.gov.) CMS charged the QIOs to help promote each of these reporting efforts. The QIOs encouraged consumers to visit the sites, answered their questions, offered providers technical assistance with improving their performance on the reported quality measures, and promoted the sites to local media. The specific required activities included:

- Development of a work plan to promote each initiative, including state and local activities;
  - Participation in CMS communications conferences;
  - Distribution of appropriate materials;
  - Coordination of media outreach;
  - Response to consumer needs; and
  - Attendance at CMS training sessions (CMS, 2002).

Task 2a Data

Figure 11.1 shows the numbers of webpage views for the Nursing Home Compare, Home Health Compare, and the Hospital Compare websites. The Dashboard section of the CMS internal website (see Chapter 13) defines a webpage view as "the number of times an entire Web page was viewed, regardless of the number of graphics, objects, or embedded objects" (QIONet Dashboard, accessed November 11, 2005). The number of webpage views per month appeared to be steady over the year-long period reflected in Figure 11.1; however, changes in the number of webpage views cannot necessarily be attributed to the activities of the QIOs. Additionally, these exposures are likely attributable to consumers as well as health care providers themselves.

Table 11.1 presents the numbers of telephone calls to 1-800-MEDICARE for nursing home–related issues. (1-800-MEDICARE is the national telephone number provided to beneficiaries and others to answer

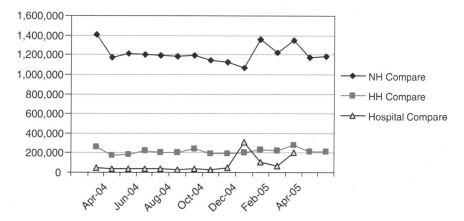

FIGURE 11.1 Numbers of webpage views (as of June 10, 2005).
NH Compare = Nursing Home Compare website; HH Compare = Home Health Compare website.
SOURCE: QIONet Dashboard (accessed November 11, 2005).

TABLE 11.1 Nursing Home–Related Calls to 1-800-MEDICARE

Date (mo-yr)	Number of Unique Calls	Total Number of Topics	Number of Referrals to a QIO	Number of Print-on-Demand Requests
Jan-04	3,126	4,029	NA[a]	100
Feb-04	2,662	3,277	69	88
Mar-04	3,156	3,811	65	72
Apr-04	2,749	3,303	82	72
May-04	1,310	1,599	29	51
Jun-04	2,373	2,898	49	67
Jul-04	2,632	3,167	45	78
Aug-04	4,998	6,027	72	111
Sep-04	3,701	4,328	63	70
Oct-04	4,044	4,672	47	45
Nov-04	4,803	5,566	84	71
Dec-04	4,919	5,741	93	78
Jan-05	6,636	7,775	121	104
Feb-05	7,115	8,290	138	80
Mar-05	7,550	8,688	118	88
Apr-05	7,013	8,069	128	78
May-05	6,747	7,805	110	57

NOTE: Data are as of June 10, 2005.

[a]NA = not available.

SOURCE: QIONet Dashboard (accessed November 11, 2005).

any Medicare-related question. It is not one of the help lines run by individual QIOs. Other issues related to 1-800-MEDICARE are discussed later in this chapter.) The data show the number of individual callers as well as the number of nursing home topics discussed. Note that each caller may discuss more than one topic. Table 11.1 also shows the numbers of callers to 1-800-MEDICARE who were referred to QIOs. Finally, the last column presents the total number of Nursing Home Compare print-on-demand requests. CMS generates these documents when a caller requests printed information from Nursing Home Compare. The data show an approximate doubling of the numbers of unique calls, the numbers of topics discussed, and the numbers of referrals made to QIOs over the entire time period.

The numbers of referrals made from 1-800-MEDICARE to individual QIOs as a result of these nursing home–related calls are shown in Figure 11.2.

Table 11.2 presents the numbers of calls to 1-800-MEDICARE related to home health topics. The table breaks down the topic areas mentioned in all calls. Again, one caller may mention multiple topics.

Interestingly, except for a sudden drop in the last 2 months of reporting, the data show gradual increases in both the total numbers of complaints and the total numbers of home health care–related topics discussed during this time period (see Figure 11.3).

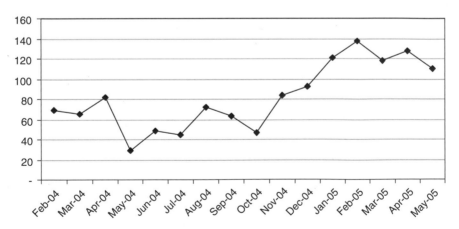

FIGURE 11.2   Referrals to QIOs from 1-800-MEDICARE for nursing home topics (as of June 10, 2005).
SOURCE: QIONet Dashboard (accessed November 11, 2005).

In the 7th scope of work (SOW), the Project Officer, the Regional Office Communications Specialist, and the Government Task Leader assessed the success of each QIO on Task 2a on the basis of the following:

- The extent to which the QIOs used information from CMS or others to alter their activities to reach their goals,
  - The timeliness of work plan submission, and
  - The timeliness of reports and deliverables (CMS, 2002).

Deliverables included:

- Submission of a work plan,
- Response to various information requests, and
- Maintenance of communications and planning tools (CMS, 2002).

In the 7th SOW, the QIOs spent $33.5 million on Task 2a, which represents approximately 4.2 percent of the QIO core contract budget (personal communication, C. Lazarus, March 17, 2005).

Experiences with Public Reporting

In telephone interviews with 20 QIO chief executive officers (CEOs), 11 CEOs independently raised concerns about public reporting. More than half of them noted difficulties with beneficiary understanding of publicly reported data and with the utility of those data for consumers when the consumers had a limited choice of providers offering Medicare services. Three CEOs commented specifically on problems in getting facilities involved in public reporting, one raised CMS's lack of timeliness as a drawback to public reporting, and three discussed the positive aspects of public reporting. Seven of the 20 CEOs mentioned problems with the utility of publicly reported data for beneficiaries and how simplification and presentation by CMS might enhance their value. Three CEOs commented on how public reporting, credentialing, and accreditation help with culture change by driving competition among providers. The mixed reaction of CEOs is evident in the variety of comments below:

- "Most of the roll out of nursing home and home health data is too complex for beneficiaries. Also, the reality is that our nursing homes are community based, and it doesn't really matter what the quality is because you go to the one in the area where your family and support system [are]."
- "The nursing home formula needs to be simplified; there are too many measures. There is no incentive for a nursing home to change because

TABLE 11.2   Home Health–Related Calls to 1-800-MEDICARE

Date (mo-yr)	Number of Calls Related to HH[a] Quality Initiative Overview	Number of Calls Related to HH[a] Quality Measures	Number of HH[a] Compare-Related Calls
Jan-04	9	11	142
Feb-04	9	3	101
Mar-04	4	4	70
Apr-04	2	1	90
May-04	4	1	72
Jun-04	5	4	110
Jul-04	NA[b]	4	86
Aug-04	9	2	144
Sep-04	2	1	109
Oct-04	8	3	107
Nov-04	9	1	124
Dec-04	8	6	133
Jan-05	10	4	156
Feb-05	9	3	131
Mar-05	10	3	156
Apr-05	25	4	NA[b]
May-05	14	2	NA[b]

NOTE: Data are as of June 10, 2005.

[a]HH = home health; [b]NA = not available.

SOURCE: QIONet Dashboard (accessed November 11, 2005).

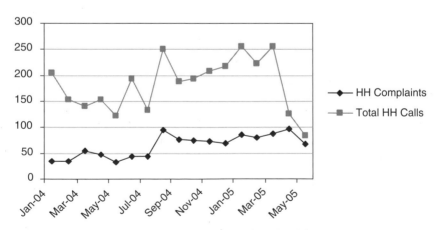

FIGURE 11.3   Home health care (HH)–related calls to 1-800-MEDICARE (complaints versus total calls) (as of June 10, 2005).
SOURCE: QIONet Dashboard (accessed November 11, 2005).

THE NATIONAL ACADEMIES PRESS

Publisher for The National Academies

National Academy of Sciences • National Academy of Engineering • Institute of Medicine • National Research Council

THE NATIONAL ACADEMIES
Advisers to the Nation on Science, Engineering, and Medicine

Visit our web site at

www.nap.edu

Use the form on the reverse of this card to order additional copies, or order online and receive a 10% discount.

ORDER CARD
(Customers in North America Only)

Use this card to order additional copies of **Medicare's Quality Improvement Organization Program**. All orders must be prepaid. Please add $4.50 for shipping and handling for the first copy ordered and $0.95 for each additional copy. If you live in CA, DC, FL, MD, MO, TX, CT, NY or Canada, add applicable sales tax or GST. Prices apply only in the United States, Canada, and Mexico and are subject to change without notice.

____ I am enclosing a U.S. check or money order.

____ Please charge my VISA/MasterCard/American Express account.

Number: _____

Expiration date: _____

Signature: _____

FOUR EASY WAYS TO ORDER

- **Electronically:** Order from our secure website at: www.nap.edu
- **By phone:** Call toll-free 1-888-624-8422 or (202) 334-3313 or call your favorite bookstore.
- **By fax:** Copy the order card and fax to (202) 334-2451.
- **By mail:** Return this card with your payment to NATIONAL ACADEMIES PRESS, 500 Fifth Street NW, Lockbox 285, Washington, DC 20001.

All international customers please contact National Academies Press for export prices and ordering information.

Medicare's Quality Improvement Organization Program: Maximizing Potential

PLEASE SEND ME:

Qty.	Title	Price
____	Medicare's Quality Improvement	$59.95
	Subtotal	____
	Shipping	____
	Tax	____
	Total	____

Please print.

Name _____

Address _____

City _____ State _____ Zip Code _____

10108

Number of Calls Concerned that the HH[a] Compare Website is Down	Number of Calls Concerned that HH[a] Compare is Moving Slowly	Number of HH[a]-Related Complaints	Total Number of Calls
3	4	35	204
4	2	35	154
7	2	54	141
11	2	48	154
9	4	33	123
31	NA[b]	43	193
NA[b]	NA[b]	44	134
NA[b]	NA[b]	95	250
NA[b]	NA[b]	77	189
NA[b]	NA[b]	75	193
NA[b]	NA[b]	74	208
NA[b]	NA[b]	70	217
NA[b]	NA[b]	86	256
NA[b]	NA[b]	81	224
NA[b]	NA[b]	87	256
NA[b]	NA[b]	97	126
NA[b]	NA[b]	68	84

the multitude of measures confuses the public and the public cannot judge what is a good and what is a bad nursing home."

• "Public reporting spurs culture change—facilities want to improve; otherwise, they might lose clients. Once the data are in front of them and they know they are so far behind they show great determination to turn around."

• "Fear of public reporting is what helps get hospitals and other providers to focus on quality and realize that they have to do something."

As of this writing, CMS had not defined any specific duties related to public reporting for the 8th SOW (CMS, 2005b).

TASK 2B: TRANSITIONING TO HOSPITAL-GENERATED DATA

In the 7th SOW, the overall purpose of Task 2b was to prepare hospitals for public reporting. Initiatives such as the National Voluntary Hospital Reporting Initiative (now known as the Hospital Quality Alliance) and the Reporting Hospital Quality Data for Annual Payment Update motivated hospitals to collect their own data using standardized measure specifications (CMS, 2002, 2004a).

The Hospital Quality Alliance is a public-private collaboration initiated by the American Hospital Association, the American Association of Medical Colleges, and the Federation of American Hospitals to begin the voluntary public reporting of certain quality measures by hospital providers. They were later joined by others, including the Joint Commission on Accreditation of Healthcare Organizations, the National Quality Forum, the American Medical Association, and the U.S. Department of Health and Human Services. This collaborative effort led to the development of a starter set of quality measures to be reported on the Hospital Compare website and encouraged beneficiaries and others to use the site to make better-informed decisions about their hospital care. The overall goals were to provide useful information to the public, align measures and reporting requirements, and ease burdens on reporting hospitals (Providence Health System, 2005).

The Reporting Hospital Quality Data for Annual Payment Update was a financial incentive established by the Medicare Prescription Drug, Improvement, and Modernization Act of 2003 (P.L. 108-173) for prospective payment system hospitals to submit performance data (see Table A.1 in Appendix A). Hospitals submitted data to the QIO Data Warehouse using the CMS Abstraction and Reporting Tool (CMS, 2005a). Qualifying hospitals that did not submit such data received a 0.4 percent lower update to their prospective payment system rates than the hospitals that did report data. As of the third quarter of 2004, 96.29 percent of qualifying providers were submitting data on these measures (QIONet Dashboard, accessed November 11, 2005). CMS did not require hospitals to participate in the Hospital Quality Alliance to receive the update but encouraged their participation in both initiatives. In the 7th SOW, the QIOs helped hospitals learn how to collect their own data on these measures. To facilitate this, the QIOs:

- Assessed the capabilities of each provider;
- Provided technical assistance on the collection, processing, and reporting of data;
- Performed data validation;
- Used data systems to collect confidential information; and
- Encouraged as many hospitals as possible to participate (CMS, 2002).

In the 7th SOW, QIO contract performance success on Task 2b was based on:

• The completion of surveys on hospitals' readiness for automated reporting (30 percent of the total score),
• The proportion of hospitals implementing data abstraction systems (50 percent of the total score), and
• Hospital satisfaction with QIO support in data abstraction activities (20 percent of the total score) (CMS, 2002).

The only deliverable for Task 2b was a survey of hospital readiness for automated reporting (CMS, 2002).

In the 7th SOW, the QIOs spent $38.3 million on Task 2b, which represents approximately 4.8 percent of the QIO core contract budget (personal communication, C. Lazarus, March 17, 2005).

TASK 2c: OTHER MANDATED COMMUNICATIONS ACTIVITIES

In the 7th SOW, CMS required the QIOs to engage in many communications activities to serve the beneficiary population, including:

• Establish a Consumer Advisory Council to advise the QIO,
• Maintain a toll-free telephone help line for beneficiaries,
• Publish an annual medical services review report (a report on all QIO review activities), and
• Reach out to hospitals and meet with medical and administrative staff (CMS, 2002).

The success of these interactions is questionable. As discussed in Chapter 7, the Consumer Advisory Council has only an advisory role on the main board and therefore may not have much of an impact in directing consumer needs. Also, studies of the effectiveness of Medicare's main toll-free number for beneficiaries (1-800-MEDICARE) as well as of carrier call centers reveal many problems. A July 2004 study by the Government Accountability Office found that only 4 percent of 300 policy-related calls made to carrier call centers received correct and complete answers (GAO, 2004a). In a December 2004 study by the Government Accountability Office, callers to 1-800-MEDICARE asked questions about eligibility, enrollment, and benefits. Only 61 percent of 420 callers received accurate answers (GAO, 2004b). The remaining answers were either inaccurate (29 percent) or unable to be provided (10 percent). Also in 2005, the Office of the Inspector General of the U.S. Department of Health and Human Services surveyed 305 callers to 1-800-MEDICARE and found that 84 percent of callers were satisfied overall (DHHS, 2005). However, 44 percent of callers related difficulty in accessing information because of difficulty with the telephone system, the lack of a full answer, or the speed of the response. Both of these studies recommend that CMS improve its help line organization and management. No information on consumer satisfaction with the QIOs' individual help lines was readily available.

Box 11.1 presents a template used by many QIOs for their Annual Medical Services Review Reports. These reports relate to case review activities (see Chapter 12).

In the 7th SOW, the Project Officer determined each QIO's success on Task 2c on the basis of the following:

- Establishment and use of a Consumer Advisory Council (see Chapter 7),
- Broadening of consumer representation on the QIO board of directors,
- Operation of a successful consumer help line (with success based on the findings of surveys of consumer satisfaction), and
- Production of an annual medical services review report (see Box 11.1) (CMS, 2002).

Deliverables included:

- Submission of a plan for the Consumer Advisory Council,
- Tracking performance of the help line, and
- An annual medical services review report (CMS, 2002).

CMS has not defined deliverables or evaluation plans for communications or beneficiary education activities because these activities are defined on a limited basis within other tasks (see Chapter 12).

In the 7th SOW, QIOs spent $32.4 million on Task 2c, which represents approximately 4.1 percent of the QIO core contract budget (personal communication, C. Lazarus, March 17, 2005).

ROLE OF QIOs IN BENEFICIARY EDUCATION: TELEPHONE INTERVIEWS

Nineteen QIO CEOs responded to questions about whether beneficiary education added value to quality improvement efforts and whether this function should continue. Almost three-quarters (14 of the 19 CEOs) favored continuation of this function. One of the 19 CEOs was unsure of its value because he believed that it depended on what CMS values, and the remaining 4 of the 19 CEOs thought that their QIOs could be successful without beneficiary education. One CEO who favored beneficiary education thought that this function could be done at the discretion of the individual QIO.

BOX 11.1 Annual Medical Services Review Report

<u>"Annual Medical Services Review Report:</u>

State:

Name of QIO:

Time Frame:

A. Beneficiary Complaints

Under Medicare law, Quality Improvement Organizations (QIOs) review complaints about the quality of care that Medicare patients receive. The complaints come from Medicare patients and/or their representatives. In reviewing a complaint, the QIO looks at the services a patient received and decides whether those services met standards of health care that are commonly accepted by physicians and others in the medical community.

"Quality of care complaints may involve more than one concern, due to the following: (1) more than one quality of care concern in a single setting; (2) the same quality of care complaint for a single patient episode of illness involving multiple settings and/or providers; (3) or more than one quality of care concern involving more than one setting and/or provider. For example, a Medicare beneficiary complaint related to a hospital stay might include several different quality of care concerns or a beneficiary who was hospitalized and then moved into a skilled nursing facility or other outpatient hospital setting might have the same quality of care concern occur in each type of setting. Consequently, for a specific Setting or Provider type, the number of quality of care concerns confirmed by the QIO may exceed the number of beneficiary cases reviewed.

"Beneficiary Complaint Cases: Number and Review Results

Number and Rate	Review Results
Total cases reviewed by the QIO:	Cases with confirmed quality concern:
Cases per 10,000 Part A Medicare beneficiaries:	Cases without confirmed quality concern:
	Cases in process (without completion date):

NOTE: Individual cases may involve more than one setting and/or provider.

continues

BOX 11.1   Continued

"Complaint Cases with Confirmed Concerns: The Setting or Provider

Care Setting or Care Provider	Total Number of Concerns	Number and Percent of Confirmed Concerns for the State	
		Number	Percent
Hospital			
Skilled Nursing Facility (SNF) (includes SNF, swing, and swing critical access)			
Home Health Agency			
Medicare Advantage			
Physician			
Other Provider			

NOTE: Individual cases may involve more than one setting and/or provider."

"Complaint Cases with Confirmed Concerns: Type of Problem

The numbers below represent only complaints by beneficiaries or their representatives. They do not include any other QIO reviews of medical services.

Type of Concern Confirmed	Total Number of Concerns	Number/Percentage of Confirmed Concerns	
		Number of Confirmed Concerns	Percent of Total Confirmed Concerns
Inappropriate or unnecessary services			
Inappropriate setting			
Services with a confirmed quality concern			

"B. Hospital Admission and Continued Stay Concerns

Under Medicare law, QIOs review the need for inpatient hospital care. They help determine whether a patient received care in the proper place or 'care setting.' This review may take place at two different times, either during or after a hospitalization. In the first instance, patients or their representatives ask the QIO to review a 'Hospital Initiated Notice of Non-Coverage,' or HINN, in which the hospital informs a patient that either an admission or a continued stay in a hospital is not needed. In such cases, the QIO conducts an 'immediate review,' whereby the QIO reviews the case (within 2 working days following the beneficiary's request for a pre-admission or admission HINN and within 30 days for review after discharge or when the beneficiary was not admitted to the hospital) and issues either a denial notice or a notice explaining that the care would be, or is, covered. In other cases where a hospital issues a HINN, but the patient does not immediately ask for a review, the QIO automatically reviews the case after the fact in what is called 'retrospective review.' In all reviews, the QIO staff looks carefully at the patient's medical record to decide if an admission or continued stay is/was needed.

"Beneficiary Notice Reviews

		Review Results	
		Appropriate Cases	Inappropriate Cases
Type/Timing of Review	Number of Cases	(Agree with notice)	(Disagree with notice)
Notice of Non-coverage FFS Preadmission Notice Concurrent Immediate Review			
Notice of Non-coverage FFS Preadmission Notice Nonimmediate Review			
Notice of Non-coverage FFS Admission Notice Concurrent Immediate Review			
Notice of Non-coverage FFS Admission Notice Non-immediate Review			
Notice of Non-coverage Continued Stay Notice			

continues

BOX 11.1   Continued

		Review Results	
"Type/Timing of Review	Number of Cases	Appropriate Cases (Agree with notice)	Inappropriate Cases (Disagree with notice)
Immediate Review— Attending Physician Concurs			
Notice of Non-coverage			
Continued Stay Notice			
Concurrent Non-immediate Review			
Notice of Non-coverage			
Continued Stay Notice— Attending Physician Does not Concur			
Notice of Non-coverage			
Continued Stay Retrospective			
Notice of Non-coverage			
Retrospective Monitoring Review			
NODMAR Immediate Review MA			
MA Appeal Review (CORF, HHA, SNF)"			

SOURCES: Georgia Medical Care Foundation (2005), Texas Medical Foundation (2005), and OMPRO (2005).

Two CEOs mentioned the indirect benefits of beneficiary education activities: "If you go to the media with just the professional side of the story, you wouldn't get any play; the beneficiary story gets the front page" and "Beneficiary education gives meaning to my staff by reinforcing the meaning of their work—quality of care for patients. If you continually only talk about systems of care, the work becomes estranged from the patient."

The reasons given for questioning the value of beneficiary education activities included the belief that limited funding is best spent on providers, that other groups could perform the function, and that most of the issues are too complicated for consumers. The one CEO who was unsure said continuation depended on what CMS wants QIOs to be accountable for:

"Are we trying to have a more satisfied beneficiary pool or are we trying to improve the value of health care? But there are some projects where involving beneficiaries would be beneficial."

Leveraging Education Funding

Among the 14 CEOs who favored continuing beneficiary education activities, three added that although they thought that this function should continue, the amount of money available allows the QIOs to do only a meager amount of education and that they did less education during the 7th SOW than during the 6th SOW. Another CEO said that working with beneficiaries does not have to be expensive; however, the costs may depend on the nature of the projects done with beneficiaries.

Seven of 19 respondents gave examples of how they leveraged their resources for beneficiary education by working with other groups in the community and statewide. These groups, in turn, communicate information on health and beneficiary rights to their memberships. In addition, some do the actual work of setting up influenza and pneumonia immunization clinics and support other QIO projects on issues like screening for depression and heart health. Two CEOs mentioned that they include beneficiaries in their work by having them on advisory councils for each of their tasks. Without involving and educating beneficiaries, the QIOs would "lose the pulse of what is on consumers' minds."

Need to Increase Beneficiary Education

Seven of the 19 CEOs argued for increased funding for beneficiary education activities. Three CEOs underscored their comments by saying that outreach to beneficiaries in underserved communities is essential in making change: Statements included, "We need to educate them to get better care and to take better care of themselves" and "As QIOs work to change systems and have more of a focus on chronic versus acute care, the need for educating consumers on patient self-management will only grow" because of the inability of physicians to spend sufficient time on education and physician shortages in some areas.

QIO SUPPORT CENTERS IN THE 7TH AND 8TH SOWs

7th SOW

Several QIO Support Centers (QIOSCs) collectively support the communications and beneficiary education activities of the 7th and 8th SOWs. First, Qualis Health (under its contract as the QIO for Washington State) acted as the lead for the Communications QIOSC, along with assistance from Primaris (Missouri's QIO) as a subcontractor. The Communications QIOSC coordinated strategic planning for all communications activities, including national initiatives and methods that promote the QIO program.

Another QIOSC strongly involved with communications activities is the Interventions QIOSC (run by the Iowa Foundation for Medical Care, Iowa's QIO), which supports the Medicare Quality Improvement Community (MedQIC) website (www.medqic.org). MedQIC (see Chapter 13) is a public website, available to both consumers and providers, that displays information about the QIO program and allows the sharing of knowledge. For providers, MedQIC presents specific stories and tools submitted by all QIOs on effective intervention programs for each of the task areas. For consumers, MedQIC supplies contact information for all the QIOs, but most of the website's content is aimed at providers or staff working in the quality improvement arena. The MedQIC website underwent a major structural overhaul in the 7th SOW. Version 2.0 was released in March 2005, and as of this writing, version 2.1 was scheduled for a November 2005 release (personal communication, J. Kelly, September 6, 2005). The redesign includes a new architecture and framework so that it is coordinated with the activities of the 8th SOW. In the 8th SOW, MedQIC strives to increase public awareness of MedQIC, including a collaboration with the Communications QIOSC and the American Health Quality Association.

Additionally, the Iowa Foundation for Medical Care supported other communications activities of the 7th SOW and held contracts to serve as a QIOSC for the following topic areas: outpatient data, hospital data collection, and the Standard Data Processing System (see Chapter 13).

Many of the other task-specific QIOSCs participated in beneficiary education activities during the 7th SOW through the supply of materials for providers to distribute to their patients, but CMS did not specifically designate a single QIOSC for beneficiary education.

8th SOW

In the 8th SOW, the QIOSC redesign (see Chapter 7) creates some restructuring of the QIOSCs' supporting communications and beneficiary education activities. Again, all task-related QIOSCs provide some degree of support to these interactions. Qualis Health continues as the Communications QIOSC in the 8th SOW, with Primaris continuing as a subcontractor. The Iowa Foundation for Medical Care continues its data-related activities under separate, restructured QIOSC contracts: the Hospital-Data Reporting QIOSC, the Outpatient Data QIOSC, the Data Reports QIOSC, and the MedQIC QIOSC. The Health Services Advisory Group (Arizona's QIO) supports communications activities as the new Measures Management QIOSC.

SUMMARY

This chapter has discussed issues related to the communications and beneficiary education activities of the QIO program. The following are some of the main themes of this chapter, which are reflected in the findings and conclusions presented in Chapter 2:

- QIOs have significant experience with the collection of data for performance measures and the promotion of publicly reported information.
- Little evidence exists to prove the effectiveness of QIOs' outreach to beneficiaries. The numbers of consumer visits to websites and the numbers of calls referred to the QIOs by Medicare are relatively low compared with the size of the entire beneficiary population. Studies have shown significant problems with CMS's main beneficiary help line (1-800-MEDICARE).
- Successive SOWs have had a decreasing direct-to-beneficiary role for the QIOs. In general, both CMS and the QIOs view providers as their primary customers.
- Beneficiary education most often occurs indirectly through providers as part of quality intervention plans or in partnership with local community organizations whose primary focus is on beneficiary concerns.

REFERENCES

CMS (Centers for Medicare and Medicaid Services). 2002. *7th Statement of Work (SOW)*. [Online]. Available: http://www.cms.hhs.gov/qio [accessed April 9, 2005].

CMS. 2004a. *The Quality Improvement Organization Program: CMS Briefing for IOM Staff*. [Online]. Available: http://www.medqic.org/dcs/ContentServer?cid=1105558772835& pagename=Medqic%2FMQGeneralPage%2FGeneralPageTemplate&c=MQGeneralPage [accessed December 26, 2005].

CMS. 2004b. *Quality Improvement Organization Manual*. September 16. [Online]. Available: http://www.cms.hhs.gov/manuals/110_qio/qio110index.asp [accessed May 11, 2005].

CMS. 2005a. *Hospital Quality Alliance: Improving Care Through Information*. [Online]. Available: http://www.cms.hhs.gov/quality/hospital/HQAFactSheet.pdf [accessed April 25, 2005].

CMS. 2005b. *8th Statement of Work (SOW)*. [Online]. Available: http://www.cms.hhs.gov/qio [accessed April 9, 2005].

DHHS (U.S. Department of Health and Human Services, Office of Inspector General). 2005. *Medicare Beneficiary Telephone Customer Service*. Washington, DC: U.S. Department of Health and Human Services.

GAO (U.S. Government Accountability Office). 2004a. *Medicare Call Centers Need to Improve Responses to Policy-Oriented Questions from Providers*. Washington, DC: U.S. Government Printing Office.

GAO. 2004b. *Accuracy of Responses from the 1-800-MEDICARE Help Line Should Be Improved.* Washington, DC: U.S. Government Printing Office.

Georgia Medical Care Foundation. 2005. *Annual Medical Services Review Report, Georgia, Georgia Medical Care Foundation.* [Online]. Available: http://www.gmcf.org/about/publications/Annual_Report_2004.pdf [accessed May 18, 2005].

OMPRO (Oregon Medical Professional Review Organization). 2005. *Annual Medical Services Review Report, Oregon, OMPRO.* [Online]. Available: http://www.ompro.org/downloads/annual_reports/0304MedQofCAnnualReport.pdf [accessed May 18, 2005].

Providence Health System. 2005. *The History of the Hospital Quality Alliance.* [Online]. Available: http://www.providence.org/alaska/quality/hqa_history.htm [accessed July 14, 2005].

Texas Medical Foundation. 2005. *Annual Medical Services Review Report, Texas, Texas Medical Foundation.* [Online]. Available: http://www.tmf.org/publicationsMedicareAnnual Report2004.pdf [accessed May 18, 2005].

12

Protection of Medicare Beneficiaries and Program Integrity

CHAPTER SUMMARY

This chapter discusses the case review activities that were under-taken by Quality Improvement Organizations (QIOs) during the 7th scope of work (SOW), including the categories and the types of reviews, the review process, and use of mediation, as well as the activities of the related QIO Support Centers (QIOSCs). Next, the chapter outlines the evaluation methodologies used for case review activities during the 7th SOW and the general case review activities of the 8th SOW, followed by an extensive discussion of the Hospital Payment Monitoring System in both the 7th and the 8th SOWs. Finally, the chapter describes the impacts of the case review activities in the 7th SOW.

During the 7th SOW, Quality Improvement Organizations (QIOs) performed tasks to protect both the beneficiaries of the Medicare program and the Medicare Trust Fund (CMS, 2002, 2004a,b). Beneficiary protection involved the review of all complaints about the quality of care or appeals of noncoverage decisions filed by Medicare beneficiaries or their representatives. These complaints and appeals could be submitted in writing or by telephone. Each complaint had to be reviewed for quality-of-care concerns, including the appropriateness of services and the appropriateness of the setting. The QIO program introduced mediation during the 7th scope of work (SOW) to replace the traditional case review process for certain beneficiary complaints. Until recently, the complainants received no information about the outcomes of their complaints. Today, the complainants receive answers concerning the confirmation of a presence or an absence of quality concerns but are not informed about the specific actions taken, if any are taken. If mediation is involved, the complainant may be aware of or involved in any subsequent actions.

QIOs helped maintain the integrity of the Medicare program by performing specific reviews related to utilization concerns, including hospital admissions and coding, to ensure that the reimbursed services were necessary and appropriate. Earlier cycles of the QIO program focused on case review, but this was primarily carried out only in the hospital inpatient setting and for fewer categories of cases. The numbers of review categories have continued to increase over the life of the QIO program, including through the 7th and the 8th SOWs.

CASE REVIEW ACTIVITIES IN THE 7TH SOW

In the 7th SOW, cases for review were generally brought to the attention of QIOs from outside sources, such as Medicare beneficiaries, intermediaries, carriers, or subcontractors; the Centers for Medicare and Medicaid Services (CMS) or the Clinical Data Abstraction Centers (CDACs) (discussed later in this chapter and in Chapter 13); and the Office of the Inspector General of the U.S. Department of Health and Human Services (DHHS) (CMS, 2002, 2004b). The Project Officer submitted each case referred by an outside agency to CMS's Central Office for approval before the QIO could conduct the review. In the 7th SOW, the QIOs performed case reviews under Tasks 3a and 3c. Task 3a—Beneficiary Complaint Response Program—required the investigation of all beneficiary complaints related to quality of care and allowed QIOs to offer mediation when appropriate. During this contract period, the QIO program adopted a new approach to the complaints process, in which a single case manager worked with the complainant throughout the entire process. In Task 3c—Other Beneficiary Protection Activities—QIOs performed all other case reviews (aside from those stemming from beneficiary complaints). Several different categories of reviews and types of review processes exist, and CMS has mandated specific requirements for each category and type of review in great detail in the *Quality Improvement Organization Manual* (CMS, 2002, 2004b). Activities related to Medicare Trust Funds protection also included the Hospital Payment Monitoring Program (HPMP) (Task 3b), in which QIOs worked to monitor and reduce the number of payments made in error in the hospital setting (HPMP is also discussed later in this chapter).

The type of review that a QIO conducted was based on the triggering event or category of review, as discussed below. Table 12.1 lists some of the most common types of reviews and the categories for which they were conducted. These include reviews related to beneficiary protection as well as protection of the Medicare Trust Fund.

TABLE 12.1   Types of Reviews for Each Mandated Category of Review

Category of Review	Type of Review	Provider Setting
Beneficiary complaints	Quality review	All settings except nursing homes (which are addressed by the state survey agency)
Potential EMTALA violations (patient dumping)	Quality review	Hospitals
Assistants at cataract surgery	Utilization review (medical necessity of a physician's assistant at cataract surgery)	Any setting, but not for Medicare managed care cases
Hospital-issued notices of noncoverage (HINNs)	Utilization review (medical necessity of admission, length-of-stay review, and appropriateness of noncoverage notice)	Hospitals
Notice of discharge and Medicare appeal rights (NODMARs)	Utilization review (medical necessity of admission, length-of-stay review, and appropriateness of noncoverage notice)	Hospitals
Fast-track appeals	Utilization review (medical necessity of admission, length-of-stay review, and appropriateness of noncoverage notice)	Skilled nursing facilities, home health agencies, and comprehensive outpatient rehabilitation facilities
Hospital-requested higher-weighted DRG adjustments	DRG validation and utilization review (medical necessity of admission)	Prospective payment system hospitals
Potential instances of gross or flagrant violations of professionally recognized standards of care	Quality review	All settings
Referrals from CDACs as part of HPMP	DRG validation and utilization review (medical necessity of admission and any procedure performed)	Acute care hospitals

NOTE: EMTALA = Emergency Medical Treatment and Labor Act; DRG = diagnosis-related group

SOURCES: CMS (2004b) and Northeast Health Care Quality Foundation (2005).

Categories of Case Reviews

The following are the required categories of case review that QIOs performed (CMS, 2002, 2004b):

1. Beneficiary complaints. Beneficiary complaints underwent either a traditional review process or the new option of mediation. Both processes are discussed later in this chapter.

2. Alleged antidumping violations of the Emergency Medical Treatment and Labor Act (EMTALA).[1] The QIOs did not determine or resolve EMTALA violations. Instead, the QIOs functioned to answer specific questions about screening, stabilization, and transfer. The QIOs performed either 5-day or 60-day reviews. The ultimate decision about EMTALA violations rested with the CMS Regional Office or the Office of the Inspector General of DHHS.

3. Requests for assistants at cataract surgery for fee-for-service beneficiaries. Ophthalmologists had to obtain preapprovals from the QIO for specific procedure codes that allow the use of and billing for assistants during cataract surgery.

4. Hospital-issued notices of noncoverage (HINNs). HINNs apply to services determined by the hospital to be medically unnecessary, custodial in nature, or provided in an inappropriate setting. Hospitals issue HINNs to beneficiaries or their representatives if the hospital determines that the current or future care of the beneficiary will not be covered by Medicare. The hospital is not required to acquire concurrence from the attending physician. QIO review of HINNs was performed upon the request of the beneficiary or his or her representative who wanted to appeal the notice and receive the services identified by the hospital as unnecessary or inappropriate.

5. Notices of discharge and Medicare appeal rights (NODMARs). NODMARs are delivered to Medicare managed care beneficiaries by a managed care organization or by a hospital on behalf of the managed care organization. NODMARs notify beneficiaries that their current hospital services will be terminated. Unlike HINNs, NODMARs can be issued only with the agreement of the beneficiary's treating physician. QIOs reviewed NODMARs immediately upon request of the beneficiary or his or her representative.

6. Medicare+Choice fast-track appeals. Medicare+Choice fast-track appeals were conducted at the beneficiary's request when the beneficiary

---

[1]Passed in 1986 as section 9121 of the Consolidated Omnibus Reconciliation Act (COBRA) of 1985 (P.L. 99-272).

received notice from the managed care organization that the services provided by a skilled nursing facility, a home health agency, or a comprehensive outpatient rehabilitation facility were being terminated. The managed care organization must issue a notice of Medicare noncoverage (also referred to as an advanced notice) at least 2 days or two visits before the services are to end. Upon receipt of the medical records, QIOs determined within 48 hours whether the services would be continued or terminated. These reviews, which were new in the 7th SOW, are also known as "Grijalva reviews," based on Grijalva v. Shalala, a class action lawsuit that challenged the managed care appeals process (CMS, 2005a).

7. Hospital requests for adjustments to a higher-weighted diagnosis-related group (DRG).[2] The QIOs performed these reviews to ensure that the diagnosis, the related clinical procedures performed, discharge status, and medical record all matched. An exemption existed for hospitals waived from the prospective payment system, in excluded geographic areas, or in the case of a beneficiary in managed care.

8. Cases of potential gross and flagrant violations or substantial violations in many cases.

9. HPMP is a specialized category of case review that is discussed in detail later in this chapter.

If a new quality concern arose during the review of a case in any one of these categories, then the QIO had to perform a separate quality review, in addition to the original review (CMS, 2002, 2004a,b). For example, from October 2002 to June 2005, the QIOs reviewed 1,950 records for EMTALA 5-day reviews and 1,196 records for EMTALA 60-day reviews (personal communication, J. Kelly, CMS, August 30, 2005). As a result, the QIOs conducted 34 reviews of the quality of care for concerns that arose during EMTALA reviews.

Types of Reviews

QIOs evaluated cases using three general types of review: quality reviews, utilization reviews, and DRG validation reviews (CMS, 2004b). In general, the QIOs performed quality reviews for cases related to beneficiary protection and performed utilization reviews or DRG validation reviews for cases related to program integrity.

---

[2]Diagnosis-related groups are codes that link diagnoses and procedures to a level of reimbursement.

Quality Reviews

Quality reviews assess whether the health care delivered to beneficiaries met professionally recognized standards, was provided economically, was medically necessary, and was supported by adequate documentation. QIOs performed quality reviews for cases of both fee-for-service and managed care beneficiaries, but managed care cases were assessed only on the basis of the appropriateness of the services provided and the setting in which they were provided and not on the basis of medical necessity. Quality review cases apply to services provided by many different types of providers, such as hospitals, home health agencies, and skilled nursing facilities (CMS, 2002, 2004b).

Utilization Reviews

Utilization reviews cover the medical necessity and the reasonableness of services provided, as well as the appropriateness of the care setting. QIOs did not conduct utilization reviews for services provided to beneficiaries in managed care. Any of the four reviews listed below might be conducted under the umbrella of utilization review (CMS, 2002, 2004b):

- Admission or discharge reviews,
- Invasive procedure reviews,
- Length-of-stay reviews, and
- Coverage reviews.

DRG Validation Review

The QIOs performed DRG validation reviews for prospective payment system hospital cases, including hospital-requested higher-weighted DRG assignments and cases in the HPMP (Task 3b of both the 7th and the 8th SOWs). The QIO did this type of review to ensure that the claims codes matched the information in the medical record. The reviewers examined diagnoses, the clinical procedures performed, and discharge status to validate the claim (CMS, 2002, 2004b).

Other Types of Reviews

In addition to quality, utilization, and DRG validation reviews, QIOs conducted additional specific case reviews on a more limited basis, as the need required. The following types of reviews were conducted only in conjunction with one of the types of reviews mentioned above (CMS, 2002, 2004b):

- Outlier reviews,
- Limitation on liability determinations,
- Readmission reviews,
- Transfer reviews,
- Circumvention of prospective payment system reviews, and
- On-site reviews.

Review Process

QIOs conducted the reviews described above with the assistance of contracted reviewers who met specified requirements (CMS, 2004b). At the initial level of review, nonphysician reviewers could be used if they had the necessary clinical education and the relevant experience to screen medical records. At least one registered records administrator or accredited records technician had to oversee the process. After the initial review, only physicians could be used for the remainder of the review process and generally had to meet the following requirements:

- Have authorization to practice medicine, surgery, osteopathy, dentistry, podiatry, or optometry;
- Be in active practice;
- Have the same medical license (as well as be in the same specialty) as the physician under review; and
- Be practicing in the same setting and state as the physician under review (if possible).

In general, the case reviews followed the structure outlined below, except for cases of potential gross and flagrant violations, for which a different, expedited process was used because of possible concerns of immediate danger. Similarly, HINNs and NODMARs had shorter processes because of time constraints (Figure 12.1).

Nonphysician Review

The nonphysician reviewer performs a first screening review, based on screening tools and professional expertise, to determine if:

- There is adequate documentation in the medical record;
- The case should be referred to a physician reviewer; and
- The medical services and items were provided economically and only when medically necessary, were provided up to professionally recognized standards, and were supported by evidence and documentation.

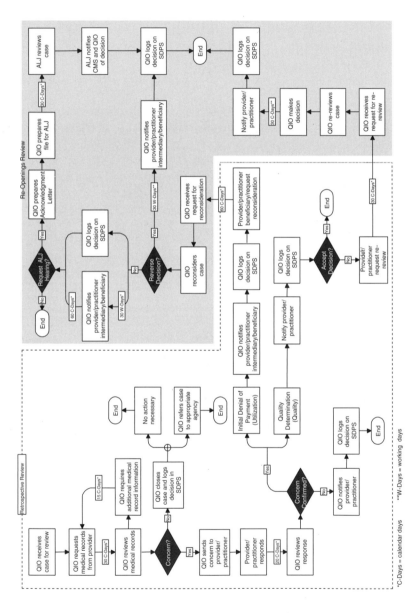

FIGURE 12.1 Standard mandatory case review process. SDPS = Standard Data Processing System; ALJ = Administrative Law Judge. SOURCE: CMS (2004b).

A second screening review is performed after any missing documentation is provided.

First Physician Review

In the first physician review, a physician reviewer determines whether the concerns of the nonphysician reviewer are valid and if other concerns not previously identified exist. If the physician reviewer determines there are valid concerns, the QIO sends a preliminary notice to the provider and offers the opportunity to discuss the case. If there is a potential gross and flagrant violation, the case follows a separate path.

Opportunity for Discussion

If the provider responds to the QIO's offer to discuss the case, the case is referred to a second physician reviewer. If there is no response, the first reviewer may make a final determination and notify the parties, or the reviewer may refer the case to a second physician if he or she is still unable to identify the source of the concern.

Second Physician Review

The second physician reviews the medical records, discusses the case with the parties involved, and makes the final decision.

Third Physician Review

When the provider under review requests reconsideration for initial utilization denials or rereview for confirmed DRG or quality concerns, a physician reviewer other than the ones from the first and second reviews examines the case.

Provider Response to Concerns

If a simple corrective action is needed (such as a DRG adjustment), the QIO can give the provider a chance to address the concern. For other issues, the provider must establish and complete a quality improvement plan (or a corrective action plan when associated with sanction activity), with assistance from the QIO as needed. Exceptions include flagrant violations and dangers to beneficiaries. No plan is needed when:

- The case is referred to a state or federal enforcement agency,
- There is a satisfactory explanation for the pattern,

- No reason for the pattern is found,
- The provider has already found the problem and taken action,
- The pattern for the case is the same as a pattern already identified and acted upon, or
- The physician is no longer in practice.

Other options are used when the provider is unwilling to formulate a plan or fails to complete the plan satisfactorily. The QIO must use the least intrusive option from among the following:

- Impose a QIO-directed plan (see Box 12.1),
- Negotiate a plan with the provider,
- Refer the case to the CMS Regional Office (or state survey agency),
- Refer the case to the state licensing board,
- Refer the case to the Medicare carrier, or

BOX 12.1   Example of Recommendation for a Quality Improvement Plan

"**Issue**: A 68-year old man underwent a total hip replacement. Postoperatively, the patient developed a deep vein thrombosis (DVT). The patient is concerned that the DVT was the result of the care he received. Per the record, the patient did not receive pharmacological anticoagulant therapy after his surgery. During the opportunity for discussion, the physician stated that he never uses pharmacological anticoagulant therapy, only mechanical.

"**Recommendation/Action**: Recommend that both the provider and the practitioner develop and implement a QIP, and also recommend initiation of intensified review activity.

"This situation warrants a QIP as there is published clinical evidence which shows that the standard of practice is to use a combination of anticoagulant medication and mechanical treatment after this type of procedure, and the physician states that he routinely chooses not to use pharmacological options. This is both the provider and physician's responsibility, since the hospital is expected to have their Chief of Staff work with a physician when accepted practice is not being followed. Intensified review of similar cases after QIP implementation can then be done to ensure the updated approach is being carried out."

SOURCE: Lumetra (2004).

• Refer the case to the Office of the Inspector General of DHHS for sanctions.

Sanctions can include a period of exclusion from the Medicare program (for a minimum of 1 year) and a monetary penalty (up to $10,000 for each instance). The provider may have the right to a preexclusion hearing, an administrative review, or a judicial review.

QIO Monitoring

The QIO monitors the provider during implementation of the quality improvement plan and must develop criteria that can be used to judge success, which may include a process or outcome assessment.

Provider Profiling Activities

On the basis of all of its review activities, each QIO was required to conduct certain profiling activities (CMS, 2002), including:

• Construction of a database consisting of data collected from all review activities for use in HPMP;
• Identification of possible interventions;
• Generation of provider profiles, when needed;
• Production of reports upon request by providers or CMS; and
• Determination of whether patterns indicative of a systemic problem exist.

If the QIO suspected a systemic problem, it could ask the provider to submit written guidelines of standard operating procedures. For example, if a communications problem between two specific departments of a hospital existed, the QIO may have asked the hospital to provide its internal guidelines on how the departments are supposed to communicate. For all review types, CMS required QIOs to maintain the Case Review Information System (CRIS), a tool used to report on activities to CMS (see Chapter 13). Through this application, the QIOs entered data related to the case review process to monitor a case's progress and ultimately produce reports on the timeliness of case review completion (CMS, 2002, 2004a,b).

MEDIATION IN THE 7TH SOW

QIOs reviewed all quality-of-care complaints filed by Medicare beneficiaries or their representatives. In any quality review, the QIO first determined whether no substantial improvement opportunities are identified or the care could have been better. Cases falling into the former designation were deemed appropriate for mediation. For the latter, the cases were further subdivided into the following categories:

- The care was grossly and flagrantly unacceptable,
- The care failed to follow accepted guidelines or usual practice, or
- The care could reasonably have been expected to be better (Lumetra, 2004).

Only the last of these three determinations represented a case appropriate for mediation.

QIOs could offer mediation in place of the traditional review process, but only if mediation was agreed to by both the complainant and the provider. Mediation tended to be recommended only in cases of a less serious nature, not in cases of grossly unacceptable care, nor when generally accepted standards of care were not provided (CMS, 2002, 2004a,b).

An example of a case appropriate for mediation might be one of miscommunication between the provider and the complainant. For example, consider a scenario in which the complainant claims that he received the wrong medication. A medical record review determines that the correct medication was given but that the instructions given to the patient were unclear. This case would be appropriate for mediation since there was no serious breach in the quality of care but the complainant should have received better information (CMS, 2002, 2004a,b; Lumetra, 2004).

MEDICARE BENEFICIARY PROTECTION QIOSC

In the 7th SOW, Lumetra (California's QIO) served as the Medicare Beneficiary Protection QIOSC (CMS, 2004a). CMS first awarded this contract in 2002 as a result of Lumetra's work on a pilot project in 1998 that sought to find alternatives to the traditional complaint process, including mediation and the use of case management approaches. In the 7th SOW, Lumetra provided assistance on protection activities by the use of various training methods and tool development. For example, Lumetra created the *Guide to Review of Quality of Care Issues for Physician Reviewers* to help standardize the review process, including the use of flowcharts for decision making (Lumetra, 2004). The two main objectives of the QIOSC were to (1) assist with the case management approach to beneficiary complaints, including mediation, and (2) develop methods for assessment of interrater reliability and evaluate interrater reliability for case reviews.

As a central source of information for case review activities, Lumetra acted to simplify and explain complaint and mediation procedures to pro-

---

BOX 12.2   Fast-Track Appeals Process

"**Step 1**: A beneficiary or his or her representative receives a *Notification of Medicare Non-Coverage* from a health care provider advising of an effective date when coverage for services will end, along with the beneficiary's appeal rights.

Step 2: By noon of the day before the effective date that Medicare coverage ends, the beneficiary or his or her representative calls Lumetra and requests an appeal.

Step 3: Lumetra informs the MEDICARE PLUS CHOICE ORGANIZATION immediately of the request for an appeal and requests copies of the Notice of Medicare Non-Coverage and the Detailed Explanation of Non-Coverage.

Step 4: Lumetra confirms the validity of the advance notice and requests the medical records to be faxed by the close of business that same day.

Step 5: Lumetra makes a decision on an appeal by close of business the day after it receives the information necessary to make the decision and notifies the beneficiary or their authorized representative, the MEDICARE PLUS CHOICE ORGANIZATION, and the provider of the outcome of the appeal.

"Your Responsibilities

The MEDICARE PLUS CHOICE ORGANIZATION is responsible for determining the appropriate effective date of termination of services and providing the advance notice. In some cases, MEDICARE PLUS CHOICE ORGANIZATIONS may choose to delegate these responsibilities to their contracting medical groups and providers.

The provider is usually responsible for delivering the Notice of Medicare Non-Coverage to all enrollees no later than two days before their covered services end. However, the production and delivery of the notices can be a collaborative effort between the MEDICARE PLUS CHOICE ORGANIZATION , the medical group, and the provider."

SOURCE: Lumetra (2005).

---

viders. Box 12.2 gives an example of the information that Lumetra shared with the Institute of Medicine (IOM) committee on how beneficiaries and providers in California experience the fast-track appeals process.

In November 2005, the Medicare Beneficiary Protection QIOSC contract for the 8th SOW was awarded to the Texas Medical Foundation (Texas's QIO).

QIO PERFORMANCE EVALUATION IN THE 7TH SOW

In the 7th SOW, CMS based a QIO's success in performing protection activities on:

- Daily updates of activities in CRIS;
- Development and implementation of a mediation plan;
- Reporting on improvement plan activities;
- Completion of beneficiary satisfaction surveys (after completion of the complaint process);
  - Collection of various contracts, reports, and other documents;
  - The timeliness of review completion (reviews should be completed within the designated time frames at least 90 percent of the time); and
  - Determination of interrater reliability (CMS, 2002).

In some specific review types, however, CMS considered only the timeliness of completion of the review (CMS, 2002). In all cases, no specific weighting was described in the QIO contract; the evaluation was mostly subjective. Deliverables included the documentation of activities related to the evaluation components listed above. HPMP is discussed separately later in this chapter.

CASE REVIEW ACTIVITIES IN THE 8TH SOW

In the 8th SOW, protective activities are combined under Task 3—Protecting Beneficiaries and the Medicare Program (CMS, 2005b). Under Task 3a—Beneficiary Protection—the QIOs continue all case review activities performed during the 7th SOW (Tasks 3a and 3c), including mediation, along with some of the communications and education activities of Task 2 of the 7th SOW (see Chapter 11). During the 8th SOW, QIOs must perform a new type of review as a result of the Medicare, Medicaid, and SCHIP Benefits Improvement and Protection Act (P.L. 106-554) of 2000 (BIPA). These "BIPA reviews" parallel the Grijalva reviews described above but apply to fee-for-service beneficiaries and include the hospice setting. QIOs conduct BIPA reviews at the beneficiary's request upon the beneficiary's receipt of a notice of noncoverage for services provided by a skilled nursing facility, home health agency, comprehensive outpatient rehabilitation facility, or hospice. The timelines are similar to those for Grijalva reviews, but BIPA reviews require certification by a physician that the termination of services will result in a risk to the beneficiary's health (Stratis Health, 2005).

In the 8th SOW, CMS will evaluate a QIO's success on Task 3a as follows (CMS, 2005b):

- Timeliness for all Task 3a reviews (24 points),
- Beneficiary satisfaction with the complaint process (21 points),
- Beneficiary satisfaction with the complaint outcome (13 points),
- Quality improvement activities resulting from case review (21 points), and
- Interrater reliability assessment (21 points).

The evaluation in the 8th SOW is even more complex because of the further definitions for conditional pass, full pass, and excellent pass for each of the elements listed above and then for the overall score. QIOs will receive an overall conditional pass if they attain 65 points, a full pass for 75 points, and an excellent pass for scores over 90 (CMS, 2005b). Deliverables for Task 3a include:

- Entry of data on all case review and helpline information into CRIS (see Chapter 13);
- Documentation of quality improvement activities resulting from case reviews, including how determinations were made and how the information was used; and
- An Annual Medical Services Review Report (see Chapter 11) (CMS, 2005b).

The Medicare Beneficiary Protection QIOSC continues to support these activities in the 8th SOW.

HOSPITAL PAYMENT MONITORING PROGRAM IN THE 7TH SOW

Under Task 3b of the 7th SOW, HPMP represented an effort by CMS to protect the Medicare Trust Funds by measuring, monitoring, and reducing improper payments for fee-for-service beneficiaries in the inpatient hospital setting. This QIO-run program sought to analyze whether the services rendered in the inpatient hospital setting were medically necessary and were provided in the proper setting and whether the DRG coding was accurate (CMS, 2002). For fiscal year (FY) 2002, the Office of the Inspector General of DHHS estimated that improper Medicare payments for fee-for-service beneficiaries totaled $13.3 billion, which represents approximately 6.3 percent of the $212.7 billion in fee-for-service payments made by Medicare (OIG, 2003). This number has been greatly reduced since FY 1996, when total improper payments were estimated to be $23.2 billion. CMS's Program Integrity Office, the DHHS Office of the Inspector General, and the Federal Bureau of Investigation, as well as the QIOs, all play significant roles in reducing these errors and in addressing fraud and abuse issues. In the 6th SOW of the QIO program, CMS addressed improper payments through utilization review and by the addition of the Payment Error Prevention Program. In the 7th SOW, the QIOs participated in HPMP, the successor to the Payment Error Prevention Program. Under HPMP, the QIOs worked to reduce (or at least maintain) the payment error rate in each state (CMS, 1999, 2002).

Clinical Data Abstraction Centers

Under HPMP, the CDACs screened claims for a random sample of inpatient hospital cases and then forwarded cases to QIOs for review, including a full medical review and DRG validation (see Chapter 13 for more information on CDACs). For HPMP, CDACs sampled for each state or jurisdiction 62 records of the discharges made each month, or approximately 38,000 to 44,000 records annually (personal communication, M. Krushat and W. Matos, CMS, October 25, 2004). Alaska and the Virgin Islands each had smaller sample sizes. QIOs reviewed CDAC-referred random samples of acute care prospective payment system hospital cases for improper payments. QIOs subsequently calculated statewide payment error rates on a quarterly basis. QIOs also assessed their case review reliability by comparing their results with CDAC's results. In addition to calculating the payment error rate, CMS also expected QIOs to monitor cases for trends in errors of admission or coding, such as:

- Inappropriate setting,
- Medically unnecessary or insufficient care,
- Incorrect DRGs, and
- Premature discharges or inappropriate transfers (CMS, 2004b).

Generating Reports for HPMP

When QIOs identified problematic patterns, they developed projects to correct those practices (after obtaining CMS approval). The QIOs used hospital-level reports developed by the HPMP QIOSC, known as the Program for Evaluating Payment Patterns Electronic Reports (PEPPER), to identify coding and admissions patterns that might be of concern because of their outlier status in comparison with statewide averages (CMS, 2002, 2004a; MassPRO, 2004; Texas Medical Foundation, 2005a). These reports included statewide comparative data that allowed the QIOs to show a hospital how it compared with its peers on certain indicators such as DRGs or 1-day stays. The QIOs then encouraged individual hospitals to participate in improvement plans (see the examples provided below).

QIOs implemented these improvement plans in the same manner as they implemented the quality improvement projects under their technical assistance duties. QIOs developed plans to target specific providers or topic areas and created project plans describing the background, purpose, and goals of the project, including what indicators and calculations were to be used to evaluate a hospital's success. CMS encouraged QIOs to collaborate with other entities, such as the Office of the Inspector General of DHHS, state agencies, intermediaries, and others to reduce the payment error rate or associated practice patterns of concern. QIOs encouraged hospitals to use the reports themselves to identify specific areas where they could concentrate their internal monitoring and improvement efforts (CMS, 2002, 2004b; MassPRO, 2004; Texas Medical Foundation, 2005a).

Table 12.2 gives an example of a report that can be used to inform a hospital of how it ranks among its peers on the use of specific DRGs. In this case, for FY 2003 the median rate for reporting one of the two indicated pneumonia-related DRGs among all pneumonia-related discharges was 21.71 percent. Therefore, an individual hospital may use the report to compare its reporting rates for individual DRGs to how its peers report those DRGs using the data provided by the QIO.

Table 12.3 shows a portion of a report that lists the number of total discharges in the state for a particular DRG, as well as the number of times that a patient had only a 1-day stay in the hospital under that DRG. A QIO may use this type of report to show individual hospitals how their 1-day-stay rates for a particular DRG compared with the state average. This is especially important because 1-day stays have been identified as a problem area and are indicative of inappropriate utilization and payment errors (Texas Medical Foundation, 2005c).

TABLE 12.2   DRG for Complex Pneumonia (DRG Code 079 and 080) Project from FY 2000 Through FY 2003

	Percentage of Hospitals Using DRG Code 079 or 080			
Parameter	FY 2000	FY 2001	FY 2002	FY 2003
10th percentile	12.25	10.65	10.91	11.11
Median	22.33	21.60	20.39	21.71
75th percentile	28.77	28.11	25.93	27.68
90th percentile	35.15	33.91	32.90	33.69

NOTE: Indicator 1 is the proportion of DRG Code 079 and 080 discharges (complex pneumonia) to total pneumonia discharges (DRG Codes 079, 080, 089, and 090).

SOURCE: Texas Medical Foundation (2005d).

TABLE 12.3   Texas 1-Day-Stay and Other Statewide Statistics for All DRGs

DRG Code	DRG Description	Number of Discharges after 1-Day Stay	Total Number of Discharges	Percent 1-Day Stays
005	Extracranial vascular procedures	2,231	6,971	32.00
006	Carpal tunnel release	13	25	52.00
066	Epistaxis	91	369	24.66
134	Hypertension	942	4,368	21.57

NOTE: The 1-day-stay count excludes deaths, transfers, and patients leaving against medical advice. Data are for all prospective payment system inpatient hospitals (n = 340), FY 2003 (October 1, 2002, through September 30, 2003).

SOURCE: Texas Medical Foundation (2005b).

Box 12.3 gives an example of how the Texas Medical Foundation (Texas's QIO) used data to identify a problem area (1-day stays for specific DRG codes) and then implemented a project to address the issue, including the use of a collaborative (see Chapter 8).

HPMP QIOSC

The Texas Medical Foundation acted as the QIOSC for the HPMP during the 7th SOW to:

- Develop and implement projects related to payment errors;
- Identify trends in payment errors;
- Advise the QIOs, hospitals, and others on the implementation of HPMP;
- Work with CDACs to produce PEPPER; and
- Develop tools, flowcharts, templates, etc., to help providers make decisions related to coding and the documentation of services (CMS, 2004a).

The Texas Medical Foundation continues as the HPMP QIOSC in the 8th SOW.

QIO Performance Evaluation

QIOs documented achievement in HPMP by comparing the statewide payment error rate at the baseline with the rate calculated at the end of the

7th SOW (CMS, 2002). The Project Officer and Government Task Leader determined the success of each QIO on the basis of the following criteria:

- The timeliness of reviews (the QIOs must meet the timelines at least 90 percent of the time),
  - The completion of a reliability assessment, and
  - Reporting of processes and findings to CRIS (CMS, 2002).

Additionally, the QIOs had to meet one of the following two criteria: (1) the follow-up payment error rate could not be more than 1.5 standard errors above the baseline error rate or (2) the QIO made effort and progress on all improvement plans (CMS, 2002). Deliverables included the development of a project related to problematic utilization or billing patterns and the determination of inter-rated reliability for review decisions (CMS, 2002).

HPMP IN THE 8TH SOW

In the 8th SOW, HPMP continues as Task 3b (CMS, 2005b). Again, the purpose of HPMP is to monitor and reduce payment error rates for fee-for-service beneficiary services in the hospital setting by looking at the accuracies of DRG codes, the medical necessity of services, and the appropriateness of the care setting. The QIOs continue with their hospital profiling activities as well as monitoring of admission and billing patterns. CMS continues to provide hospital-level reports, and subsequently, the QIOs must submit a project proposal to work on an inappropriate or incorrect utilization pattern or billing or coding pattern in either the short-term or the long-term acute care setting. Again, all projects are subject to the approval of the Project Officer and Government Task Leader and are funded as special projects under Task 4 of the 8th SOW (CMS, 2005b).

QIO success on the HPMP task in the 8th SOW is based on the following:

- Absolute and net payment error rates (no more than 1.5 standard errors above the baseline error rate) (1 point for each rate),
- The timeliness of reviews (2 points),
- Approval of the project (or justification for exclusion) and project implementation (3 points), and
- Documentation of monitoring activities (1 point) (CMS, 2005b).

If the QIO has an article about an HPMP project accepted for publication in peer-reviewed journals, it earns 1 extra-credit point. If the QIO does not publish its results anywhere (including the QIO's newsletter), 1 point is deducted. If no project is approved and no justification has been submitted,

BOX 12.3   Texas Medical Foundation One-Day-Stay Project

"Details

According to analysis performed by the Texas Medical Foundation (TMF), there was a 51 percent increase in one-day stay discharges between fiscal year (FY) 1999 and FY 2001, with a 164 percent increase in TMF-issued admission denials for one-day stay claims during the same period. In FY 2002, one-day stay discharges comprised 10.5 percent of total Medicare discharges in Texas; of these discharges, 17 percent were associated with diagnosis related groups (DRGs) 127 (heart failure & shock), 143 (chest pain), 182/183 (esophagitis, gastroenteritis and miscellaneous digestive disorders age >17 with/without CC [complication and comorbidity]) and 296/297 (nutritional and metabolic disorders age >17 with/without CC). Because one-day stays are known to be associated with medically unnecessary admissions, TMF chose to develop a Hospital Payment Monitoring Program (HPMP) project in this area. The goal of the One-Day Stay Project is to reduce inappropriate admissions for the following target DRGs: 127, 143, 182/183, and 296/297.

"Primary criteria for hospital inclusion in the project:
- At least 500 total one-day stay claims in FY 2002 and
- At least a 20 percent increase in one-day stay claims from FY 2000 to FY 2002.

"Secondary criteria for hospital inclusion in the project:
- Three or more target DRGs with at least 25 one-day stay claims each or
- A proportion of one-day stay claims to total claims greater than or equal to 12.8 percent (the 75th percentile for the proportion of one-day stay claims to total claims) and one target DRG with at least 25 one-day stay claims.

Of the 341 Texas PPS hospitals included in the claims data in FY 2002, 20 hospitals met the criteria for inclusion in the project. These 20 hospitals combined had 20,262 one-day stays, which represented 24.7 percent of the total one-day stays in Texas for FY 2002. The 20 hospitals had 2,969 one-day stays billed to the target DRGs, which represented 18.1 percent of the total one-day stays for the 20 hospitals.

"TMF is requesting that all hospitals:
• Analyze comparative data related to the project indicator provided by TMF as well as one-day stay data provided periodically by TMF in the Program for Evaluating Payment Patterns Electronic Report (PEPPER) to determine if problems might exist.

• Provide feedback to the medical staff on concerns related to inappropriate admission/discharge/quality of care and provide education on alternatives to inpatient admission when appropriate.

• Review TMF's educational information and distribute educational materials and tools provided by TMF to medical staff and other staff as appropriate.

"TMF is requesting that project hospitals:
• Perform an audit of randomly selected one-day stay cases identified by TMF in order to determine if a problem related to one-day stays exists.

• Develop an improvement plan if the internal audit identifies problems.

• Notify TMF of audit findings and any improvement plan initiated.

• Participate in TMF's One-Day Stay Collaborative (see below).

"TMF will:
• Perform case review of project hospital medical records to collect initial baseline data and later remeasurement data.

• Evaluate project hospital action taken regarding improvement plans and the quality of hospital-developed improvement plans and provide feedback as needed.

• Perform on-site hospital visits to project hospitals as needed to provide education.

• Provide one-day stay data and improvement tools to hospitals statewide.

• Conduct a One-Day Stay Collaborative over a one-year period based on the Institute for Healthcare Improvement's Breakthrough series. First face-to-face session will be held October 16, 2003.

• Conduct teleconferences on coding of DRGs associated with Medicare coding payment errors and other relevant topics.

• Disseminate educational newsletters."

SOURCE: Texas Medical Foundation (2005c).

the QIO loses 2 points. The QIO will receive an excellent pass for attaining 7 or more points, a full pass for 6 points, a conditional pass for 5 points, and a not pass for a score of 4 points or less (CMS, 2005b).

Deliverables for the HPMP task include a project proposal (or justification for exclusion) and monitoring reports via the Program Activity Reporting Tool (CMS, 2005b).

IMPACT OF PROTECTIVE ACTIVITIES IN THE 7TH SOW

Interaction with Providers

On the IOM committee's site visits to 11 QIOs, 3 QIOs mentioned that they have lingering difficulties in terms of their reputations as punitive organizations stemming from the history of the QIO program as one of pure utilization review. Additionally, during the IOM committee telephone interviews with the chief executive officers (CEOs) of the QIOs, 7 of 19 QIO CEOs noted that the QIOs were perceived as punitive enforcers. These 7 CEOs believed that that perception is currently more of an issue among nursing homes and home health agencies but that there is some residual feeling that the QIOs are punitive enforcers in the physician community in some states. One CEO indicated, "Perception as a punitive regulator is a problem. We are not generally viewed that way by hospitals, but it has taken a long time to convince nursing homes that we are not a Survey and Certification entity. Home health agencies are similarly concerned. Physicians don't care because they won't see any value or incentive until pay for performance." Another CEO commented, "Some older physicians still have the historical PSRO [Professional Standards Review Organization] mindset. We have a huge educational push to educate on quality assurance."

However, general consensus exists among QIOs (as exhibited during multiple site visits, interviews, and other personal interactions by the IOM committee) that this reputation has improved. Conversations with hospital CEOs confirm this perception (NORC, 2004; Bradley et al., 2005).

Case Review and Quality Improvement

In the telephone interviews, 19 QIO CEOs were asked whether the QIOs should continue the case review function and whether the performance of the case review function added to quality improvement. Only one CEO was not sure that the QIOs need to be the entity performing Medicare case reviews and appeals, but even he was not sure who else would do it well and believed that there is a need for the function to be continued by a qualified entity. The remaining 18 CEOs believed that case review was an integral part of the QIOs' overall quality improvement efforts because of its ability to protect beneficiaries and identify systemic quality problems. They strongly expressed their feelings about the need to keep case review as part of their repertoire and about the direct connections to quality improvement work:

- "Quality improvement is often predicated on the [basis of the] findings of case review. The connections between these functions should be strengthened if anything—not separated. Separation would be a disaster. We would no longer have a system."
- "Case review identifies problems that often reflect a systemic problem. It is essential to have a feedback component from case review to QI [quality improvement]."
- "Case reviews give us an opportunity for more oversight, and if it is not done, then poor practices will creep back up. Someone has to watch."
- "Performing case review gives us an opportunity to observe trends. This was a good change in the 7th SOW because it allows us to do something constructive rather than be a whistleblower. We actually educate providers, and this is positive in changing patterns."

Three of the 18 CEOs supporting case review additionally emphasized the important role of case review in knowledge transfer. For example, one CEO stated, "Certainly, case review is not a population-based exercise but it brings us closer to the daily practice of patient care, obstacles to delivering care, and problems with education level of both provider and patient. While the focus is on changing individual physicians, we incorporate lessons to a broader audience as part of knowledge transfer."

Case Review Activities

From October 2002 through September 2004, the QIOs received 5,921 separate complaints (i.e., complaints only and not appeals) by telephone or letter from beneficiaries (personal communications, S. Blackstock, April 29, 2005, and February 11, 2005). These complaints required the examination of 11,372 sets of medical records because of many complaints involving treatment by more than one provider during the episode of care. From September 2003 through July 2004, of the 2,321 completed examinations of beneficiary complaints, 357 were deemed appropriate for the mediation process. Of those, detailed data were available for 172. The data revealed that 79 cases had reached agreement, whereas the remaining 93 were still in progress or were withdrawn from the process or the provider had refused mediation. Thirty-one QIOs have handled at least one case deemed appropriate for mediation, and 15 QIOs have completed at least one mediation case (Rollow, 2005).

In all complaint cases, regardless of the use of mediation, the QIOs surveyed beneficiaries on their satisfaction with the complaint review process. This survey was implemented nationally in April 2003. From April 2003 through July 2004, there were 3,378 beneficiary complaint cases (personal communication, S. Blackstock, February 11, 2005). Of those, 357 entered the mediation process. The QIOs administered 1,964 satisfaction surveys for completed cases. For the traditional process, 93.4 percent of respondents expressed that they were satisfied or very satisfied overall. The rate of satisfaction with the case manager was 92 percent and, the rate of satisfaction with the QIO response was 93 percent., However, only 39 percent of respondents were satisfied with the review outcome. The QIOs used the survey results to alter their review processes. After they made adjustments to the process, a comparison of the levels of satisfaction levels for the period from April to June 2003 with the levels of satisfaction from April to June 2004 showed improvements in the satisfaction levels for both the process (from 93 to 95 percent) and the outcomes (39 to 60 percent).

During FY 2004 (October 2003 to September 2004), the QIOs conducted 8,168 reviews of appeals (HINNs, NODMARs, and Grijalva reviews), plus retrospective reviews of an additional 3,084 cases of HINNs (Rollow, 2005). All other review types (such as EMTALA, CMS referrals, and higher-weighted DRGs) accounted for an additional 46,062 case reviews during this time period. Comparatively, only 14 reviews for assistants at cataract surgery were performed during the same time period, and all cases were approved (personal communication, S. Blackstock, April 29, 2005).

HPMP

In the 7th SOW, opportunities to save costs by preventing payment errors were generally the result of the prevention of unnecessary admissions, as underpayment and upcoding of cases tended to cancel each other out (Rollow, 2005). The baseline absolute payment error rates for individual states at the beginning of the 7th SOW ranged from 1.19 to 8.00 percent, with a mean payment error rate of 4.33 percent and a median payment error rate of 4.24 percent (QIONet Dashboard, accessed November 11, 2005). The exact time frame for each QIO's baseline differed, depending on what round of the SOW in which it started. For the second quarter of FY 2004, the state error rates ranged from 0.32 to 10.84 percent, with a mean error rate of 4.24 percent and a median error rate of 4.25 percent. However, the states with the highest and lowest rates of error in 2004 were not necessarily the same as those at the baseline (QIONet Dashboard, accessed November 11, 2005).

TABLE 12.4 Trends for National Weighted Payment Error Rates

Period	Error Rate (percent)
FY 2001	4.7
FY 2002	4.82
FY 2003 (overall)	4.64
FY 2003 Q2	4.06
FY 2003 Q3	4.37
FY 2003 Q4	4.64
FY 2004 Q1	4.97
FY 2004 Q2	4.81
FY 2003 Q3 through FY 2004 Q2 (overall)	4.70

NOTE: Q = quarter.

SOURCE: QIONet Dashboard (accessed April 13, 2005, and November 11, 2005).

For FY 2001, the national weighted rate (the total amount of money paid in error divided by the total reimbursements) was 4.7 percent (QIONet Dashboard, accessed November 11, 2005). The most recent data cover the period from the third quarter of FY 2003 through the second quarter of FY 2004. For this time period, the national weighted rate was again 4.7 percent. Table 12.4 lists the national weighted payment error rates for FY 2001 to FY 2003, with the rates for individual quarters for FY 2003 to FY 2004 provided when the data were available. Although individual quarters show minor variations, the overall national rate since the baseline in FY 2001 has remained steady.

Telephone Interviews

In the telephone interviews, when 16 QIO CEOs were asked whether the QIOs should continue their payment error review function, only 1 CEO responded with a definitive negative: "It is not essential; we have found in the past as many payment errors to the good as to the bad." The remaining 15 said that the function is compatible with their mission; however, 6 of those 15 expressed less passion for QIOs' need to continue the payment error review function than their passion for their need to continue the case review function; for example, one CEO stated, "Payment error is an important part of the care program. The functions go hand in hand, but I could live without this one if forced to." Another CEO commented, "I don't have as strong a feeling about payment error as case review. Our payment error rates are pretty low."

The remainder of the CEOs (9 of 15) said that that payment error reviews are definitely useful to quality improvement by providing leverage, enhanced access to provider staff for educational interventions, and monetary savings to Medicare. One CEO commented, "Payment error gives us one more reason to walk through the hospital doors, and as a result, we develop closer relationships by offering chances to educate. We have the opportunity to talk to different staff segments than we usually do." Another CEO stated, "It is useful to maintain the payment error function because it gives us better credibility. Appropriate utilization and appropriate quality go hand in hand. Also, having this function helps sell the QIO as a resource to facilities. Most of the payment errors are a result of bad reporting that the QIO can help the facility to address."

Financial Costs

At the end of calendar year 2004, CMS expected the QIOs to spend $45.5 million on the beneficiary complaint response program in the 7th SOW (Task 3a). This represents approximately 5.8 percent of the QIO core contract budget. CMS estimated expenditures for HPMP (Task 3b) at $41.2 million, or approximately 5.2 percent of the core contract budget. The cost of all other protection activities (Task 3c) was estimated at $161.7 million on Task 3c, which represents approximately 20.5 percent of the QIO core contract budget (personal communication, C. Lazarus, March 17, 2005).

SUMMARY

This chapter has discussed issues related to the case review activities of the QIO program. The following are some of the main themes of this chapter, which are reflected in the findings and conclusions presented in Chapter 2:

- The QIO program's origins are based on case review activities that focused on identifying utilization outliers in the hospital setting. The QIOs have significant experience with these activities.
- The categories of review have increased over the life of the QIO program, but the focus of the program itself has shifted away from utilization review and toward collaboration to improve the quality of care. This is reflected in the development of a mediation process to address beneficiary complaints through better communication with the provider and the use of quality improvement plans by providers to address inadequate practice patterns found during review.
- Although the QIO program has shifted toward performing a collaborative role, some providers still have a lingering perception that QIOs

are punitive organizations. Despite this perception, many QIOs argue that the dual roles can be synergistic.

• Some categories of review may have very low value, such as reviews for assistants at cataract surgery. Reviews for payment errors showed fairly equal numbers of over- and underpayments. In general, payment error rates are currently low (less than 5 percent) and remain steady.

REFERENCES

Bradley EH, Carlson MDA, Gallo WT, Scinto J, Campbell MK, Krumholz HM. 2005. From adversary to partner: Have quality improvement organizations made the transition? *Health Services Research* 40(2):459–476.

CMS (Centers for Medicare and Medicaid Services). 1999. *6th Statement of Work (SOW)*. [Online]. Available: http://www.cms.hhs.gov/qio [accessed April 9, 2005].

CMS. 2002. *7th Statement of Work (SOW)*. [Online]. Available: http://www.cms.hhs.gov/qio [accessed April 9, 2005].

CMS. 2004a. *The Quality Improvement Organization Program: CMS Briefing for IOM Staff.* [Online]. Available: http://www.medqic.org/dcs/ContentServer?cid=1105558772835& pagename=Medqic%2FMQGeneralPage%2FGeneralPageTemplate&c=MQGeneralPage [accessed December 26, 2005].

CMS. 2004b. *Quality Improvement Organization Manual.* September 16. [Online]. Available: http://www.cms.hhs.gov/manuals/110_qio/qio110index.asp [accessed May 11, 2005].

CMS. 2005a. *Medicare Managed Care, Appeals and Grievances.* [Online]. Available: http:// www.cms.hhs.gov/healthplans/appeals [accessed May 31, 2005].

CMS. 2005b. *8th Statement of Work (SOW), Version #080105-1.* [Online]. Available: http:// www.cms.hhs.gov/qio [accessed November 4, 2005].

Lumetra. 2004. *Lumetra QIOSC Background Materials.* Unpublished. San Francisco, CA: Lumetra.

Lumetra. 2005. *Fast Track Appeals Process.* [Online]. Available: http://www.lumetra.com/ appeals/process/index.asp [accessed April 26, 2005].

MassPRO. 2004. *PEPPER: Program for Evaluating Payment Patterns Electronic Report.* Unpublished. Waltham, MA: MassPRO.

NORC (A National Organization for Research at the University of Chicago). 2004. *Final Report: Physician Meetings on Take-Up of Electronic Health Records.* Unpublished. Washington, DC: NORC.

Northeast Health Care Quality Foundation. 2005. *Required Review Activities.* [Online]. Available: http://www.nhcqf.org/Review/QIO/11_RequiredReviewActivities.html [accessed April 27, 2005].

OIG (Office of the Inspector General, U.S. Department of Health and Human Services). 2003. *Improper Fiscal Year 2002 Medicare Fee-for-Service Payments.* Washington, DC: Office of the Inspector General, U.S. Department of Health and Human Services.

Rollow WC. 2005. *The Medicare Quality Improvement (QIO) Program 7th SOW and Results.* PowerPoint Presentation to the Committee on Redesigning Health Insurance, June 13, Washington, DC.

Stratis Health. 2005. *Comparison of Termination of Service Appeal Process: Grijalva versus BIPA.* [Online]. Available: http://www.stratishealth.org/health-care/documents/Appeal ProcessComparison_000.pdf [accessed July 25, 2005].

Texas Medical Foundation. 2005a. *Hospital Payment Monitoring Program (HPMP).* [Online]. Available: http://www.tmf.org/hpmp [accessed April 13, 2005].

Texas Medical Foundation. 2005b. *Texas One-Day Stay and Other Statewide Statistics for All DRGs, All PPS Hospitals (340 Hospitals) FY2003 (October 1, 2002 through September 30, 2003).* [Online]. Available: http://www.tmf.org/hpmp/data/TX_DRGs1Day AllFY2003-by-DRG.pdf [accessed April 13, 2005].

Texas Medical Foundation. 2005c. *TMF One-Day Stay Project Details.* [Online]. Available: http://www.tmf.org/hpmp/projects/One-Day%20Stay%20Project%20Details.htm [accessed April 28, 2005].

Texas Medical Foundation. 2005d. *Update on Statewide Percentiles for PEPPER 3 Measures Through Fourth Quarter, FY2003 (July–September 2003).* [Online]. Available: http://www.tmf.org/hpmp/data/Updated_PEPPER3_Q4FY2003.pdf [accessed April 13, 2005].

13

CMS Oversight

CHAPTER SUMMARY

This chapter examines how the Centers for Medicare and Medicaid Services (CMS) oversees and manages the Quality Improvement Organization (QIO) program as a whole. First, the integration of the program into CMS's organizational structure is discussed, including the use of personnel who help with oversight. Next, communications, information technology, and data services are discussed both in the context of how they are used in the operations of the program and how they are used as a resource for management. Then, contract issues are presented, including how contracts are competed, awarded, implemented, and monitored. Finally, there is an examination of how CMS provides overall guidance to the Quality Improvement Organization program through strategic planning, policy decision making, coordination, and overall program evaluation.

ORGANIZATIONAL STRUCTURE OF QIO PROGRAM IN CMS

Oversight of the Quality Improvement Organization (QIO) program involves coordination of the efforts of multiple personnel in several offices within the Centers for Medicare and Medicaid Services (CMS), each of which has distinct roles. The administrative office of CMS, located in Baltimore, Maryland, is commonly referred to as the "Central Office." Two offices within CMS's Central Office share the responsibility for management of the QIO program: the Office of Clinical Standards and Quality, the "Program Office," and the Office of Acquisition and Grants Management, the "Contracts Office." Other groups have indirect roles in the management of the QIO program. The QIO and End-Stage Renal Disease Steering Committee manages the daily operations of the QIO program. The membership on the QIO and End-Stage Renal Disease Steering Committee comprises the Associate Regional Administrator for each of the four Regional

325

Offices affiliated with the QIO program and both the director and the deputy director of each of three groups within the Office of Clinical Standards and Quality: the Quality Improvement Group, the Information Systems Group, and the Quality Measurement and Health Assessment Group. The committee, currently chaired by the director of the Quality Improvement Group, meets weekly and primarily discusses operational issues (personal communication, J. V. Kelly, June 28, 2005).

Program Office

Overall responsibility for the QIO program lies in CMS's Office of Clinical Standards and Quality, with direct oversight provided by the Quality Improvement Group (Jost, 1991; CMS, 2004c) and with support provided by other groups within that office. The Program Office monitors the QIO program, coordinates with the Office of Internal Customer Support on financial matters, and creates and interprets policy related to the QIO program's operations. The office is divided into six groups, each of which may have one or more of the following divisions:

- Quality Improvement Group,
- Quality Measurement and Health Assessment Group,
- Information Systems Group,
- Quality Coordination Team,
- Coverage and Analysis Group, and
- Clinical Standards Group.

In the Institute of Medicine (IOM) committee's web-based data collection tool, 52 QIOs rated the Program Office on several functions. Overall, the office received higher scores on "clarity" than on "timeliness" (Table 13.1).

Concerns over clarity and timeliness also arose during the IOM committee and staff site visits. Four QIOs mentioned that the information that they receive is often ambiguous, and eight related frustration with the timeliness of access to information or data related to their tasks (referred to here as data lags). Data lags, however, may also be attributable to the measurement process, based on claims (this is discussed more later in this chapter).

Contracts Office

Many groups contribute to the development of a QIO contract, including the Office of Clinical Standards and Quality, the Office of Acquisition and Grants Management, and Regional Office Divisions of Quality Improvement (CMS, 2004b). However, responsibility for the QIO contract ultimately rests with the Acquisition and Grants Group of the Office of

TABLE 13.1 QIO Ratings of CMS Program Office

Ratings	Clarity of Overall Program Direction	Overall Support of QIO Work	Clarity of Information on Core Tasks	Timeliness of Information on Core Tasks
Excellent	2	3	1	0
Good	33	33	26	8
Fair	15	9	22	30
Poor	2	7	3	14

NOTE: The data in the table represent the number of QIOs responding as indicated. Data are for a total of 52 QIOs.

SOURCE: IOM committee web-based data collection tool.

Acquisitions and Grants Management. The Contracting Officer, a representative of the Acquisition and Grants Group, is the only person with the authority to release the contract or make modifications to the contract. The Contracting Officer oversees all contracts for the QIO program, and several contract specialists are each assigned to specific QIOs. As of June 2005, nine contract specialists were each assigned to work directly with between five and seven QIOs (personal communication, J. V. Kelly, June 30, 2005).

The QIOs expressed frustration with their interactions with the Contracts Office. During the site visits, two QIOs raised issues about conflicting messages between the Program and Contracts Offices. Additionally, at CMS's annual technical conference for the QIO program (QualityNet 2004), many QIO staff related difficulties with being asked to perform duties not specified within their contracts. They were asked to perform these duties by different sources, such as their Program Officer or Government Task Leader, or through a Transmittal of Policy System (TOPS) document (all of these are described later in this chapter). Although CMS presenters clarified that the Contracting Officer has the final say on required duties, the QIOs expressed frustration with conflicting messages from different individuals and groups at CMS (Hughes, 2004).

The QIOs rated the contracts office on many functions. Thirty-five of 52 QIOs stated that they had interaction with the Contracts Office only on an as-needed basis. The majority of QIOs rated the Contracts Office as "good" or "fair" on all questions (Table 13.2).

Regional Offices

CMS has 10 Regional Offices around the country. In four of these Regional Offices (Boston, Dallas, Kansas City, and Seattle), CMS established

TABLE 13.2   QIO Ratings of CMS Contracts Office

Ratings	Overall Clarity of Communications	Overall Timeliness of Communications	Timeliness of Contract Modifications	Expertise/ Understanding of QIO Tasks
Excellent	6	6	3	4
Good	26	25	27	19
Fair	14	17	15	19
Poor	6	4	7	10

NOTE: The data in the table represent the number of QIOs responding as indicated. Data are for a total of 52 QIOs.

SOURCE: IOM committee web-based data collection tool.

Divisions of Quality Improvement that act as liaisons between the QIOs and CMS's Central Office (Jost, 1991; CMS, 2004b). The remaining six CMS Regional Offices do not have any direct responsibility for the QIO program. The four Regional Offices with Divisions of Quality Improvement (referred to in the QIO program as "Regional Offices") assist QIOs with technical issues on a daily basis by interpreting CMS policy, monitoring finances, and providing feedback.

The staff of the Divisions of Quality Improvement include an Associate Regional Administrator, Project Officers, and Scientific Officers. The Associate Regional Administrator oversees daily operations, including development and the implementation of goals, participation in consortium meetings, maintenance of stakeholder relationships, and management of funds (CMS, 2004b). Before the 7th SOW, Divisions of Quality Improvement existed in all 10 CMS Regional Offices and were generally staffed only by Project Officers. As the program focus shifted toward quality improvement, oversight was condensed into the four Regional Offices mentioned above, as new skills were needed to parallel the skills needed at the QIO level. New staff included epidemiologists, clinicians, biostatisticians, data managers, and communications specialists (CMS, 2004b). Today, staffing at each Regional Office varies in terms of both the numbers of personnel and the skill sets of those personnel (CMS, 2004b).

CMS also divided the country into four consortiums that correlated with the four Regional Offices with Divisions of Quality Improvement. These consortiums (Northeast, Midwest, Southern, and Western) include the one Regional Office's with QIO oversight in that area and any other Regional Offices in that area that are not directly involved in the QIO program. The consortiums act to improve communications and share resources among the 10 Regional Offices and enhance consistency in the QIO program as a whole (CMS, 2004b).

Project Officers

Project Officers monitor technical aspects of the QIO core contract (CMS, 2004b). All Project Officers participate in a week-long basic training session, with some officers completing optional advanced Project Officer training or performance-based contracting training. Each QIO is assigned one Project Officer, but a single Project Officer works with multiple QIOs. The QIOs reported that they have frequent contacts with their Project Officers: half (26 of 52) reported weekly contact, and 92 percent (48 of 52) reported at least monthly contact (Figure 13.1).

The Project Officer provides direct technical assistance to each QIO, serves as the advocate for the QIO within CMS, and is an expert resource for the QIOs in terms of contract content and CMS policy. The Project Officers manage QIO contracts by monitoring the progress of the QIOs, acting as a direct liaison to the Contracting Officer at CMS, and participating in strategic planning. Monitoring activities include scheduled calls with individual QIOs and review of the data on the Dashboard section of CMS's intranet site (see below). Official monitoring visits are discussed in greater detail later in this chapter. The Project Officers also have communications and coordination responsibilities at both the local and the national levels. Table 13.3 shows the number of full-time Project Officers at each Regional

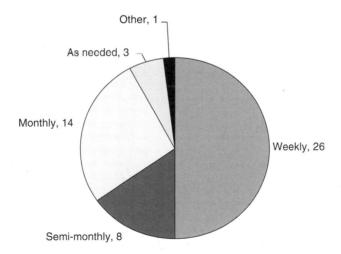

FIGURE 13.1 Frequency of Project Officer contact with QIOs reported by 52 QIOs. The numbers in the figure represent the number of QIOs responding as indicated. SOURCE: IOM committee web-based data collection tool.

TABLE 13.3 Numbers of Project Officers and Contracts for Each CMS Regional Office

Regional Office	Number of Project Officers	Number of QIO Contracts	Average Number of Contracts per Project Officer
Boston	5	16	3.2
Dallas	4.6	11	2.4
Kansas City	4	13	3.25
Seattle	4	13	3.25

SOURCE: CMS (2004b).

TABLE 13.4 QIO Ratings of Project Officers

Rating	Clarity of Responses[a]	Timeliness of Responses[a]	Expertise/ Understanding of Review Tasks	Expertise/ Understanding of HCQIP Tasks
Excellent	34	36	25	21
Good	13	13	19	24
Fair	4	3	7	6
Poor	1	0	1	1

NOTE: The data in the table represent the number of QIOs responding as indicated. Data are for a total of 52 QIOs. HCQIP = Health Care Quality Improvement Program.

[a]Responses to questions raised or issues posed by the QIO.

SOURCE: IOM committee web-based data collection tool.

Office, as well as the total number of QIO contracts monitored in that region as of June 2004 (CMS, 2004b).

The QIOs rated the Project Officers on various functions. Overall, the Project Officers received high ratings in all areas, with the majority of QIOs rating their Project Officers as "excellent" or "good" in each area (Table 13.4).

Scientific Officers

The Scientific Officers support the Project Officers by providing scientific and clinical expertise (CMS, 2004b). Scientific Officers are not assigned to specific QIOs but, instead, assist all QIOs in the region covered by the Regional Office with specific technical needs. They also assist the

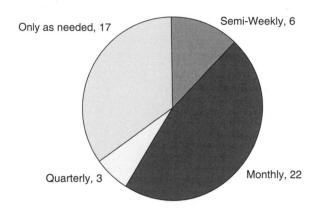

FIGURE 13.2 Frequency of Scientific Officer contact with QIOs reported by 48 QIOs. The numbers in the figure represent the number of QIOs responding as indicated.
SOURCE: IOM committee web-based data collection tool.

QIOs in other regions, if they are requested to do so. As of June 2004, the Boston Regional Office had five Scientific Officers on staff, and the three other Regional Offices each had four Scientific Officers (CMS, 2004b). The QIOs reported extremely variable interactions with the Scientific Officers (Figure 13.2).

Scientific Officers evaluate measurement methodologies and surveys, analyze QIO data, review manuscripts, provide clinical expertise, and manage special studies (CMS, 2004b). Scientific Officers possess specific skills in areas such as statistics, epidemiology, clinical science (Medical Officer), and data management. Scientific Officers may complete any of the training sessions described for Project Officers, but they are not required to do so. Scientific Officers also participate in official monitoring visits, described later in this chapter. In addition to their basic duties, Scientific Officers often serve as Government Task Leaders (see below).

Table 13.5 shows the QIO ratings of Scientific Officers on a variety of functions. In general, QIOs rated Scientific Officers highly in all areas, with most QIOs providing "excellent" or "good" ratings for their Scientific Officers.

Government Task Leaders

Each task of the QIO contract and each special study are assigned a single Government Task Leader to provide direct oversight. The Govern-

TABLE 13.5 QIO Ratings of Scientific Officers

Rating	Clarity of Responses[a]	Timeliness of Responses[b]	Timeliness of Manuscript Reviews[c]
Excellent	17	17	18
Good	24	29	14
Fair	6	2	1
Poor	0	0	2

[a]Data are for a total of 47 QIOs.
[b]Data are for a total of 48 QIOs.
[c]Data are for a total of 35 QIOs.

SOURCE: IOM committee web-based data collection tool.

ment Task Leader may be located in either the Regional or Central Office. In the IOM committee telephone interviews, 11 of 20 QIO chief executive officers (CEOs) expressed problems with Government Task Leaders. Three CEOs, including two with QIO support center (QIOSC) contracts, specifically mentioned, unprompted, that many Government Task Leaders lack substantive expertise in their topic areas. Some of their comments were as follows:

• "What QIOSCs need to do the best job are exceptional CMS Government Task Leaders. They blend a knowledge of breaking research with pragmatism and good political instincts."
• "There should be better coordination among the Government Task Leaders at CMS. They tend to get siloed in their specialties and do not understand the scope of what QIOs are doing."
• "You can usually attribute the difference [in timeliness] to the relationship with the CMS Government Task Leader; if it is positive, you get things approved in a timely manner."

Difficult relationships with Government Task Leaders were echoed in interviews with staff from five organizations representing seven QIOSCs. All of them believed that the relationship often depended on the Government Task Leader's experience in the topic area. One staff member stated that the Government Task Leader used the QIOSC as an extension of his or her personal staff. Two staff members indicated that the rate of turnover of their Government Task Leaders was high and that their skills and experience with their assigned topic areas varied.

TABLE 13.6 Full-Time CMS Employees for the QIO Program

Area of CMS		FTE[a] Count	Percentage of Total
Regional Offices	Total count	42.45	32
	Dallas	9.2	
	Boston	11.25	
	Seattle	11.0	
	Kansas City	11.0	
Quality Improvement Group (Office of Clinical Standards and Quality)	Total count	36.5	28
	Division of Contract Operations and Support	14.5	
	Division of Quality Improvement Policy for Acute Care	14.0	
	Division of Quality Improvement Policy for Chronic and Ambulatory Care	4.5	
	Front office staff	3.5	
Information Systems Group (Office of Clinical Standards and Quality)		24.0	18
Quality Measurement and Health Assessment Group (Office of Clinical Standards and Quality)		20.5	16
Office of Acquisition and Grants Management	8.5		6

[a]FTE = full-time equivalent.

SOURCE: Personal communication, J. V. Kelly, September 8, 2005.

Full-Time Employees

As of September 2005, the full-time employee count for the QIO program was 131.95 (personal communication, J. V. Kelly, September 8, 2005). This includes all CMS employees who work on the core contract, special studies, or developmental work. Most employees (62 percent) work in one of the groups of the Office of Clinical Standards and Quality. The breakdown is presented in Table 13.6.

COMMUNICATIONS AND INFORMATION TECHNOLOGY SERVICES

Communications

QIO Manual and Contract

Many conduits of communication exist within the QIO program (CMS, 2004b). A primary source of program information is the QIO manual, which lays out basic program policy on the basis of legal and agency requirements and which is unlikely to change during the course of a contract. The QIO contract itself is another source of information for QIOs. The contract includes a statement of work, a document that delineates detailed work requirements, a list of deliverables, evaluation criteria, and a budget. The scope of work (SOW) is a section of the statement of work that provides an overall nontechnical description of the required activities during the contract cycle. According to the J-1 attachment of the QIO contract (the glossary), the abbreviation "SOW" can be used to refer to either the scope of work or statement of work but declares that the terms themselves are not interchangeable (CMS, 2002).

Memos and Letters

CMS uses TOPS documents to inform the QIOs quickly about anticipated changes in policy, including draft statements (Jost, 1991; CMS, 2004b). Although TOPS documents deal with policy changes, Standard Data Processing System (SDPS) memos inform QIOs about operational concerns. Examples include one-time requests for information, emergency alerts, and administrative announcements (CMS, 2004b). SDPS memos may come from different sources, but all memos must be cleared by the Information Systems Group of the Office of Clinical Standards and Quality.

CMS uses contractor clarification letters to inform QIOs of alterations or additions to their contracts. The letters may also clarify requirements or respond to specific questions. Two types of clarification letters are used. The first type is an unofficial letter that explains an issue or question but does not result in a contract modification (personal communication, J. V. Kelly, May 31, 2005). The second type is one that is a precursor to a contract modification, informs QIOs of forthcoming contract changes, and ultimately, results in a contract modification. No matter the source, all letters must be cleared by the Contracting Officer in the Acquisition and Grants Group. For day-to-day work and specific questions, CMS may use e-mail or conference calls to communicate with the QIOs. These formal letters and memos are all sent by e-mail to each QIO and are also posted in appropriate sections of QIONet, CMS's internal intranet website (described later in this chapter).

Figure 13.3 shows QIO satisfaction with the clarity and the timeliness of TOPS memos. Overall, most QIOs believe that clarity was "good" but that timeliness was "fair."

Regional Office Communications

The Regional Offices coordinate much of the communication between CMS and the QIOs (CMS, 2004b). Informal interactions often occur daily

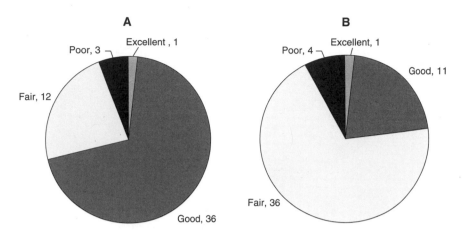

FIGURE 13.3 Clarity (A) and timeliness (B) of TOPS memos reported by 52 QIOs. The numbers in the figure represent the number of QIOs responding as indicated. SOURCE: IOM committee web-based data collection tool.

via e-mail and telephone. Formal interactions occur at the 9- and 18-month evaluations (discussed later in this chapter). Some Project Officers expressed frustration that limited travel budgets do not permit more than two on-site evaluation visits. Finally, the Regional Offices interact with each other as well as with CMS Regional Offices that do not oversee the QIOs. The Project Officers of the four Regional Offices that oversee QIOs participate in a monthly community-of-practice call; this is a regularly scheduled tele-conference that allows officers to exchange ideas and information. Interaction with CMS Regional Offices not associated with the QIO program is less formalized but still occurs, especially when national programs (like Nursing Home Compare) are launched.

Medicare Quality Improvement Community

The Medicare Quality Improvement Community (MedQIC) (formerly known as the Medicare Quality Improvement Clearinghouse) is a public website available to anyone via the Internet at http://www.medqic.org (CMS, 2004b). MedQIC currently features support for seven areas: structural and systems change, physicians' offices, hospitals, home health agencies, nursing homes, underserved populations, and managed care organizations. These areas are subject to change with the evolution of the SOWs and refinement of the website. The site serves as a resource for quality improvement efforts and includes bibliographies, tool kits, flowcharts, and sugges-

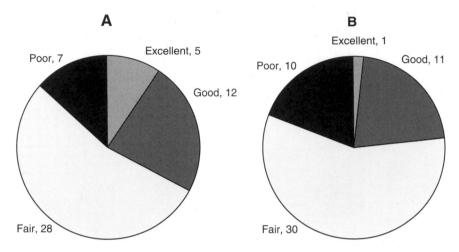

FIGURE 13.4   Value (A) and ease of use (B) of MedQIC reported by 52 QIOs. The numbers in the figure represent the number of QIOs responding as indicated. SOURCE: IOM committee web-based data collection tool.

tions. The site also provides information for consumers, including lists of all QIOs and activities of the QIO program, but it does not divulge provider- or beneficiary-specific information (CMS, 2003). As discussed in Chapter 11, in the 7th SOW, the Iowa Foundation for Medical Care (Iowa's QIO) acted as a virtual QIOSC for the operation of MedQIC. Figure 13.4 shows QIO assessments of the value and the ease of use of MedQIC. More than half of the QIOs rated MedQIC as "fair" in each case. As MedQIC was redesigned in early 2005, an effort spearheaded by the 7th SOW's Quality Improvement Interventions and Related Resources QIOSC, Figure 13.4 does not reflect the value or ease of use of the new version of MedQIC.

QIONet

QIONet is a protected intranet website of CMS used by the QIO community to share task-specific information, provide forums and training resources, archive memos, and display data and progress reports (CMS, 2004b). Only preapproved users may gain access to the site. The Iowa Foundation for Medical Care (Iowa's QIO) maintains QIONet. All the tools of the SDPS (see later in this chapter) may be accessed via QIONet. The majority of QIOs rated QIONet as "excellent" or "good" on the dimensions of value and ease of use (Figure 13.5).

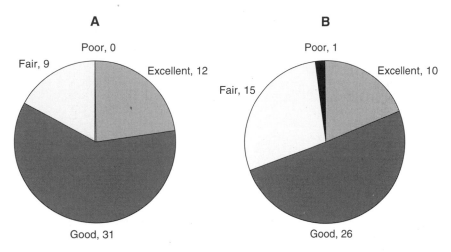

FIGURE 13.5   Value (A) and ease of use (B) of QIONet reported by 52 QIOs. The numbers in the figure represent the number of QIOs responding as indicated. SOURCE: IOM committee web-based data collection tool.

Information and Communication Technology Systems and Tools

SDPS is the information system for the QIO program and includes hardware and software developed by the SDPS team for use by the QIO community (CMS, 2004b). MedQIC and QIONet (described above) also fall under the umbrella of SDPS. SDPS became operational in May 1997 in response to the needs of the QIO program and interfaces with the Central Office, the 53 QIOs, and the Clinical Data Abstraction Centers (CDACs) (CMS, 2003). As mentioned above, the Iowa Foundation for Medical Care (Iowa's QIO) acted as the QIOSC for data collection and SDPS issues.

In the web-based data collection, the QIOs rated the value of SDPS to their core contract work. Thirty-three of 52 QIOs (63 percent) rated its value as "excellent" or "good." The QIOs also rated SDPS on timeliness and overall ease of use, with slightly higher ratings for ease of use than timeliness (Table 13.7).

Dashboard

Data from the CMS Dashboard, a part of QIONet, show the results of each QIO's work on the contract tasks (CMS, 2004b). Many Dashboard reports include quarterly trends and provider participation rates. Project Officers use the Dashboard to monitor the progress of the QIOs under their

TABLE 13.7   QIO Ratings of SDPS

Rating	Value	Timeliness of Support	Overall Ease of Use
Excellent	8	4	6
Good	25	19	21
Fair	12	18	20
Poor	7	11	5

NOTE: The data in the table represent the number of QIOs responding as indicated. Data are for a total of 52 QIOs.

SOURCE: IOM committee web-based data collection tool.

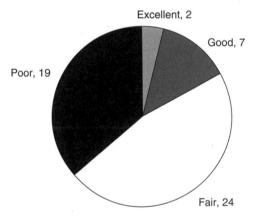

FIGURE 13.6   QIO satisfaction with timeliness of Dashboard data reported by 52 QIOs. The numbers in the figure represent the number of QIOs responding as indicated.
SOURCE: IOM committee web-based data collection tool.

management, and QIOs may use it to compare their results with those of other QIOs around the country. As described above, however, many QIOs express frustration with the time delays that they encounter when they try access to different types of data, including data presented on Dashboard. Forty-three of 52 QIOs (83 percent) rated the timeliness of Dashboard data as "fair" or "poor" (Figure 13.6).

Program Activity Reporting Tool

The Program Activity Reporting Tool (PARTner) is an application that QIOs use to report on their deliverables (CMS, 2004b), including regular

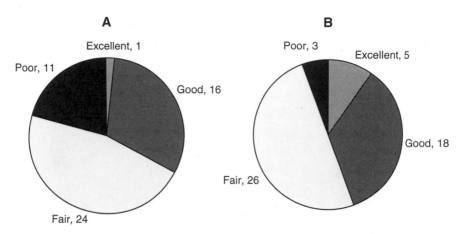

FIGURE 13.7   Value (A) and ease of use (B) of PARTner reported by 52 QIOs. The numbers in the figure represent the number of QIOs responding as indicated. SOURCE: IOM committee web-based data collection tool.

reports on activities and projects, information on publications, data on identified participants, and project proposals. CMS Central and Regional Office staff use PARTner to monitor these deliverables or approve the project plans submitted by QIOs. CMS staff warned the IOM, however, that some of the data sets were not complete and consistent enough for analytical purposes (personal communication, J. V. Kelly, January 11, 2005). Figure 13.7 shows the QIO ratings of the value and ease of use of PARTner. More than half of the QIOs rated PARTner as "fair" or "poor."

Case Review Information System

The Case Review Information System (CRIS) is an application that the QIOs use to track and report data on case review activities (CMS, 2003, 2004b). The QIOs also use CRIS to describe other activities, such as the number or type of helpline calls recived. CRIS allows the QIOs and CMS to organize and monitor these activities. Project Officers use CRIS to monitor the timeliness of the case review activities of each QIO. Figure 13.8 shows the QIO ratings of the value and ease of use of CRIS. Thirty-two of 52 QIOs (62 percent) rated CRIS as "excellent" or "good" on CRIS's value, but 35 of 52 (67 percent) rated its ease of use as "fair" or "poor."

CMS Abstraction and Reporting Tool

Providers, QIOs, and CDACs use the CMS Abstraction and Reporting Tool (CART) to collect and analyze data on quality indicators related to the

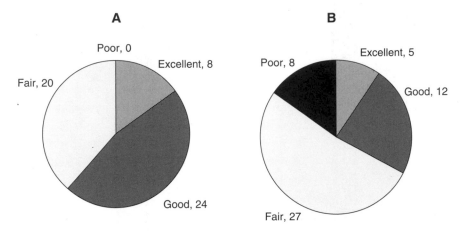

FIGURE 13.8   Value (A) and ease of use (B) of CRIS reported by 52 QIOs. The numbers in the figure represent the number of QIOs responding as indicated.
SOURCE: IOM committee web-based data collection tool.

hospital tasks (CMS, 2004b). The tool was developed by a team that included CMS, the Joint Commission on Accreditation of Healthcare Organizations, and the QIOs themselves. Figure 13.9 shows the QIO ratings of the value and ease of use of CART. The QIOs appear to be evenly divided as to its value and ease of use, with about half of the QIOs rating CART as

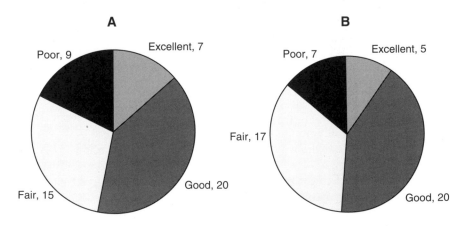

FIGURE 13.9   Value (A) and ease of use (B) of CART reported by 51 QIOs for value and by 49 QIOs for ease of use. The numbers in the figure represent the number of QIOs responding as indicated.
SOURCE: IOM committee web-based data collection tool.

"excellent" or "good" and half rating it as "fair" or "poor" for both parameters.

DATA FLOW

Clinical Data Abstraction Centers

In the 7th SOW, CMS contracted with two CDACs, AdvanceMed and DynKePRO, to abstract clinical data from medical records (CMS, 2004b). CMS contracted with these companies directly on behalf of the QIOs for the Hospital Payment Monitoring Program (see Chapter 12) as well as for other surveillance and validation needs (described later in this chapter). The contracts with the CDACs lasted for 5-year periods (personal communication, M. Krushat and W. Matos, CMS, October 25, 2004). The most recent contract period began in September 2004 and was granted to DynKePRO alone. This contract is for 5 years at a cost of $74 million. The previous 5-year contract was for $125 million. The contract cost was reduced for several reasons, including the availability of improved data collection and reporting tools, decreased abstraction needs, and the fact that the use of only one CDAC will lead to more efficient operations (personal communication, W. Matos, CMS, July 7, 2005).

Nursing Homes and Home Health Agencies

In the 7th SOW, CMS obtained performance data for nursing homes and home health agencies from the Center for Medicaid and State Operations, which generated nursing home measures from data collected with the Minimum Data Set tool and home health agency measures from data collected with the Outcome and Assessment Information Set tool. In the 7th SOW, the measures were available to QIOs and CMS in two ways. First, the measures were available through an internal electronic information system. Second, the Office of Clinical Standards and Quality of CMS received a date file containing the measures, which was posted onto Dashboard for use by the QIOs. In the 8th SOW, the Information Systems Group is working on a tool (modeled after CART) to track clinical processes associated with positive outcomes. The data will be submitted to a warehouse and comparative performance feedback will be provided back to the nursing home to help them target areas for improvement.

Hospitals

In the 6th SOW, the CDACs collected data on performance measures for the hospital setting, but these data were collected only at the baseline and the time of remeasurement. If the QIOs wanted information at earlier intervals, they had to collect their own data. QIOs interested in interim data used various tools, which led to inconsistent results. For the baseline and final measurements, the data flowed from the CDACs to the Clinical Area Support Peer Review Organization (the predecessor to the QIOSCs) to the QIO. In this case the data were often too old to be helpful to the QIOs for their interventions. Furthermore, the sample size was targeted at the state level and not the provider level. By the beginning of the 7th SOW, CDACs increased data collection to a quarterly basis. However, there was still a lag from the time of service to the time of data availability, in part because the sample relied on claims filed by the provider and processed before abstraction. Efficiency was improved through the creation of the CART tool and the creation of a centralized data repository (instead of the use of the QIOSCs as intermediaries). Also, under Task 2b of the 7th SOW, Hospital Public Reporting, hospitals began to collect and report their own data via the CART tool directly to the warehouse on a quarterly basis (see Chapter 11).

In the 7th SOW, CDACs abstracted a surveillance sample of records for hospital quality measures (~52,000 records annually), stroke and atrial fibrillation measures (~3,800 records annually), and patient safety measures (~27,000 records annually) (personal communication, M. Krushat and W. Matos, CMS, October 25, 2004). The average cost of a single record abstraction in 2003 was $56 per chart, with a range (depending on the type of review) of $47 to $103 per chart. Surveillance samples were not large enough to allow users to assess individual providers.

In the 8th SOW, due to the duplicative efforts of the Hospital Quality Alliance and the reporting requirements of the Medicare Prescription Drug, Improvement, and Modernization Act of 2003 (P.L. 108-173), abstractions for surveillance have been eliminated or greatly reduced because data are available from public reports. Instead, the CDACs perform validation for a number of records sampled by SDPS. Patient safety measures are abstracted and validated separately.

Although there has been a centralization of the data collection efforts and a standardization of the tools and processes in the hospital setting, CMS does not believe that there will be a significant improvement in the data lag (personal communication, W. Matos, CMS, July 7, 2005). As part of measures alignment among stakeholders, CMS and the Joint Commission on Accreditation of Healthcare Organizations agreed to collect measures using the same timeline, which limits the availability of the information reported. Hospitals do have the ability to concurrently submit their data and generate their own reports. The QIOs and hospitals are able to look at these results in real time if the hospital does immediate reporting, but they would be unable to compare those data with statewide or national results. In the hospital setting, the data lag is mostly attributable to the chart abstraction process.

Physicians' Offices

CMS currently collects claims-based measures for physicians' offices (personal communication, W. Matos, CMS, July 7, 2005). Some of these measures lack reliability because of reporting issues, such as incomplete records and services delivered but not billed separately. In the 8th SOW, a Doctor's Office Quality–Information Technology warehouse has been established, and the QIOs will help physicians with the reporting of measures data.

DATA LAG ISSUES

In the IOM committee telephone interviews with the QIO CEOS, all the CEOs commented that the timeliness of the data available for the different settings is a problem. Most CEOs focused on how a lack of timeliness generally hindered improvement because of a lack of availability of up-to-date baseline data and rapid feedback to QIOs so that they could alter their interventions or motivate providers to continue their system changes. A lack of timeliness also affected their views on contract length and the fairness of the evaluation process. This was confirmed during the IOM site visits, in which 8 of 11 QIOs independently cited data lag as a problem in their work. Many CEOs claimed that the data were often too old to reflect the effects of the quality improvement interventions and did not reflect the QIOs' efforts during their 3-year contracts due to the timing of evaluations (see later in this chapter for more on the evaluation period).

Other studies also confirm the CEOs' concerns over data lag times. A random national sample of hospital quality improvement managers interviewed in 2002 raised concerns about the use of data for quality improvement interventions because physicians perceived questions of validity and substantive problems with the data and because the data were too old (several months to a year old) to be helpful (Bradley et al., 2005). However, a recent study of hospitals not participating in specific quality improvement interventions showed no difference in performance measures between hospitals that received immediate feedback and those that received data that were delayed 17 months (Beck et al., 2005).

Many CEOs expressed the need for QIOs to supplement CMS data with more timely data for feedback to providers. Fourteen of 20 CEOs mentioned the continuing need to collect data themselves, although they recognize that they cannot abstract information at all facilities or for all providers because of limited resources.

Nursing Homes and Home Health Agencies

Five of 20 CEOs mentioned problems with nursing home data, and four mentioned delays with home health data. In general, because of the tools used for data collection in these settings, data lag is not a major issue.

Hospitals

Thirteen of the 20 CEOs mentioned problems with hospital data timeliness. Ostensibly, with hospitals collecting their own data, the burden would be lifted from the QIOs, feedback would be more immediate, and the tracking of changes in the hospital setting would be easier. However, seven CEOs said that data availability was more timely under the 6th SOW. Four CEOs specifically mentioned problems with CART. However, others affirmed progress in the hospital arena: "If three years ago you would have said that every hospital in the state would report to CMS, I would have been surprised." One CEO said that CART data are "a good first step for facilities."

The CEOs had different opinions on the ability to get data more frequently. One stated, "Hospitals might scream, but if they can provide it quarterly, they can do it monthly and that would allow even more timely evaluation of improvement." However, another CEO said that getting CMS data more often than quarterly was not realistic because in some states the provider pool and sample of patients would be too small on a monthly basis. Also, he was not sure the QIO or the hospitals could deal with the process of getting and sharing data monthly or the emotional gear up and reaction to data.

Physician's Office and Outpatient Settings

Half of the CEOs related that they encountered problems with lags in data from physicians' offices and outpatient practices. They considered these settings to be the most difficult from which to obtain data, both from CMS claims and directly from provider offices. Two CEOs offered specific comments about the CMS data. One CEO stated, "Physician office data [were] nonexistent, and we were already 18 to 24 months into the 7th SOW." Another CEO indicated, "In physician offices, the evaluation strategy for 7th SOW was seriously flawed. At 14 months we had at most a couple of weeks of data that would reflect anything we had done in the 14 months. There [were] no data early on to show us to correct our course. We had to use proxy measures like the number of improvement plans drawn up; CMS does not give enough credit for these proxy measures."

With respect to gaining access to data directly from physicians' offices, one CEO believed that "CMS doesn't trust QIOs with physician data, but the CMS data [are] old when we get [them]; QIOs have the capacity to handle the physician data." Another stated, "It is difficult to get into physician offices to abstract data; physicians do not have the space or the time to accommodate persons collecting data." Data lag in this setting is often attributable to confidentiality restrictions or abstraction issues; however, future public reporting efforts and requirements will ameliorate these difficulties.

QIO CONTRACTS

Competition for Contracts

QIOs that qualify as in-state organizations (CMS, 2004d) may have their contracts automatically renewed upon successful completion of the previous contract, known as a "noncompetitive renewal." If the organization holding the contract does not qualify as in state, CMS must announce the contract's expiration date in the *Federal Register* at least 6 months before the end of the contract. In-state organizations that express interest in the contract are given priority, even if they did not hold the previous contract. Noncompetitive renewals are not allowed for out-of-state organizations, even if they are successful in the completion of the previous contract, unless no qualified in-state organization applies (CMS, 2002, 2004d, 2005a).

If a QIO fails to successfully complete all parts of the contract, it may present arguments to a CMS review panel as to why it was not successful. CMS may elect to renew the contract noncompetitively if it finds exceptional circumstances; or it may decide to not renew the contract, which will go out for competition, known as a "competitive renewal" (CMS, 2004b).

At the end of the 6th SOW, the CMS panel reviewed 16 contracts, and for the 7th SOW recommended that a recompetition be conducted for 9 of them. Of those 9, CMS reversed the decision for 2 of them, which were renewed noncompetitively. CMS put the remaining 7 contracts up for competition, but only 2 contracts were awarded to new organizations. Of the five organizations that ultimately regained their contracts, three had no other bidders, one won the contract against other bidders, and one had only one other bidder that ended up not qualifying (CMS, 2004b).

At the end of the 7th SOW, CMS determined that six QIOs had unsuccessfully completed their contracts. After three of the six QIOs went before the evaluation panel in the first round of QIO contracts, CMS decided that a recompetition would be conducted for all failing QIOs unless there were extremely unusual circumstances. Competition, per se, was highly valued; and the potential of bringing new organizations into the program or stimulating creative changes in the current QIOs apparently outweighed the possible loss of long-established working relationships with providers and stakeholder groups (personal communication, W. Rollow and E. Freund, CMS, March 9, 2005). The incumbent QIOs retained the contracts for the three Round 1 QIO contracts up for competition (personal communications, C. Lazarus, November 1, 2005, and November 9, 2005; personal communication, J. V. Kelly, October 25, 2005). Two of the contracts received only one proposal each, and the third received three proposals, all of which came from organizations that held at least one QIO contract in the 7th SOW. Of the two Round 2 contracts that were put up for competition, one was retained by the incumbent and had no other competitors. The second contract had three proposals and was won by an organization that holds other QIO contracts. The contract that was up for competition in Round 3 was retained by the incumbent QIO and had no other competitors (personal communications, J. Kelly, January 31, 2006, and March 27, 2006).

QIO View of Competition

In the IOM committee telephone interviews, the QIO CEOs responded to questions about automatic recompetition for each new QIO contract and what impact that might have on their operations.

CEO views on routine recompetition   Twelve of 19 CEOs opposed recompetition for any reason other than nonperformance of contract requirements. They reiterated that the CMS evaluation needed to be fair, and many expressed concern that the QIOs are called before the CMS panel to address matters beyond their control (see the discussion of program evaluation later in this chapter). The major reasons against routine competition that the CEOs cited were the potential for the loss of momentum in quality improvement, the loss of knowledgeable staff, the length of time needed to develop relationships with the provider community, decreased sharing, and perhaps even less innovation. The following are the specific comments of three of the CEOs:

- "It is appropriate to compete if the evaluation is a fair one and the QIO does not pass, but to compete all QIOs is a waste of resources and a diversion from our work. There would be a loss of momentum, as we would be acting in survival mode rather than continuing to improve in the later part of the contract."

- "Gaining trust and knowing the right people in the medical community is a time-consuming process and if you changed every 5 years, you lose momentum."
- "QIOs will not be as innovative because they would be less inclined to take risks."

Decreased sharing Of the seven CEOs asked about the impact on sharing, all believed that recompeting each contract would have a dampening effect. However, one CEO qualified that by saying, "Competition will not impair sharing on best practices for quality improvement but will impact sharing on organizational operations." Two of the seven CEOs said that some of their peers were already cautious about sharing, "You may not want to share something with a neighbor QIO that you think is going to try to take your work away." Some QIOs are perceived as having a growth philosophy with a "predatory" design on other QIO territories.

Timeline Seven of 19 CEOs said that they could accept recompetition at each contract cycle, as long as there was a longer contract period. Of those seven, three favored having everyone competing on a 5-year basis. The other four said that they could accept competition but believed that the QIO program is better off with the incumbent, as long as there is not a nonperformance issue. One of these CEOs commented that a "Baldrige award winner said winning is a culmination of a 10-year journey; it is not something that happens overnight. The same is true for QIOs."

Nine- and 18-Month Monitoring Visits

Much of the monitoring of QIOs occurs on a regular basis through official memos, e-mails, teleconferences, and interactions with project officers, as discussed above; but CMS performs formal monitoring visits at the 9- and 18-month points in the contract cycle (CMS, 2004b). A group of Regional Office staff visit each QIO. This group generally includes the Project Officer in charge of that QIO, a second Project Officer, and one Scientific Officer; but the makeup of the team may vary and can include other Regional or Central Office staff. In general, the 9-month visit serves to clarify contract requirements and to ensure that the QIOs are heading in the right direction. At the 18-month visit, the QIO's performance on the contract thus far is evaluated; and input on how it may improve on activities in those areas on which it is not performing well may be given. Project and Scientific Officers work to develop standardized monitoring forms and streamline these visits. The officers also undergo training by teleconference or webex before the visit cycles.

Before the visits, QIOs complete extensive standardized monitoring reports, and the Project Officers and Government Task Leaders subsequently comment on those reports (CMS, 2004b). During the visit, CMS and QIO staff may discuss items from the report or the difficulties with the performance of the contract that that QIO faced. The visiting team also assesses samples of cases that the QIO reviewed. After the visit, the Project Officer (with input from other team members) finishes the report and prepares a letter with the team's observations and findings. The letter is ultimately reviewed by the Associate Regional Administrator and is sent to the QIO and the Contracting Officer.

During the IOM site visits, many QIOs stated that they believed that the 9- and 18-month visits were not well timed, as the 9th month was too late to change any work already initiated and the 18th month was too late to do anything if it looked like the QIO might fail on a task. However, the IOM committee's web-based data collection tool showed that the QIOs believe that there is intrinsic value in the process of preparation for these monitoring visits, as well as in the feedback that they receive. Forty-two of 52 QIOs (81 percent) rated the value to the QIO of its own preparation for the 9-month monitoring visit as either excellent or good. Forty-three of 52 QIOs (83 percent) said the same about the preparation for the 18-month visit. Forty-two of 52 QIOs (81 percent) rated the value of the feedback received from the 9-month visit as excellent or good, and 43 of 52 QIOs (83 percent) said the same for the value of the feedback received from the 18-month visit.

Contract Implementation and Length

CMS divides the QIO contracts into three rounds for staggered implementation over a 6-month period, from August 2005 to February 2006. For the 8th SOW, Round 1 QIO contracts had an official start date of August 1, 2005; however, the QIOs whose contracts were to begin in Round 2 and Round 3 also began working on 8th SOW activities on the same date by the use of modifications to their contracts for the 7th SOW (personal communication, S. Pazinski, November 14, 2005). If a QIO contract is up for competition but the decision has not yet been made to award the contract to that QIO (as is the case for the one Round 3 QIO contract up for competition as of this writing), the incumbent QIO begins 8th SOW activities along with all the other QIOs. If the contract is eventually awarded to a different organization, the incumbent assists the successor by use of a transition plan that familiarizes the new contractor with state activities, including the provision of materials for case review and quality improvement activities. CMS also adjusts the contracts for new contractors to allow extra time for the delivery of certain deliverables.

During the IOM committee site visits, 7 of 11 QIOs indicated that they believed that the contract cycle was too short. Some believed that a longer contract cycle would help address some of the difficulties associated with the monitoring visits and data lag (as discussed above), which they believed limited their abilities to prove success during the time period of the contract cycle. Three of those QIOs independently suggested the use of a 5-year cycle. Thus, the QIOs also expressed concern that the evaluations focused too much on quantitative results and that the evaluation guidelines were too rigid. (See the discussion on program evaluation later in this chapter.)

In the telephone interviews, the QIO CEOs related that a lack of provision of data in a timely manner has implications for the length of the QIO contract and the perceived unfairness of the CMS evaluation. Eleven of the 20 CEOs mentioned that the lack of timeliness made the 3-year contract time frame inappropriately short because, first, it did not allow sufficient time for the provision of feedback data on quality improvement changes by providers and, second, the data that CMS uses to monitor whether the QIOs had met their performance requirements did not reflect the work that they had done. The QIOs in the first round believed that they were at a particular disadvantage. Some CEOs commented:

- "The way things are structured now, we don't have data that [reflect] but a short intervention period. We should really be doing an intensive 3-year period of intervention. We'd do better if we had feedback on identified participants sooner so we could adapt."
- "We need a longer time horizon; with a longer contract we would have time to use our data to course correct."
- "We really need 24 months of actual intervention which is impossible within a 3-year contract; we need at least a 4-year contract."

QIOSC Contracts

In the IOM committee telephone interviews, 7 of 20 QIO CEOs raised the question of whether the QIOSCs can ever be ahead of the curve if they are trying to sort out task content at the same time that implementation of the QIO contract is required. CEOs suggested that QIOs need a head start by having their contract tasks 6, 9, or even 12 months before the QIOs start new tasks or that all new tasks need to be the subject of pilot tests before the QIOs are assigned the new tasks. As one CEO put it, "Timeliness is a problem because we [QIOs and QIOSCs] are working on the same issue in a parallel time frame." Another CEO said, "Given the time constraints of our own contracts, we need quick answers. Sometimes, if we are trying to get a new project off the ground, we can't get direction from QIOSCs." All CEOs indicated that if the QIOSC is not ready to go on day one, the QIO must move ahead on its own. The QIOs in the first round were particularly affected and had to start the new tasks with no QIOSC materials.

Award Fees

In the QIO contract for the 8th SOW, the Award Fee Plan involves a combination of cost plus fixed fee and cost plus award fee mechanisms. CMS also built in several types of incentives in addition to the base fee. The base fee is 1 percent of contract costs, excluding pass-through costs (reimbursable expenses) and special studies (CMS, 2005a). The Full Pass Performance Award Fee is an award of 1 percent of contract costs per applicable subtask (excluding pass-through and special studies costs) for QIOs that meet all full pass performance expectations. The Excellent Pass Performance Award Fee is an additional award of 1 percent of contract costs per applicable subtask (excluding pass-through and special studies costs) for QIOs that meet the excellent pass criteria. Finally, a Group Award Fee of 2 percent of contract costs per subtask is awarded to QIOs that meet the following three criteria:

- the QIO receives a full pass on evaluation standards for that subtask,
- no more than five QIOs have failed to achieve at least a conditional pass on that subtask, and
- the composite scores for all QIOs meet or exceed specific achievement standards delineated for each subtask in the J-2 attachment of the QIO contract for the eighth.

The Group Award Fee is designed to encourage sharing and collaboration among QIOs, for it is in the best interest of each QIO to ensure that all QIOs pass so that all will receive the additional fee. The contract also specifies that the QIOs will be paid a fixed fee for information systems, contractual requirements, and special studies costs.

In the 8th SOW, QIOs may also qualify for an interim award fee based on performance as of January 2007 (CMS, 2005c). This includes up to 50 percent of the Full Pass Performance Award Fee and up to 50 percent of the Group Award Fee. QIOs that do not qualify for Interim Award Fee payments may receive full award amounts in November 2007. QIOs qualifying for an Interim Award Fee may receive the remainder of the fee at that time as well. In the QIO contract for the 8th SOW, CMS presents detailed information on the measures and calculations used to assess performance for these payments.

OVERALL PROGRAM GUIDANCE

For a public program as diverse and multifaceted as the QIO program, some of the most important functions at the federal level include strategic planning, broad policy guidance and priority setting, coordination with other programs of the U.S. Department of Health and Human Services (DHHS), and evaluation of the whole program. In a federal program, even one that does not require an annual appropriation, these guidance functions take place in the context of the federal budget. That context inevitably creates some uncertainties. Also, as the QIO program becomes more integrated with other CMS activities, the independence of the program's planning and operations will likely be affected.

Strategic Planning

In the months preceding the start of the 8th SOW, CMS began an ambitious long-range planning process for the QIO program with the help of a consultant and the Process Improvement QIOSC (Qualis Health, under its contract as the QIO for Washington state). CMS was looking well beyond the 8th SOW and considering the program over the next 10 to 12 years. After considerable internal discussion, external stakeholder groups offered advice on how transformational change could be achieved. The meetings of the stakeholder groups, including representatives of QIOs, were organized according to the main provider settings addressed by the QIO program: home health agency providers, hospitals, nursing homes, and physicians' practices. The discussion at the physicians' meeting was wide ranging and touched on many of the issues raised by the 8th SOW, such as the role of QIOs in promoting the use of health information technology in physicians' practices. Discussions among the stakeholders and CMS indicated much uncertainty about the roles of QIOs in the 8th SOW, as well as in the future. CMS planned to prepare a report on the substance of the meetings and to provide feedback to the participants.

Policy Direction

As described in the evolution of the QIO program in Chapter 2, there have been significant changes in policy direction with each new contract, including occasional additional changes within a 3-year contract period. In the past, CMS released a version of the new QIO contract well in advance of the request for proposal for the first contract cycle so that the QIOs had time to plan their work and respond to the request for proposal. The transition from the 7th to the 8th SOW was not easy because negotiations within DHHS and among DHHS, CMS, and the Office of Management and Budget over the new QIO contract and funding took longer than it did in previous years. The contract for the 8th SOW, which had been expected to be available in the summer of 2004 for implementation on August 1, 2005, was not formally released until April 2005; and all of the final budget figures were not available until May 20, 2005. Subsequent altered versions of the contract were released in June, September, and November 2005. All QIOs bidding in the first round received guidance from CMS on most but not all of the QIO budget before their responses were due to CMS (personal communication, D. Adler, American Health Quality Association, May 16, 2005).

In the 8th SOW, the tasks of the QIO program reflect a major change from measurement-based quality improvement to assisting providers with achieving transformational change (Rollow, 2004). Early summaries of the 8th SOW, as well as the request for proposal, raised many questions. The QIOs speculated about what "transformational change" really meant and how it would be accomplished (CMS, 2004a; AHQA, 2005). CMS had to post questions and answers on its website to clarify its intent for the QIO contract bidders. The long-range strategic planning meetings mentioned above, which were held after the release of the QIO contract for the 8th SOW, defined the goal as soliciting advice from the stakeholders on how to achieve transformational change in their care settings, how to measure it, and how CMS and QIOs could support that change.

Priority setting is also a key need for the QIO program; beyond the goal of "transformational change" and the six quality aims for health care established by IOM (safety, timeliness, effectiveness, efficiency, equity, and patient-centeredness), it is difficult to discern priorities within the 8th SOW. Compared with the 7th SOW, the 8th SOW involves considerably more tasks, more measures for evaluation, and more identified participant groups. The evaluation formulas are complex, with many different subscores and many different weights, making it impossible to determine where a QIO should focus its time and resources (see Table A.6 in Appendix A). Because failure on any one task could jeopardize noncompetitive renewal for the next SOW, one might assume that all tasks are of equal priority.

The QIOs voiced concerns about CMS's priorities and focus in the 7th SOW. During the IOM committee site visits, 6 of 11 QIOs described frustration with CMS's inconsistent or changing priorities, including contract changes in the middle of an SOW. One QIO specifically criticized the lack of continuity between SOWs, describing difficulty with a "stop-start" effect. Several QIOs expressed a desire for fewer, more well-defined priority areas so that the QIOs could focus their efforts on just a few priorities.

The participants of a focus group held by the IOM committee discussed the direction that the QIO program is taking in the 8th SOW. Themes of concern included the challenge of working with an increased number of identified participants with limited resources, overly complex evaluation formulas, and the lack of flexibility in the contract. The participants also believed that increased competition might lead to decreased collaboration among QIOs, that the contract length was too short to create culture change, and that administrative reporting requirements should be decreased. Overall, the focus group participants believed that DHHS as a whole needs to align its priorities to provide incentives for quality improvement, such as through the implementation of regulatory requirements and pay for performance.

Program Coordination

The QIO program is only one of several health care quality–related efforts under way within CMS, which increases the need for coordination within Medicare and CMS as a whole. Some of that coordination may take place when other offices within CMS desire to use the QIO apportionment to fund their research or other activities or to use the apportionment for policy planning at broader levels.

Support Contracts and Special Studies

Chapter 7 described the various review and funding mechanisms for the special studies and support contracts. At the beginning of the SOW, the program indicates priorities for special studies, but unsolicited proposals may be considered and funded later in the contract period for the SOW. However, no apparent mechanism exists for coordinating projects and funding priorities among those projects. Also, it is unclear how CMS shares information about ongoing studies with the QIO community or what it does with the results of all studies. As one QIOSC representative stated in an interview, "I have no idea what CMS does with special studies' results."

In the IOM committee telephone interviews, 8 of 20 QIO CEOs commented on the pros and cons of pilot testing. All found pilot testing to be favorable from the standpoint of having experience with the task at hand before all QIOs approach that task. However, two CEOs cautioned that sometimes pilot studies are not always the answer, as they can be too state specific and may not have been translated for a wider audience. One CEO commented further that the oversight of special projects is sometimes assigned to a middle manager at CMS with no expertise in the topic area of the project.

Quality Coordination Team

Recently, CMS made efforts to coordinate the quality improvement efforts across all programs of CMS. On September 14, 2004, CMS announced the creation of a new Quality Coordination Team to support and act as staff to the redesigned Quality Council (CMS, 2004c). The administrator of CMS, Mark McClellan, chairs the Quality Council; and its members include the director of each major CMS office. The Quality Council strives to coordinate all CMS efforts related to quality as well as to align those efforts with the quality improvement activities of other public and private organizations (Jencks, 2004). The Quality Coordination Team is led by Steve Jencks, former director of the Quality Improvement Group. Almost all team members are staff from CMS.

In July 2005, CMS released the Quality Council's Quality Improvement Roadmap to improving the quality of care (CMS, 2005b). This roadmap included five major strategies: working through partnerships, public reporting, paying for quality performance, promoting efficient systems (such as electronic health systems), and increasing the availability and improved use of innovative technologies. Major activities of the Quality Coordination Team include direct support of the Quality Council, such as monitoring of work groups, facilitation of partnerships and collaboratives, and participation in breakthrough projects. Topics chosen for focus in the work groups include performance measures and pay for performance, health information technology, the Medicare Part D prescription drug benefit, and CMS Regional Office–Central Office communications. Breakthrough projects include Fistula First, which seeks to improve vascular access in patients with end-stage renal disease; a project that seeks to raise immunization rates in specific settings; and the Institute for Healthcare Improvement's 100,000 Lives campaign (personal communication, S. Jencks, CMS, July 21, 2005). The Quality Coordination Team strives to facilitate partnerships within CMS, with other federal agencies (such as the Centers for Disease Control and Prevention and the Agency for Healthcare Research and Quality), and with nongovernmental organizations (such as the Institute for Healthcare Improvement). The Quality Council and Quality Coordination Team have no direct responsibility for the QIO program, but many CMS staff on the team are directly responsible for the operation of the QIO program.

Measures Selection and Coordination

Some QIO functions, such as the selection of quality measures, require coordination with national stakeholder organizations as well with various offices in CMS. CMS identified four criteria for the selection of measures:

- the measures must be scientifically and clinically sound,
- the measures must be reproducible,
- the measures should not add burden to the provider, and

- the measures should use existing data sources (CMS, 2004b).

CMS worked collaboratively with the CMS Survey and Certification program as well as with the Joint Commission on Accreditation of Healthcare Organizations, the American Medical Association, and the National Committee for Quality Assurance to align measure specifications to minimize reporting burdens on providers. Ultimately, the groups seek endorsement of selected measures by the National Quality Forum. In the 7th SOW, CMS contracted with the Health Services Advisory Group (Arizona's QIO) to maintain measures by the identification, standardization, and endorsement of measures with updating and retirement of the measures as needed (CMS, 2004b). The QIO program also funded work through other parts of CMS that contributed to the development and refinement of other measures, such as the support contract for the Consumer Assessment of Healthcare Providers and Systems (CAHPS) family of surveys ($33.4 million during the 7th SOW) (personal communication, C. Lazarus, March 17, 2005).

Roles and Relationships

Overall, the QIOs express great concern about the relationships between and among QIOs, Program Officers, Government Task Leaders, QIOSCs, and CMS. The QIOs want better definitions of the roles of each of these individuals or groups and streamlining of the management process. During the IOM committee's site visits, the QIOs discussed many challenges related to CMS oversight of the QIO program. Seven of 11 QIOs expressed concerns over the relationship between CMS and the QIOs and communications problems. Specific examples included references to isolation of groups within CMS and poor communication between CMS, the Regional Offices, and the QIOs. The QIOs referred to "tension" in these interactions. Three QIOs specifically mentioned difficulties with ambiguous or poorly defined information, and three were frustrated with "micromanagement" of the program. Five QIOs wanted more flexibility in the program in terms of either quality improvement topic areas or how goals are achieved.

In interviews with five organizations representing seven QIOSCs, QIO staff members also mentioned difficulties in their relationships with CMS's Central Office and with their Government Task Leaders. As described above, all QIOs believed that the relationship with their Government Task Leaders was key, and they provided a range of responses as to whether or not that relationship was positive. QIOSC staff believed that they had limited to no direct interaction with CMS's Central Office and wanted to see a reduction of silos and increased communication among and between the Government Task Leaders and CMS's Central Office.

Elaborating on this issue, during the telephone interviews, one QIO CEO said, "CMS develops these contracts to develop expertise in an area, but then CMS doesn't listen to or take the advice of experts, so we end up with a program directed by Government Task Leaders rather than experts. This structure could use improvement." To get better service, this CEO stated, "There should be direct knowledge transfer [to QIOs] rather than having to get approval by a Government Task Leader at every step." The CEO asserted that "the Government Task Leaders don't seem to have any great urgency in approving materials, so lots of time can transpire. Government Task Leader delay cuts into the time available for technical assistance to QIOs." Another CEO reported that "there is often lack of clear direction from CMS on desired outcomes or that expectations change during the project. Sometimes change is inevitable as information is gathered, but that can substantially change the QIOSC resources. Reasons for change are more palatable if they are clinical rather than political."

In these telephone interviews, the QIO CEOs also expressed concern about the interaction between the QIOSCs and CMS. CEOs pointed out that the QIOSCs have dual audiences, both the QIOs and CMS, and thus have a sense of being caught in the middle. Four respondents whose organizations held QIOSC contracts mentioned having difficulty in being able to respond to QIOs as a direct consequence of CMS delay. One said, "QIOSCs are caught between a rock and a hard place, with CMS being the rock that they have to be responsive to over the QIOs. What the QIOs want goes nowhere until CMS wants it to."

Overall Program Evaluation

Compared with the considerable effort that CMS put into designing complex formulas to evaluate the contract performance of each QIO (see Chapter 10), creating the databases necessary to evaluate their performance, and monitoring the progress of each QIO, it appears to have spent little time on evaluating other aspects of the program and the program as a whole. Although priorities for special studies are set by the Science Council of the Office of Clinical Standards and Quality, as described in Chapter 7, CMS has not developed a system for tracking all the various special study and support contracts, considering the balance of topics and spending, and determining how they might serve program priorities. Also, no system exists for broadly sharing the knowledge acquired through the studies or even letting all the QIOs and other Project Officers and Government Task Leaders know which QIO is working on a particular special study topic.

The Quality Improvement Group was unable to provide the IOM committee with information on the various contracts at a level of detail sufficient for the committee to know what the contracts are supposed to accomplish and whether accomplishments have been made, although individual Project Officers are required to assess their own projects. This lack of information prevents an assessment of the overall value and impact of the spending on special studies and support contracts. In the 7th SOW, nearly 31 percent ($355 million) of the total program's apportionment ($1,154.3 million) was spent on special studies and support contracts (personal communication, C. Lazarus, March 17, 2005).

CMS does not have a mechanism or formula with which it can evaluate individual QIOs overall. Although the program can determine whether a specific QIO has achieved a passing score on its contract performance, it cannot distinguish outstanding QIOs from mediocre QIOs in a holistic sense. Although the QIOs vary widely on many organizational criteria, it is unclear which, if any, of those factors contribute to better performance, as it was not feasible to identify the better-performing QIOs. For example, at the end of the 7th SOW, one of the three QIO contracts for which recompetition was conducted in the first round was held by an organization that had been awarded one of the highest number of special study contracts. Also, as mentioned in Chapter 10, the committee's attempts to group QIOs according to their overall performance on the quality improvement subtasks were unsuccessful. The web-based data collection tool attempted to gather opinions about other QIOs by the QIO community itself, but the results were inconclusive.

More importantly, neither CMS nor independent researchers have performed a conclusive evaluation of the impacts of the 53 QIOs on quality improvement nationally. Also, CMS has not performed a programwide evaluation to examine in detail the synergy, or lack thereof, between the spending on special studies, QIOSCs, and support contracts and the spending on the core contracts.

During the IOM committee's site visits, 4 of 11 QIOs independently related frustration with the contract evaluation process. They believed that the goals were too stringent and that too much emphasis was placed on short-term quantitative results. In the web-based data collection tool, 52 QIOs rated the clarity and timeliness of the evaluation process. Overall, the process did not receive high marks, with only one QIO giving a score of "excellent" on one of the three dimensions indicated in Table 13.8. More than half of the QIOs answered "fair" or "poor" for each of the three dimensions.

In contrast to the QIO evaluations of the 7th SOW, QIOSC evaluations were informal and were primarily based on the completion of a set of deliverables, according to interviews with five organizations representing seven QIOSCs. All believed that their "success" was very subjective and based on the personal satisfaction of their Government Task Leaders.

TABLE 13.8   QIO Ratings of Evaluation Process

Rating	Clarity of Quantitative Portion of Evaluation	Clarity of Qualitative Portion of Evaluation	Overall Timeliness of Information About Evaluation (methodology, process, etc.)
Excellent	1	0	0
Good	18	21	10
Fair	19	19	19
Poor	14	12	23

NOTE: The data in the table represent the number of QIOs responding as indicated. Data are for a total of 52 QIOs.

SOURCE: IOM committee web-based data collection tool.

SUMMARY

This chapter has discussed CMS's oversight of the QIO program. The following are some of the main themes of this chapter, which are reflected in the findings and conclusions presented in Chapter 2:

• Multiple offices and divisions within CMS have responsibility for the QIO program. QIOs expressed frustration with the lack of coordination and communication between and among personnel and with the timeliness of the information provided to them. They criticized the lack of coordination by CMS, which leads to competing agendas for different managers within the QIO program.

• One of the greatest concerns for QIOs was the time lag to the receipt of performance data because it affects their quality interventions as well as their contract performance assessments.

• QIOs oppose routine recompetition for the core contract because of the loss of momentum that it causes, the decreased incentive that QIOs have to share knowledge, and the chance that they might lose their contract.

• Overall, QIOs believe that the 3-year contract period is too short to achieve measurable change and is complicated by the concurrent lag in the time to receipt of performance data. They also believe that the timeline for QIOSC contracts should begin earlier so that the QIOSCs may help the QIOs immediately upon the start of a new SOW.

• Although CMS is developing a strategic plan for the QIO program 12 years into the future, the program still lacks distinct, focused priorities. Neither the core contracts nor the associated evaluation schemes prioritize the QIO activities.

- Evaluations of the QIO core contract are based on overly complex formulas. They hold the QIO accountable for provider improvements on specified measures for short-term quantitative results. In contrast, QIOSC evaluations are mainly subjective and are based primarily on the satisfaction of the Government Task Leader and completion of a set of deliverables.
- CMS lacks any formal means of evaluation of the whole QIO program, its success on improving quality, or the distinction of the performance of one QIO over another.

REFERENCES

AHQA (American Health Quality Association). 2005. *Proceedings of the AHQA Annual Meeting and Technical Conference.* San Francisco, CA: American Health Quality Association.

Beck C, Richard H, Tu J, Pilote L. 2005. Administrative data feedback for effective cardiac treatment: AFFECT, A Cluster Randomized Trial. *Journal of the American Medical Association* 294(3):309–317.

Bradley EH, Carlson MDA, Gallo WT, Scinto J, Campbell MK, Krumholz HM. 2005. From adversary to partner: have quality improvement organizations made the transition? *Health Services Research* 40(2):459–476.

CMS (Centers for Medicare and Medicaid Services). 2002. *7th Statement of Work (SOW).* [Online]. Available: http://www.cms.hhs.gov/qio [accessed April 9, 2005].

CMS. 2003. *HHS Privacy Impact Assessment (PIA)* November 18. [Online]. Available. www.cms.hhs.gov/privacyact/hcqis.pdf [accessed April 21, 2005].

CMS. 2004a. *Proceedings of the QualityNet 2004 Conference.* Washington, DC: Centers for Medicare and Medicaid Services.

CMS. 2004b. The Quality Improvement Organization Program: CMS Briefing for IOM Staff. [Online]. Available: http://www.medqic.org/dcs/ContentServer?cid=1105558772835& pagename=Medqic%2FMQGeneralPage%2FGeneralPageTemplate&c=MQGeneralPage [accessed December 26, 2005].

CMS. 2004c. *Notice from CMS Concerning Positions of Steve Jencks and Bill Rollow.* Unpublished. Baltimore, MD: Centers for Medicare and Medicaid Services.

CMS. 2004d. *Quality Improvement Organization Manual.* September 16. [Online]. Available: http://www.cms.hhs.gov/manuals/110_qio/qio110index.asp [accessed May 11, 2005].

CMS. 2005a. *8th Statement of Work (SOW).* [Online] Available: http://www.cms.hhs.gov/qio [accessed April 9, 2005].

CMS. 2005b. Executive Summary. In: *Quality Improvement Roadmap.* [Online]. Available: http://www.cms.hhs.gov/quality/quality%20roadmap.pdf [accessed September 30, 2005].

CMS. 2005c. *8th Statement of Work (SOW), Version #080105-1.* [Online]. Available: http:// www.cms.hhs.gov/qio [accessed November 4, 2005].

Hughes E. 2004. *8th SOW Contract Issues.* Presentation at QualityNet 2004 Conference. Washington, DC: Centers for Medicare and Medicaid Services.

Jencks SF. 2004. *The Health Care Quality Improvement Partnership.* Powerpoint Presentation to Quality Improvement Organization Subcommittee, October 4, Baltimore, MD.

Jost TS. 1991. Policing cost containment: The Medicare Peer Review Organization Program. *University of Puget Sound Law Review* 3:483–526.

Rollow WC. 2004. *Evaluating the HCQIP Program.* Powerpoint Presentation to Quality Improvement Organization Subcommittee, October 4, Baltimore, MD.

Appendixes

A

Supporting Tables

TABLE A.1 Literature Review on Impact of Quality Improvement[a]

Reference	Data Source, Sample Size, and Time Frame
Barr J, et al. "A Randomized Intervention to Improve Ongoing Participation in Mammography." *The American Journal of Managed Care.* 2001.	• 1,908 women aged 50–75 enrolled in a northeast HMO who had a mammogram with no subsequent visits for next 18–21 months • 1994–1996
Berner, et al. "Do Local Opinion Leaders Augment Hospital Quality Improvement Efforts?" *Medical Care.* 2003.	• Unit of analysis: acute care hospitals in Alabama with more than 100 patients with unstable angina (UA) as the primary or secondary diagnosis; 22 hospitals were willing to participate • Baseline: 1997–1998 Follow-up: 1999–2000
Bradley E, et al. "A Qualitative Study of Increasing Beta-blocker Use After Myocardial Infarction." *JAMA.* 2001.	• Interviews with hospital staff • 45 respondents of various disciplines, staff levels, and hospitals • October 1996–September 1999

Study Purpose, Methodological Approach, and Outcome Measures	Findings
• Effectiveness of various interventions for breast cancer screening guidelines • Randomized control trial with three groups: (1) received mailings, (2) telephone call with option to schedule appointment, and (3) regular publicity campaign • The number of mammograms received after the intervention period and within 2 years of the initial mammogram	• Telephone with option to schedule appointment was the most effective intervention (relative risk = 1.39) Researchers suspect that its success was due to convenience of scheduling and personal aspect • Mailings were not found to be useful • Limitations: this group of women may have been hard to motivate or had mammograms outside of the health plan

• Assess whether or not physician opinion leaders (OL) helped implementation of CMS's HCQIP
• Three-armed randomized control trial (no intervention, HCQIP-CMS's quality improvement plan only, and OL-HCQIP plus addition of physician OL); HCQIP and OL administered change through education of guidelines, presentation of hospital-specific data, and clinical reminders
• Measured adherence to five of AHRQ's UA guidelines (electrocardiography within 20 minutes, antiplatelet medication at discharge, antiplatelet medication within 24 hours, use of heparin, and use of beta-blockers)
• Outcome measure: percent change in compliance with guidelines before and after the intervention for all five interventions
	• Use of OLs results in small, inconsistent effects
	• Use of OLs resulted in significant improvement only with the intervention of antiplatelet medication within 24 hours
	• Many caveats and reasons why the OLs did not show more influence were presented:
	  – Study was limited to chart review data
	  – A physician leader may have stepped up in no-intervention and HCQIP groups
	  – Hospital type may lead to bias
	  – Hospital may concurrently participate in other QI projects
	  – The quality-of-care indicators chosen

• Identify factors that may improve beta-blocker use (i.e., hospital size, geographic region, and changes in beta-blocker use rates). Develop method for classifying it • Qualitative study based on interviews with hospital staff, data analyzed via qualitative coding techniques • Methods to improve care, coded qualitative data	• Importance of physician leadership • Similar initiatives were used to enhance use among hospitals with various MI volumes • No factors were found to directly correlate to higher performance

continues

TABLE A.1   Continued

Reference	Data Source, Sample Size, and Time Frame
Bradley E, et al. "From Adversary to Partner: Have Quality Improvement Organizations Made the Transition?" *Health Services Research*. 2005.	• Primary data in the form of interviews • 105 randomly selected hospital quality management directors • 2002
Burwen D. "National and State Trends in Quality of Care for Acute Myocardial Infarction Between 1994–1995 and 1998–1999." *Archives of Internal Medicine*. 2003.	• Medicare patients with AMI without contraindications per state guidelines • 1994–1995: 234,754 patients 1998–1999: 35,713 patients • Baseline: 1994–1995 Follow-up: 1998–1999

Study Purpose, Methodological Approach, and Outcome Measures	Findings
• Describe impact of QIOs on AMI quality of care • Created survey instrument asking about the following: amount of contact between hospital quality departments and QIO, number of AMI-related QIO-supported or -led interventions, and whether QIO interventions had affected AMI quality	• Interviews generally found the QIOs' quality improvement efforts to be useful (more than 60% of interviewees rated interventions as helpful or very helpful) • Many thought the impact of QIOs was low in that quality of care would not be different in the absence of QIO efforts (only 25% thought care would be worse without QIOs) • QIOs are seen more as collaborative partners than as adversaries, as they were stigmatized in the past • Many believed that QIOs could be more effective at attaining more support from physicians and senior management of hospitals
• Determine improvement in quality of care for AMI • Analyzed data from CCP. Quality indicators studied: early administration of aspirin, aspirin prescribed at discharge, early administration of beta-blockers, beta-blocker prescribed at discharge, ACE prescribed at discharge, and smoking cessation counseling. Used r^2 and chi-squared analyses • Probability of patients studied for whom quality indicators were documented	• Quality improved overall between the two periods • In practice, some types of quality indicators are more readily improved than others (i.e., reperfusion therapy and smoking cessation counseling) due to challenges in implementation (e.g., improvements in an indicator cannot always be accomplished through behavioral changes initiated by a single physician) • Improvement was not due to geographic or regional differences or patient characteristics • Diffusion of evidence-based therapies into practice is not optimal

continues

TABLE A.1   Continued

Reference	Data Source, Sample Size, and Time Frame
Centor R. "Diffusion of Troponin Testing in Unstable Angina Patients: Adoption Prior to Guideline Release." *Journal of Clinical Epidemiology.* 2003.	• Medicare patients with suspected cardiac ischemia in 22 volunteer Alabama hospitals • Baseline: 1,272 patients Follow-up: 1,302 patients • Baseline: March 1997–February 1998 Follow-up: January 1999–December 1999
Chu L, et al. "Improving the Quality of Care for Patients with Pneumonia in Very Small Hospitals." *Archives of Internal Medicine.* 2003.	• Medical record abstraction • 36 hospitals, mostly rural community hospitals, in Oklahoma • Cycle 1: April 1995–June 1995 Cycle 2: November 1996–March 1997

Study Purpose, Methodological Approach, and Outcome Measures	Findings
• Determine status of quality indicators before implementation of guidelines • Examined changes in troponin use before implementation of ACC/AHA presented their clinical guidelines in 2000; quality measures: receipt of aspirin within 24 hours of admission, receipt of aspirin at discharge, receipt of beta-blocker during hospitalization, receipt of heparin during hospitalization for patients at moderate to high risk of AMI or death, performance of EKG within 20 min after arrival, and admission to hospital bed with cardiac monitoring; logistic regression analyses were used to determine appropriateness of troponin use • Troponin ordered, troponin positive when ordered, previously developed quality measures for unstable angina, use of ACE inhibitors, and procedure rates	• Guidelines released in 2000 reflected already accepted practice and not dissemination of new knowledge • Troponin tended to be ordered for higher-risk patients, which may have been an indicator for more aggressive clinical management
• Demonstrate that QIO can be effective external change agent driving improvement of pneumonia treatment guidelines • Hospitals split into two groups. Two intervention cycles. Interventions consisted of QIO providing hospitals feedback via face-to-face meetings with medical staff and individual hospital profiles; hospitals had to provide QIO with quality improvement plans. Cycle 1: first group of hospitals received intervention, results were compared with those for a control (Group 2) Cycle 2: second group (control group in Cycle 1) received intervention • Chi-squared test for proportions, two-tailed t-tests, ANOVA, regression coefficients; $p < 0.05$	• Intervention versus control groups (Cycle 1): – Intervention group found to be more likely to show statistical improvement in process measures than control group – No statistically significant differences in outcomes measures (unadjusted mortality, $p = 0.39$; length of stay, $p = 0.47$) – During Cycle 1, no significant differences from results in control group found, maintaining that differences in process measures not due to external confounders related to the condition • Intervention in control group (Cycle 2): – Statistically significant improvement made in four of five measures after intervention • Results may not be duplicated in large hospitals • CMS policy did not allow randomization of hospitals

continues

TABLE A.1 Continued

Reference	Data Source, Sample Size, and Time Frame
Coleman E, et al. "Preparing Patients and Caregivers to Participate in Care Delivered Across Settings: The Care Transitions Intervention." *Journal of the American Geriatrics Society*. 2004.	• Colorado integrated delivery system • Patients age 65+ with at least one of nine conditions Control: 1,235 patients Intervention: 158 patients • July 2001–September 2002
Cortes L. "The Impact of Quality Improvement Programs in Long Term Care." Texas Department of Human Services. 2004.	• MDS reports of restraint use • Population statewide in LTC facilities, 69,590–70,814 patients • 2002–2003
Daniel D, et al. "A State-Level Application of the Chronic Illness Breakthrough Series: Results from Two Collaboratives on Diabetes in Washington State." *Joint Commission Journal on Quality and Safety*. 2004.	• 47 teams (representing public health delivery system, community care, large clinics, hospitals systems, and private practices) • Collaborative I: October 1999–November 2000 Collaborative II: February 2001–March 2002

Study Purpose, Methodological Approach, and Outcome Measures	Findings
• Determine if transitions between health care settings can be enhanced by more active roles of patients and caregivers • Intervention: designate a transition coach to work with patient and caregiver via visits and phone calls; coaches also teach patients about personal health records; patient records are tracked for rehospitalizations 6 months after discharge • Postdischarge hospital use rates at 30, 90, and 180 days (rehospitalization and emergency room)	• Use of transition coach and personal health record is promising to reduce rehospitalization rates postdischarge • OR at 30 days: 0.52 OR at 90 days: 0.43 OR at 180 days: 0.57 • Actual cost of transition coach over 8 months: $47,133
• Determine the extent to which the Texas Dept. of Human Services (DHS) program and QIO program each contributed to reduced use of restraints among LTC residents • Attributable fraction: 139 facilities enrolled in QIO TA program, all 1,050 facilities in state received TA from DHS. The difference in observed improvement between the QIO subgroup and the remaining facilities is the fraction attributable to the QIO intervention • Change in restraint prevalence among facilities receiving QIO TA and those receiving DHS TA only	• Facilities receiving both DHS and QIO assistance showed a 55.1% reduction in restraint use • Facilities receiving only DHS assistance showed a 35.3% reduction in restraint use • Estimated excess fraction of improvement attributable to the QIO program: 19.8% • Statewide, 90% of improvement is attributable to the DHS program; 10% is attributable to QIO because QIO served only 13% of facilities statewide • Conclusion: state and QIO programs are not redundant and the programs are complementary

• Assess effect of collaboratives at state level; test what efforts may be associated with quality improvement
• Teams independently collected data on process and outcomes of clinical indicators of diabetes care; over 13-month test period, teams congregated at four conferences, sharing lessons learned
• Indicators of success: absolute improvement (from baseline to remeasurement) and improvement in remeasurement values
	• State-level collaboratives effective
	  – Provided more technical support
	  – Increased participation
	• Higher absolute improvement associated with teams with lower baseline levels
	• Process measures had greater absolute improvement, perhaps due to behavioral changes, which are necessary by both providers and patients

continues

TABLE A.1   Continued

Reference	Data Source, Sample Size, and Time Frame
Ellerbeck E, et al. "Quality of Care for Medicare Patients with Acute Myocardial Infarction: A Four-State Pilot Study from the Cooperative Cardiovascular Project." *JAMA*. 1995.	• Medicare's National Claims History File • All Medicare hospitalizations with AMI as primary diagnosis • June 1, 1992–February 28, 1993
Ellerbeck E, et al. "Impact of Quality Improvement Activities on Care for Acute Myocardial Infarction." *International Journal for Quality in Health Care*. 2000.	• 117 acute care hospitals in Iowa • Baseline: June 1992–December 1992 Follow-up: August 1995–November 1995

Study Purpose, Methodological Approach, and Outcome Measures	Findings
• Test the CCP quality-of-care indicators for AMI • Compare data abstracted from medical records for 26 quality indicators; physicians dealing with AMI were asked to check the validity of care received based on each indicator; ideal patients for CCP (those without contraindication) were identified • Percentage of patients who received appropriate care according to quality indicators, based on ACC and AHA guidelines (i.e., aspirin during hospitalization, heparin doses, timing of medication delivery)	• Seventeen to 72% of Medicare patients who should ideally receive therapies for AMI did not receive them either at all or in a timely manner • Treatments are underused for those who do receive them • Many Medicare AMI patients are not "ideal" • Need to improve medical record documentation • Cannot fully validate the measures used due to a lack of standard criteria • CCP quality indicators showed areas for improvement, but quality indicators need to be refined

• Assess relationship between PRO-involved quality improvement activities and improvement in quality of care of AMI treatment
• Two groups:
  – Hospitals with no plan or no systematic change to improve AMI care (73 hospitals)
  – Hospitals undergoing systems change and measurement (44 hospitals)
• Indicators: reperfusion, thrombolytics <60 minutes; aspirin treatment during hospital stay, aspirin treatment at discharge; treatment with beta-blockers, ACE inhibitors, and calcium blockers; smoking cessation counseling
• Change from baseline of percentage of patients receiving indicated treatment
	• Found significant ($p < 0.05$) improvement only for three indicators from baseline (aspirin treatment during stay, aspirin treatment at discharge, and beta-blocker treatment at discharge)
	• Systems change and measurement hospitals tended to have higher values at baseline
	• Suggested caveats: control group was not completely devoid of PRO activities, QI activities were not reported to PRO, process measures instead of outcomes measures were measured

continues

TABLE A.1   Continued

Reference	Data Source, Sample Size, and Time Frame
Gould B, et al. "Improving Patient Care Outcomes by Teaching Quality Improvement to Medical Students in Community-Based Practices." *Academic Medicine*. 2002.	• 77 second-year medical students • 1999–2000
Halm E, et al. "Limited Impact of a Multicenter Intervention to Improve the Quality and Efficiency of Pneumonia Care." *Chest*. 2004.	• Medical record abstraction • Preintervention: 1,013 patients Postintervention: 1,081 patients • Preintervention: December 1999–April 2000 Postintervention: November 2000–March 2001
Holman W, et al. "Alabama Coronary Artery Bypass Grafting Project." *JAMA*. 2001.	• Medical record abstraction • Alabama: 5,784 patients Comparison state: 3,214 patients National sample: 3,758 patients • Baseline: July 1995–June 1996 Follow-up: July 1998–December 1998

Study Purpose, Methodological Approach, and Outcome Measures	Findings
• Determine impact of implementing quality improvement as a component of medical school curriculum • Students used chart abstraction and continuous quality improvement methods in community practice sites; measured improvement in quality of care and surveyed students on their perspectives of the program • Quality of care: improvement in rate of documentation from baseline Students were surveyed using qualitative, open-ended questions	• Quality of care: rate of documentation increased ($p < 0.001$) • Students were more aware of CQI efforts but did not necessarily find value in CQI programs
• Impact of multidisciplinary team in four academic medical centers in New York City to enhance care for community-acquired pneumonia • Matched pre- and postintervention patients; intervention: opinion leaders formed teams to develop guidelines, run educational sessions, produce pocket reminder cards, and promote standardized orders; analyzed antibiotic use, discharge rates prior to clinical stability, length of stay, timely switch to oral antibiotics, and timely discharge • Statistical difference from pre- and postinterventions of process and outcomes measures	• Slight increase in adherence to process measures • No change in outcomes measures • Change in academic medical centers may require more systems-based approach. Process measures may have been more successful due to more evidence and fewer confounders
• Assess quality improvement efforts for CABG in 20 Alabama hospitals • Held meetings with all hospitals in Alabama that performed CABG to provide peer-based feedback and share care processes; measured process and outcomes indicators from baseline to follow-up and compared them with those from a national sample and a comparison state • Mean change from baseline to follow-up; ORs calculated for mortality	• Significant differences were seen in Alabama's improvement in comparison with those of both the comparison state and the national standard ($p < 0.02$ for all measures, $p < 0.001$ for some) • Risk-adjusted mortality OR: 0.72 and 0.76 compared with comparison state and national sample, respectively

continues

TABLE A.1   Continued

Reference	Data Source, Sample Size, and Time Frame
Jamtvedt G, et al. "Audit and Feedback: Effects on Professional Practice and Health Care Outcomes." *Cochrane Library.* 2004.	• Reviewed 85 studies of randomized control trials published between 1997 and 2001
Jencks S, et al. "Quality of Medical Care Delivered to Medicare Beneficiaries." *JAMA.* 2000.	• Medical record abstraction, Medicare hospital claims, and BRFSS • Random sample of all Medicare fee-for-service populations diagnosed with particular conditions • 1997–1999
Jencks S, et al. "Change in the Quality of Care Delivered to Medicare Beneficiaries, 1998–1999 to 2000–2001." *JAMA.* 2003.	• Medical record abstraction • Results from 52 QIOs (does not include Virgin Islands) • Data collection: 1998–1999 and 2000–2001
Joseph A, et al. "Results of a Randomized Controlled Trial of Intervention to Implement Smoking Guidelines in Veterans Affairs Medical Centers." *Medical Care.* 2004.	• Patient surveys, medical record review, surveys of site leaders and pharmacy benefit managers. • 20 Veterans Affairs centers; 5,678 people • 2000–2001

Study Purpose, Methodological Approach, and Outcome Measures	Findings
• Assess whether audit and feedback (a summary of clinical performance over a period of time returned to responsible party in written, electronic, or verbal form) to health care professional and patients was effective • Meta-analysis	• Audit and feedback can be useful but yield inconsistent results (from negative effects to strong positive effects) • Coupling of audit and feedback with other quality improvement efforts does not necessarily enhance effectiveness
• Describe and report baseline values on 24 QIO measures. Focus on processes of care, not outcomes. • Measure performance of the median state (not the national average), rank of states for each measure, and average overall ranking, with geographic trends also evaluated; clinical topics were chosen for their potential for substantial effect on quality • Percentage of people receiving appropriate care for 22 indicators of heart failure, stroke, pneumonia, breast cancer, and diabetes, as defined by CMS, ACC/AHA, ATS, BRFSS, HEDIS, DQIP, and CDC	• No state consistently performs highly or poorly on quality measures • Much room for improvement, according to the 24 measures • Need to focus on systems change, not individual practitioner • General geographic trend: higher-quality ranking associated with northern and less populated states • Impossible to attribute changes in indicators to QIO activities
• Track changes for 22 quality measures at state and national levels • Compared results in 1998–1999 per state per measure with results in 2000–2001; states were also ranked based on performance improvement. • Relative improvement (reduction in failure rate = (change in performance from baseline to follow-up)/(baseline performance – perfect performance))	• Care for Medicare fee-for-service and outpatient beneficiaries increased for 20 of 22 measures • Generally, states with lower baselines yielded greater relative improvements compared with those with higher baselines • National patterns of care were found: northern states generally had higher state rankings and larger relative improvement rates than southern states
• Improve guideline implementation for tobacco use cessation by randomized control trial using AHRQ guidelines • Intervention: training to improve documentation of tobacco use status in medical record, presentation of intervention to all smokers, and liberal use of smoking cessation medications • Odds ratios calculated for pre- and postintervention	• Interventions had little effect on smoking cessation (smoking cessation or increase in medication use) ($p > 0.51$)

continues

TABLE A.1 Continued

Reference	Data Source, Sample Size, and Time Frame
Kiefe C, et al. "Improving Quality Improvement Using Achievable Benchmarks for Physician Feedback." *JAMA.* 2001.	• Medical chart review • 70 community physicians treating 2,978 fee-for-service Medicare patients with diabetes in Alabama • December 1996–December 1998
Luthi J, et al. "Variations among Hospitals in the Quality of Care for Heart Failure." *Effective Clinical Practice.* 2000.	• 2,077 heart failure patients in 69 hospitals in Colorado, Connecticut, Georgia, Oklahoma, and Virginia • June 1995–September 1996
Marciniak T, et al. "Improving Care for Medicare Patients with AMI." *JAMA.* 1998.	• Medical records from hospitals and PROs with ICD-9 code 410 (AMI) • Base group: Medicare patients in Alabama, Connecticut, Iowa, and Wisconsin whose primary discharge diagnosis was AMI • Comparison group: Random sample of Medicare patients from the other 46 states with AMI as the primary diagnosis • Mortality comparisons of all Medicare patients with claims of AMI • June 1992–July 1996

Study Purpose, Methodological Approach, and Outcome Measures	Findings
• Determine if providing feedback to physicians for quality improvement is enhanced by use of benchmarking • Randomized controlled trial where the control group physicians received feedback based on chart review and the intervention group feedback also included benchmarking • Odds ratios were calculated	• Physician performance improved when feedback was combined with benchmarks • Significant improvements were made by the experimental group over the control group in reception of flu vaccine (OR = 1.57), foot exams (OR = 1.33), and long-term HbA1c management (OR = 1.33)
• Determine if care for heart failure varies among hospitals • Calculated percentage of patients receiving care matching the following indicators: assessment of left ventricular function, use of ACE inhibitors for systolic dysfunction, prescription of target dose, consumption of low-sodium diet, and daily weight monitoring • Interquartile range, overall range, and extremal quotient (ratio of highest and lowest values)	• Large variations exist in accordance with quality-of-care guidelines for patients with heart failure • Extremal quotient reached a high of 5.5 (assessment of left ventricular function) and low of 1.7 (use of ACE inhibitors for systolic dysfunction)
• Improve quality of care for AMI patients via CCP in Alabama, Connecticut, Iowa, and Wisconsin • Compare measures for Medicare AMI patients in four CCP states with those in all other states; looked at rates for eligible patients, as well as ideal patients (those with no contraindication) • Quality improvement for 13 clinical guidelines (i.e., reperfusion, aspirin treatment during hospitalization), length of stay, and mortality, all measured by percent difference between pilot group and comparison group	• Measures for CCP patients improved significantly more than those for the other patients • CCP results were significantly different for aspirin use at discharge, beta-blocker use at discharge, and mortality • Results for eligible and ideal patients were not statistically different; therefore, results for the eligible group (for which it is easier to gather data) can be used • Lowered length of stay was probably not due to CCP

continues

TABLE A.1 Continued

Reference	Data Source, Sample Size, and Time Frame
Mark B, et al. "A Longitudinal Examination of Hospital Registered Nurse Staffing and Quality of Care." *Health Services Research.* 2004.	• Previous research findings on five variables: hospital characteristics, market characteristics, financial performance, staffing, and quality of care (American Hospital Association Annual Survey, CMS surveys, HCUP, OSCAR, Solucient, InterStudy, Area Resources) • 442 hospitals (from 1990–1995 HCUP National Inpatient Survey) • 1990–1995
Massing M. "Prevalence and Care of Diabetes Mellitus in the Medicare Population of North Carolina." *NC Medical Journal.* 2003.	• 83,913 Medicare patients with diabetes • Baseline: July 1997–June 1999
McClellan W, et al. "Improved Diabetes Care by Primary Care Physicians: Results of a Group-Randomized Evaluation of the Medicare Health Care Quality Improvement Program." *Journal Clinical Epidemiology.* 2003.	• 22,971 Medicare diabetes patients; 477 PCPs in 123 counties in rural Georgia • Baseline: January–December 1996 Follow-up: January 1998–December 1999
Ornstein S, et al. "A Multimethod Quality Improvement Intervention to Improve Preventive Cardiovascular Care." *Annals of Internal Medicine.* 2004.	• Data extracted from electronic medical records • 87,291 patients from 20 different primary care settings in 14 states • January 2001–January 2003

Study Purpose, Methodological Approach, and Outcome Measures	Findings
• Find effects of change in nursing staffing on changes in quality of care • Used first-difference transformation procedure to analyze data (the procedure studies relationships between changes in the five variables [Anderson and Hsiao, *Journal of the American Statistical Association*, 1981]), as well as ordinary least-squares regression • Changes in nursing staffing, changes in quality of care	• Increases in staffing of registered nurses correlate to lower mortality rates • Increased staffing has broad relationship with decreased mortality rates • Increases in staffing have diminishing marginal effects • The relationship between increased staffing and lowered mortality is not causal; confounders cannot positively be identified
• HbA1c test, eye exam, lipid profile • Percentage of diabetic population claiming one of the indicators; data abstracted from Medicare Part A and B claims	• Treatment levels for target indicators do not meet guidelines, leaving much room for improvement: HbA1c = 77%, lipid profile = 53%, eye exam = 70% • African Americans disproportionately received less diabetes care
• Determine whether feedback reports from claims-based data enhance quality improvement activities, similar to QIO function • Random comparison groups: control group versus intervention group; intervention group received mailings with information about clinical guidelines and implementation tools for HbA1c, urine protein, and dilated eye tests; measured difference in percentage of patients receiving test at baseline and follow-up for both groups • Absolute difference in rates of improvement for each indicator	• PCPs in intervention group had higher rates of improvement than control group • Clinical guidelines were not met by either group • Absolute difference in rate of improvement for HbA1c was 4% (95% confidence, $p = 0.02$). Results were not significant for other indicators • Physician disagreement with clinical guidelines cited as potential reason for not meeting guidelines
• Assess if intensity of quality interventions influences physician adherence to 21 clinical practice guidelines for stroke and cardiovascular disease • Distributed practice guidelines and performance reports quarterly to all providers; randomized controlled trial: half of the practices participated in quarterly visits and annual meetings to share best practices • Percentage of indicators meeting target of 90% adherence for each indicator	• Only marginal change associated with intervention group. Absolute difference = 6% ($p > 0.2$) • 22.4% and 16.4% improvement by intervention and control groups, respectively • Limitation of small n and lack of true control group *continues*

TABLE A.1 Continued

Reference	Data Source, Sample Size, and Time Frame
Pai C, et al. "The Combined Effect of Public Profiling and Quality Improvement Efforts on Heart Failure Management." *Journal on Quality Improvement.* 2002.	• 30 hospitals in southeast Michigan • Baseline: 5,871 patients Follow-up: 4,716 patients • Baseline: January 1998–December 1998 Follow-up: March 2000–August 2000
Schade C, et al. "Using Statewide Audit and Feedback to Improve Hospital Care in West Virginia." *Joint Commission Journal on Quality and Safety.* 2004.	• 44 acute care hospitals in West Virginia • Preintervention: July 1998–June 2000 Postintervention: July 2000–December 2001
Sheikh K, et al. "Evaluation of Quality Improvement Interventions for Reducing Adverse Outcomes of Carotid Endarterectomy." *Medical Care.* 2004.	• Medical record abstraction • 14 states (7 control states, 7 intervention states) matched by number of beneficiaries and procedure rates • Intervention: 1997–1998 Time series: 1991–2001

Study Purpose, Methodological Approach, and Outcome Measures	Findings
• Assess effectiveness of public disclosure of performance data and quality improvement activities on heart failure management • Quality indicators for management of heart failure: documentation of ejection fraction for patients with LVSD, patients prescribed ACE inhibitors after LVSD profiling indicator, patients with LVSD prescribed ACE or used ACE in hospital. Public reporting to employees in November 1999; hospitals were reported by name for those with above or below average rates at 95% confidence • Change in quality indicators (measured in proportions of patients) from the baseline	• Public profiling and quality improvement efforts not indicative of changes in clinical practice • Indicators for ACE inhibitor use showed regression toward the mean (hospitals with high baseline rates had showed declines from the baseline rates, whereas hospitals with low baseline rates showed improvements from baseline rates). • Potential lack of physician understanding and support of quality improvement efforts
• Evaluate effectiveness of audit and feedback systems in improving care in hospitals for five conditions: AMI, heart failure, pneumonia, stroke, and atrial fibrillation • Three groups, based on number of discharges of target conditions; intervention: audit and feedback through reports released after collection of data every 6 months • Pooled pre- and postintervention data from all hospitals' quality indicator rates using simple and weighted paired t-tests, with significance being a p value <0.05; chi-squared tests performed for trend data	• Improvement of quality indicators were achieved in most hospitals; improvement could not be entirely attributable to audit and feedback • Improvement trends were identified mostly in postintervention period • 20% average improvement of quality indicator performance
• Determine effectiveness of quality interventions in reducing mortality rates and adverse outcomes of CEA • PRO provided clinical guidelines and quality indicators to hospitals and physicians, aided in development of improvement plans, and facilitates dissemination of best practices among physicians • Comparison of in-hospital and 30-day post-CEA stroke and mortality rates by using t-tests and chi-square tests; time series from 1991 to 2001 was used to analyze trends	• No decrease found in 30-day mortality and stroke rates • No change in trends studied by the 1991–2001 time series • Lack of improvement may be due to little opportunity for change (i.e., hospitals and physicians already made improvements to CEA procedure before PRO intervention) • Recognizes importance of provider-led change

continues

TABLE A.1 Continued

Reference	Data Source, Sample Size, and Time Frame
Sutherland D, et al. "Diabetes Management Quality Improvement in a Family Practice Residency Program." *Journal of the American Board of Family Practice*. 2001.	• Iowa Medicare patients diagnosed with diabetes • 1997: 313 patients 1998: 268 patients • 1997–1998
Thomson O'Brien, M, et al. "Local Opinion Leaders: Effects on Professional Practice and Health Care Outcomes." *Cochrane Library*. 2005.	• Reviewed eight randomized control trials from a search spanning from 1966 to 1998

[a]This table was used in the committee's analysis of the QIO program; analyses are presented in Chapter 9.

ABBREVIATIONS: ACC = American College of Cardiology; ACE = angiotensin-converting enzyme; AHA = American Heart Association; AHRQ = Agency for Healthcare Research and Quality; AMI = acute myocardial infarction; ANOVA = analysis of variance; ATS = American Thoracic Society; BRFSS = Behavioral Risk Factor Surveillance System; CABG = coronary artery bypass grafting; CCP = Cooperative Cardiovascular Project; CDC = Centers for Disease Control and Prevention; CEA = carotid endarterectomy; CMS = Centers for Medicare and Medicaid Services; DQIP = Diabetes Quality Improvement Project; EKG = electrocardiography;

Study Purpose, Methodological Approach, and Outcome Measures	Findings
• Determine if use of quality interventions at a local level targeting resident physicians improves quality of care • Retrospective cohort with the use of chi-square and t-tests; p values <0.05 were significant. Compared local results to statewide results • Utilization rate of accepted diabetes care indicators	• Significant improvement ($p < 0.001$) in documenting target indicators for diabetes care achieved at local level • Statewide results also indicated improvement in diabetes care but not in other indicators
• Determine the impact of local opinion leaders (educationally influential peer-nominated providers) • Meta-analysis	• The roles and definitions of opinion leaders are largely vague and without consensus, making determination of effectiveness difficult • Can be effective in combination with other types of interventions (e.g., audit and feedback, mailings, etc) and by itself; may be more effective than audit and feedback • Results are mixed

HbA1c = hemoglobin A1c; HCQIP = Health Care Quality Improvement Program; HCUP = Healthcare Cost and Utilization Project; HEDIS = Health Plan Employer Data and Information Set; HMO = health maintenance organization; ICD-9 = International Classification of Diseases-9; LTC = long term care; LVSD = left ventricular systolic dysfunction; MDS = Minimum Data Set; OR = odds ratio; OSCAR = Online Survey, Recertification, and Reporting; PCP = primary care provider; PRO = Peer Review Organization; QI = quality improvement; QIO = Quality Improvement Organization; TA = technical assistance.

TABLE A.2　Literature Methodology Table

Methodology and Reference	Quality Improvement or QIO Study	Conclusion About Effectiveness on Quality		
		Yes	Maybe	No
Systematic review				
Jamtvedt	QI		x	
Thomson O'Brien	QI		x	
Randomized controlled trial				
Barr	QIO	x		
Berner	QIO		x	
Joseph	QI			x
Kiefe	QIO	x		
McClellan	QIO		x	
Ornstein	QI		x	
Quasiexperimental				
Coleman	QI		x	
Holman	QIO	x		
Sheikh	QIO			x
Snyder	QIO			x
Cohort study				
Burwen	QIO		x	
Chu	QIO	x		
Cortes	QIO		x	
Daniel	QIO	x		
Dellinger	QI	x		
Ellerbeck (2000)	QIO		x	
Gould	QIO	x		
Halm	QI		x	
Marciniak	QIO	x		
Mark	QI		x	
Pai	QIO			x
Schade	QIO		x	
Sutherland	QIO	x		
Cross-sectional study				
Centor	QIO			x
Jencks (2000)	QIO		x	
Jencks (2003)	QIO		x	
Luthi	QIO			x
Massing	QIO			x
Ecologic study				
Ellerbeck (1995)	QIO		x	
Qualitative study				
Bradley (2005)	QIO		x	
Bradley (2001)	QI			x

NOTE: QI = quality improvement; QIO = Quality Improvement Organization.

TABLE A.3a Comparison of Quality Improvement Organization (QIO) Performance Measures and Measures Recommended by Institute of Medicine[a] for Task 1a—Nursing Homes

Performance Measure	QIO—8th SOW Statewide	QIO—8th SOW CPOCC IPG	QIO—7th SOW Statewide and Identified Participants	Performance Measure[b] Starter Set
Chronic care				
Basic tasks				
Toileting			$\checkmark^R$	$\checkmark$
Transferring			$\checkmark^R$	$\checkmark$
Eating			$\checkmark^R$	$\checkmark$
Mobility decline			$\checkmark^R$	$\checkmark$
Bedfast				$\checkmark$
Pain	$\checkmark^R$ (optional)	$\checkmark^R$ (optional)	$\checkmark^R$	$\checkmark$
Infections			$\checkmark^R$	
Pressure sores				
High risk	$\checkmark^R$	$\checkmark^R$	$\checkmark^R$	$\checkmark$
Low risk			$\checkmark^R$	$\checkmark$
Restraint use	$\checkmark^R$	$\checkmark^R$	$\checkmark^R$	$\checkmark$
Depression or anxiety worsening	$\checkmark^R$	$\checkmark^R$		$\checkmark$
Incontinence				$\checkmark$
Urinary tract infections				$\checkmark$
Indwelling catheters				$\checkmark$
Weight loss				$\checkmark$
Post acute care				
Pain			$\checkmark^R$	$\checkmark$
Pressure sores	$\checkmark^R$			$\checkmark$
Delirium symptoms			$\checkmark^R$	$\checkmark$
Improved in walking			$\checkmark^R$	

NOTE: $\checkmark$ = required performance measure; $\checkmark^R$ = required performance measure that is reported to the public by the Centers for Medicare and Medicaid Services (CMS); CPOCC IPG = Clinical Performance and Organizational Culture Change Identified Participant Group.

[a]See the *Performance Measurement* report of this series. IOM (Institute of Medicine). 2006. *Performance Measurement: Accelerating Improvement.* Washington, DC: The National Academies Press.

[b]The performance measure set recommended by the *Performance Measurement* report of this series (see footnote *a*).

TABLE A.3b   Comparison of Quality Improvement Organization (QIO) Performance Measures and Measures Recommended by Institute of Medicine[a] for Task 1b—Home Health

Performance Measure	QIO— 8th SOW Statewide and Clinical Performance IPG[b]	QIO— 7th SOW Statewide and Identified Participants	Performance Measure[c] Starter Set
Chronic care			
Activities of daily living			
Stabilization in bathing		✓R	✓
Post acute care			
Activities of daily living			
Improvement in dressing upper body		✓R	✓
Improvement in bathing	✓R	✓R	✓
Management of oral medications	✓R	✓R	✓
Getting around			
Improvement in toileting		✓R	✓
Improvement in ambulation/ locomotion	✓R	✓R	✓
Improvement in transferring	✓R	✓R	✓
Improvement in pain interfering with activity	✓R	✓R	✓
Physical health			
Improvement in dyspnea	✓		
Improvement in status of surgical wounds	✓		
Improvement in urinary incontinence	✓		
Mental health			
Improvement in cognitive functioning		✓	
Improvement in confusion frequency			✓
Staying at home without home care			
Discharged to community	✓		
Prevalence measures			
Acute care hospitalization	✓R	✓R	✓
Emergent care		✓R	✓

NOTE: ✓ = required performance measure; ✓R = required performance measure that is reported to the public by the Centers for Medicare and Medicaid Services (CMS).

[a]See the *Performance Measurement* report of this series. IOM (Institute of Medicine). 2006. *Performance Measurement: Accelerating Improvement.* Washington, DC: The National Academies Press.

[b]IPG = Identified Participant Group.

[c]The performance measure set recommended by the *Performance Measurement* report of this series (see footnote a).

TABLE A.3c Comparison of Quality Improvement Organization (QIO) Performance Measures and Measures Recommended by Institute of Medicine[a] for Task 1c—Hospital Setting

| Performance Measure | QIO—8th SOW | | | | QIO—7th SOW | |
	Statewide	Task 1c1: ACM IPG	Task 1c1: SCIP IPG	Task 1c2: CAH	Statewide and Identified Participants	Performance Measure[b] Starter Set
Surgical complications						
Infection						
On-time prophylactic antibiotic administration	✓		✓*		✓	✓
Appropriate selection of prophylactic antibiotics	✓		✓*			✓
Prophylactic antibiotics discontinued within 24 hours after surgery	✓		✓*		✓	✓
Controlled perioperative serum glucose (<201 mg/dL) among major cardiac surgery patients			✓*			
Postoperative wound infection diagnosed during index hospitalization			✓			
Appropriate hair removal			✓*			
Perioperative normothermia among colorectal surgical patients			✓*			
Controlled perioperative serum glucose (<201 mg/dL) among noncardiac major surgery patients			✓			
Major surgical patients without planned hypothermia who maintained normothermia during the perioperative period			✓			

continues

TABLE A.3c Continued

Performance Measure	QIO—8th SOW				QIO—7th SOW	
	Statewide	Task 1c1: ACM IPG	Task 1c1: SCIP IPG	Task 1c2: CAH	Statewide and Identified Participants	Performance Measure[b] Starter Set
Cardiovascular						
Major noncardiac surgery patients received beta-blockers during perioperative period			✓*			
Major surgery patients received beta-blocker perioperatively if they were maintained on a beta-blocker prior to surgery			✓*			
Intra- or postoperative acute myocardial infarction diagnosed during index hospitalization and within 30 days of surgery			✓			
Intra- or postoperative cardiac arrest diagnosed during index hospitalization and within 30 days of surgery			✓			
Thromboembolic						
Thromboembolism prophylaxis			✓*			
Appropriate venous thromboembolism prophylaxis			✓*			
Intra- and postoperative pulmonary embolism			✓			
Intra- and postoperative deep venous thrombosis			✓			

TABLE A.3c Continued

Performance Measure	QIO—8th SOW				QIO—7th SOW	
	Statewide	Task 1c1: ACM IPG	Task 1c1: SCIP IPG	Task 1c2: CAH	Statewide and Identified Participants	Performance Measure[b] Starter Set
Respiratory						
Postoperative orders and documentation of elevation of Head of Bed			✓*			
Postoperative ventilator associated pneumonia during index hospitalization		✓				
Peptic ulcer disease prophylaxis received			✓*			
Ventilator-weaning protocol			✓*			
Vascular access						
Permanent hospital end-stage renal disease vascular access procedures that are autogenous arteriovenous fistulas		✓				
Global						
Mortality within 30 days of surgery		✓				
Readmission within 30 days of surgery			✓			
Acute myocardial infarction						
Aspirin at arrival	✓	✓*		✓*	✓	✓
Aspirin prescribed at discharge	✓	✓*		✓*	✓	✓
Angiotensin-Converting Enzyme for left ventricular systolic dysfunction (LVSD) at discharge	✓	✓*		✓*	✓	✓
Smoking cessation	✓				✓	✓
Beta-blocker at arrival	✓	✓*		✓*	✓	✓

continues

TABLE A.3c Continued

Performance Measure	QIO—8th SOW Statewide	Task 1c1: ACM IPG	Task 1c1: SCIP IPG	Task 1c2: CAH	QIO—7th SOW Statewide and Identified Participants	Performance Measure[b] Starter Set
Acute myocardial infarction *(continued)*						
Beta-blocker prescribed at discharge	✓	✓*		✓*	✓	✓
Thrombolytic agent within 30 min of arrival	✓			✓	✓	✓
Percutaneous Coronary Intervention within 120 minutes of arrival	✓				✓	✓
Time to EKG	✓			✓*		
Heart failure						
Left ventricular function assessment	✓	✓*		✓*	✓	✓
ACE therapy for LVSD at discharge	✓	✓*		✓*	✓	✓
Detailed discharge instructions	✓	✓*			✓	✓
Smoking cessation advice/ counseling	✓				✓	✓
Pneumonia						
Blood culture performed within 24 hours prior to or after arrival at the hospital					✓	
Blood culture collected prior to first antibiotic administration	✓				✓	✓
Patients with pneumonia who receive influenza screening or vaccination	✓				✓	✓
Patients with pneumonia who receive pneumococcal screening or vaccination	✓	✓*		✓*	✓	✓
Antibiotic treatment timing	✓	✓*		✓*		✓
Oxygenation assessment	✓	✓*		✓*	✓	✓
Initial antibiotic treatment consistent with current recommendations	✓				✓	✓

TABLE A.3c Continued

Performance Measure	QIO—8th SOW				QIO—7th SOW	
	Statewide	Task 1c1: ACM IPG	Task 1c1: SCIP IPG	Task 1c2: CAH	Statewide and Identified Participants	Performance Measure[b] Starter Set
Pneumonia *(continued)*						
Smoking cessation advice/ counseling	✓				✓	✓
Smoking cessation advice/ counseling for pediatric pneumonia patients					✓	

NOTE: ✓ = required performance measure; ✓* = required performance measure; the Centers for Medicare and Medicaid Services (CMS) evaluates the QIOs only on these particular measures in assessing identified participant groups of Task 1c1 and all providers for Task 1c2. ACM IPG = Appropriate Care Measure Identified Participant Group (Task 1c1); SCIP IPG = Surgical Care Improvement Project Identified Participant Group (Task 1c1); CAH = Critical Access Hospital/Rural Hospital Quality Improvement Measures (Task 1c2).

[a]See the *Performance Measurement* report of this series. IOM (Institute of Medicine). 2006. *Performance Measurement: Accelerating Improvement.* Washington, DC: The National Academies Press.

[b]The performance measure set recommended by the *Performance Measurement* report of this series (see footnote *a*).

TABLE A.3d Comparison of Quality Improvement Organization (QIO) Performance Measures and Measures Recommended by Institute of Medicine[a] for Task 1d—Physician Office

Performance Measure	QIO—8th SOW			QIO—7th SOW	
	Task 1d1: Statewide	Task 1d1: IPG (1 and 2)[b]	Task 1d2: UP	Statewide and Identified Participants	Performance Measure[c] Starter Set
Preventive care					
Tobacco cessation counseling				✓	
Tobacco use				✓	
Prevention					
Cholesterol screening		✓R			
Blood pressure		✓R			
Colorectal cancer screening		✓R			✓
Breast cancer screening	✓R,V	✓R	✓	✓	✓
Cervical cancer screening				✓	
Pneumococcal vaccine	✓R,V	✓R	✓		✓
Influenza vaccine	✓R,V	✓R	✓		✓
Prenatal Care					
Anti-D immune globulin				✓	
Screening for human immunodeficiency virus				✓	
Acute care					
Acute myocardial infarction					
Aspirin treatment at arrival for acute myocardial infarction	✓V				
Beta-blocker treatment at time of arrival for acute myocardial infarction	✓V				
Pneumonia					
Antibiotic administration timing for patient hospitalized for pneumonia		✓V			
Surgery					
Antibiotic prophylaxis	✓V				
Thromboembolism prophylaxis	✓V				
Use of internal mammary artery in coronary artery bypass graft (CABG) surgery	✓V				
Preoperative beta-blocker for patient with isolated CABG	✓V				

TABLE A.3d Continued

Performance Measure	QIO—8th SOW			QIO—7th SOW	
	Task 1d1: Statewide	Task 1d1: IPG (1 and 2)[b]	Task 1d2: UP	Statewide and Identified Participants	Performance Measure[c] Starter Set
Prolonged intubation in isolated CABG	✓V				
Surgical reexploration in CABG	✓V				
Aspirin or clopidogrel treatment on discharge for isolated CABG	✓V				
Chronic disease care					
Diabetes[d]					
Hemogloblin A1c (HbA1c) test	✓R	✓R	✓	✓	✓
HbA1c control	✓V	✓R			✓
Urine protein testing		✓R			
Lipid profile	✓R	✓R	✓	✓	✓
Low-density lipoprotein (LDL) cholesterol screening					✓
LDL control	✓V				
Adults diagnosed with diabetes with most recent blood pressure <140/90 mm Hg					✓
High blood pressure control	✓V				
Eye exam	✓R	✓R	✓	✓	✓
Foot exams		✓R			
End-stage renal disease					
Dialysis dose	✓V				
Hematocrit level	✓V				
Receipt of autogenous ateriovenous fistula	✓V				
Coronary Artery Disease[e]					
Antiplatelet therapy	✓V	✓R			✓
Drug therapy for lowering LDL cholesterol		✓R			✓
LDL control	✓V				
Beta-blocker therapy— prior myocardial infarction	✓V	✓R			✓
Angiotensin-Converting Enzyme inhibitor therapy		✓R			

continues

TABLE A.3d　Continued

Performance Measure	QIO—8th SOW			QIO—7th SOW	
	Task 1d1: Statewide	Task 1d1: IPG (1 and 2)[b]	Task 1d2: UP	Statewide and Identified Participants	Performance Measure[c] Starter Set
Heart failure					
Weight measurement		✓R			
Patient education		✓R			
Beta-blocker therapy	✓V	✓R			
Warfarin therapy for patients with atrial fibrillation	✓V	✓R			
Left ventricular ejection fraction testing		✓R			
Left ventricular function assessment					✓
ACE inhibitor/Angiotensin II-Receptor Blocks therapy for left ventricular systolic dysfunction	✓V				✓
Asthma					
Use of appropriate medications					✓
Pharmacologic therapy					✓
Depression					
Acute					
Antidepressant medication management	✓V				✓
Chronic					
Antidepressant medication management	✓V				✓
Osteoporosis					
Screening in elderly female patient	✓V				
Prescription of calcium and vitamin D supplements	✓V				
Antiresorptive therapy or parathyroid hormone treatment, or both, in patients with newly diagnosed osteoporosis	✓V				
Bone mineral density testing and osteoporosis treatment and prevention following osteoporosis-associated nontraumatic fracture	✓V				

TABLE A.3d Continued

Performance Measure	QIO—8th SOW			QIO—7th SOW	
	Task 1d1: Statewide	Task 1d1: IPG (1 and 2)[b]	Task 1d2: UP	Statewide and Identified Participants	Performance Measure[c] Starter Set
Osteoarthritis					
Annual assessment of function and pain	$\checkmark^{V}$				
Chronic obstructive pulmonary disease					
Smoking cessation intervention	$\checkmark^{V}$				
Long term care					
Screening of elderly patients for falls	$\checkmark^{V}$				
Screening of hearing acuity in elderly patients	$\checkmark^{V}$				
Screening for urinary incontinence in elderly patients	$\checkmark^{V}$				
Quality measures addressing overuse or misuse					
Appropriate treatment for children with upper respiratory infection					$\checkmark$
Appropriate testing for children with pharyngitis					$\checkmark$

NOTE: UP = underserved populations; $\checkmark$ = required performance measure; $\checkmark^{R}$ = required performance measure that is reported to the public by the Centers for Medicare and Medicaid Services (CMS); $\checkmark^{V}$ = measure included in the Physician Voluntary Reporting Program.

[a]See *Performance Measurement* report of this series. IOM (Institute of Medicine). 2006. *Performance Measurement: Accelerating Improvement.* Washington, DC: The National Academies Press.

[b]Identified Participant Groups are responsible for reporting these measures to CMS.

[c]The performance measure set recommended by the *Performance Measurement* report of this series (see footnote *a*).

[d]Identified participant groups are evaluated in part on the basis of having met target levels of performance for diabetes.

[e]Identified participant groups are evaluated in part on the basis of having met target levels of performance for coronary artery disease.

TABLE A.3e   Crosscutting Performance Measures and Other Settings

Patients' reports of care
    CAHPS family of surveys, as they become validated
        Hospital CAHPS
        Ambulatory CAHPS
End-stage renal disease
    Dialysis patients registered on a waiting list for transplantation
    Patients with treated chronic kidney failure receiving transplant within 3 years of
        renal failure
    Patient survival rate
    Hemodialysis patients with urea reduction ratio of 65 or greater
    Patients with hematocrit of 33 or greater
Efficiency measures
    After diagnosis of acute myocardial infarction
        One-year mortality rate
        Resource use
        Functional status
Health plans and accountable health organizations
    HEDIS integrated delivery system measures
        Effectiveness
        Access/availability of care
        Satisfaction with experience of care
        Health plan stability
        Use of service
        Cost of care, informed health care choices, health plan descriptive information
Structural measures
    Computerized physician order entry
    Intensive care unit intensivists
    Evidence-based hospital referrals

NOTE: Measures recommended by the *Performance Measurement* report, but not in Quality Improvement Organization measure sets. IOM (Institute of Medicine). 2006. *Performance Measurement: Accelerating Improvement.* Washington, DC: The National Academies Press.

CAHPS = Consumer Assessment of Healthcare Providers and Systems; HEDIS = Health Plan Employer Data and Information Set.

TABLE A.4a Support Contracts for the 7th SOW

Project Title	QIO	Award
Task 1a—Nursing Home Support QIO	RI	$4,229,692
Task 1a—Working with Nursing Home Chains	CO	$2,331,171
Task 1b—Home Health Support QIO	MD	$6,350,000
Task 1b—Home Health Public Reporting Pilots	CO, WA	$2,223,521
Task 1c—Infectious Disease/Surgical Site Support QIO	OK	$3,000,000
Task 1c—Infectious Disease QIOSC for Surgical Care Improvement	OK	$543,896
Task 1c—Qualis Health IHI Collaborative Project (SIP)	WA	$914,468
Task 1c—Cardiovascular Support QIO	CO	$2,971,390
Task 1d—Physician Office Support QIO	VA	$2,400,000
Task 1d—Communities of Practice	VA	$506,092
Task 1d and f—Data Support QIO	IA	$2,367,468
Task 1d and f—Outpatient Data Additional Funding	IA	$440,000
Task 1e—Task 1e Support QIO	TN	$2,731,607
Task 1f—Task 1f Support QIO	VA	$502,773
Task 2a—Task 2a Support QIO	WA	$3,100,000
Task 2b—Hospital-Generated Data Support	IA	$2,698,628
Task 3a and c— Medicare Beneficiary Protection Support QIO	CA	$3,760,032
Task 3b—Hospital Payment Monitoring QIO	TX	$2,303,910
Hospital Payment Monitoring Program (HPMP) Projects	Multiple	$9,257,769
MedQIC Website—Transition from Delmarva to IFMC	IA	$3,980,548
Quality Improvement Interventions Support QIO	VA, MD	$1,263,774
Training QIOs in human factors	UT	$350,000
Nursing Home Initiative Ads	IA	$2,800,000
Home Health Initiative Ads	IA	$3,000,000
Hospital Initiative Ads	WA	$3,000,000
TOTAL SUPPORT SEVENTH SOW CORE WORK		$67,026,739
Learning from innovative quality improvement approaches in nursing homes	WI	$975,000
Health Care Collaborative Network Project	CO	$200,000
Doctor's Office Quality—Information Technology	CA	$11,000,000
HHA Outcomes-Based Quality Improvement Evaluation	UT	$350,000
Surgical Complications	OH, KY	$3,009,672
Achievable NH targets for pressure ulcers & restraints	RI	$218,008
Depression projects	NY, MI	$1,046,000
CMS colorectal cancer screening	NC	$58,914
Physician's office registry development	MD	$35,000
Health outcomes survey	AZ	$3,600,000
Hospital public reporting pilot projects	AZ	$3,131,453
Patient safety learning pilot projects: IN, NV, UT, WI	Multiple	$1,874,056
Medicare Patient Safety Monitoring System (excluding CDACs)	CT	$786,031
Medicare Patient Safety QIOSC	CT	$1,998,290
Rural Antibiotic (RADAR) Project	ID	$33,107
Doctor's office quality	CA, IA, NY	$4,249,864

continues

TABLE A.4a   Continued

Project Title	QIO	Award
Chronic Kidney Disease Pilot Intervention	GA	$299,957
Rural Hospital Quality Measures	MN	$351,436
Quality of Care in Community Health Centers Using Health Care Facilitators	TN	$146,377
Identify New Areas of Disparity Work for Eighth SOW	TN	$131,104
Information Collection on Past/Potential Disparity Projects	TN	$118,380
Cervical Cancer Mortality	TN	$18,161
Physician Office Registry Development	MT	$4,000,000
Rebuild MedQIC Website like IHI's QHC.org	IA	$910,000
Best Practices in QIOs to Help Providers Improve Quality Measures	WA	$2,795,610
Case Studies—High Performers	AZ	$800,000
Statistical Support	IA	$636,710
Process Improvement QIOSC	WA	$1,287,910
New England Complex Systems Institute	UT	$100,000
Negative or Positive Public Reporting of Measures	MD	$93,979
Review of Managed Care Organization Required National Quality Projects	NY, CA, MD	$1,032,526
BIPA Notice of Proposed Rulemaking Grijalva	IN	$403,000
ESRD Facility Specific Reports (Dialysis Compare)	WA	$1,449,000
CAHPS Nursing Home	AZ	$1,300,000
Presenting Accurate Nursing Home Staffing Ratios	CO	$671,049
Continue Hospital Core PM Project	MS	$553,360
Measures Management	AZ	$1,301,638
Continuation of Pharmaceuticals Project	MS	$1,200,000
Development of Robust Measure Set Phase I	NY	$412,722
Voluntary Hospital Reporting (Setting Priorities)	CT, MD	$315,000
Risk Adjustment for HF outcomes	CO	$247,082
ESRD Facility Specific Reports	CO	$803,207
Admission Decisions: Developing Best Practices—NV/MO/CA	Multiple	$2,378,628
Continuing Medical Education	IA	$10,491
Continuing Medical Education	CO	$13,441
Process improvement—additional funds	WA	$125,375
Evaluating the framing of Publicly Reported Quality Performance Measures	MD	$65,000
Dev. Risk Adj. Models ($40,000 to cover shortfall)	CO	$40,000
Quality Improvement Recommendations	MA, OH	$420,969
Hospital Leadership's Impact on Performance	MD	$82,400
Dave squared	RI	$75,000
Culture Change Pilot/Workforce Study	RI	$985,494
SFF Study	OK	$100,000
Hopital PrU Cross-Setting Project	CO	$115,791
Supplemental Funding for the Task 2B QIOSC (Total $1,288,265 less $819,000 existing IA funds)	IA	$469,265
Alternative Methods for Resolving Beneficiary Complaints	CO, NY	$366,738
Development of Risk Adjustment Models	CO	$200,000

TABLE A.4a Continued

Project Title	QIO	Award
Field Testing of the HSPREAT (Human Subjects Protection Research Exemption Assessment Tool)	VA	$50,000
Quality Expert Panel	VA	$99,679
Call for Proposals for Creating an Enviornment for Quality (projects must support transitional work for Task 2 under eighth SOW using $800,000 IA Surplus transferred to Qualis)	IA	$821,075
Hospital Leadership and Systems Improvement	IN	$784,925
OBQI Web-Based Training ($250,000 to come from existing HH QIOSC)	MD	$200,000
Accelerating Hospital QI through Team Based Organizational Culture	MD	$128,000
Spreading Team Based Organization Culture to QIOs	MD	$98,500
Academic Medical Centers and Chronic Kidney Disease Collaboration	GA	$560,448
Rural Hospital Measure Development	MN	$196,547
Remaking American Medicine Website (PBS)	WA	$100,000
Cross-Setting Collaborative to Enhance Home Health Service Utilization	MD	$330,000
Spreading the Patient Safety Learning Pilot—IN/WI	IN, WI	$425,000
Optimizing the HCQIP Strategic Plan—Process Improvement Training	WA	$249,222
Determination of payment errors for improper billing of short-stay outliers for long-term acute care stays	Multiple	$209,876
Emergency Department Quality Measures Pilot Test	WA	$150,000
TOTAL DEVELOPMENTAL/SPECIAL PROJECTS		$63,795,467
TOTAL APPROVED DEVELOPMENTAL/SUPPORT QIO PROJECTS		$130,822,206

SOURCE: Personal communication, C. Lazarus, March 17, 2005.

TABLE A.4b   Special Studies for the 7th SOW

Contract Number	Proposed Activity/Project	3-Year Total
27	QIO Standard Data Processing System	$31,003,638
28	Clinical Data Abstraction Centers	$50,237,606
32	Medicare Surveillance System Data Collection	$2,844,134
33	Health Care Quality Improvement Prog (HCQIP)	$1,683,146
37	Quality Improvement and Evaluation System (QIES)	$29,623,860
74	Facilities Management Contract Support	$6,000,000
79	QIES MDS MDCN Charges	$3,014,568
193	Health Plan Management System (HPMS)	$3,173,948
331	Project to Integrate the ESRD System	$6,428,030
5004	Seventh SOW Training/Development Meetings	$31,660
5006	CDAC Pass-Thru	$4,854,997
5026	Hospital Core Measurement Set	$2,989,859
5029	Medicare HEDIS Quality-of-Care Performance Measures	$3,849,519
5032	Measurement Indicators & Improvement Quality of Life in NHs	$695,220
5038	MEGA QI Project	$2,133,000
5046	QIO Audit Support	$1,627,498
5059	Technology Assessment	$4,800,000
5061	Usefulness of Quality Indicators in Survey Process	$1,199,100
5077	Quality Forum Membership	$47,250
5079	Immunization Remeasurement (Telesurvey)	$534,240
5080	Healthy Aging Project	$5,886,150
5081	Citizen Advocacy Center Training and Support	$266,978
5082	Study and Development of QIO Best Practices	$1,489,678
5083	PRO Mediation Training & Internal Quality Control	$792,238
5084	Vista	$100,000
5085	Clinical Data Abstraction Center (CDACs) Abstraction for CHF QAPI	$1,107,250
5086	HL7 Standards Setting Process	$100,000
5087	QIO Subtask Certification	$149,986
5100	Data Accuracy and Verification	$1,766,593
5200	ESRD CAHPS	$165,000
5202	CAHPS	$33,439,343
5217	Prevention Initiatives	$799,993
5218	Website Quality Support	$3,087,000
5220	Promotion, Quality, Consumer Research	$5,381,777
5402	Influenza/Pneumococcal Vaccination Campaign	$1,708,164
5403	Mammography Campaign	$1,523,745
5501	National Quality Forum Collaboration	$749,524
5502	Doctors Office Quality Improvement Project Collaboration with AMA	$20,000
5503	Physician Measurement in Managed Care and Fee for Service	$1,422,803
5505	ESRD Performance Measures	$2,061,236
5506	Home Health Outcomes Based Quality Improvement	$300,000

continues

TABLE A.4b   Continued

Contract Number	Proposed Activity/Project	3-Year Total
5507	Home Health Quality Measurement & Refinement	$1,299,673
5508	Minimum Data Set (MDS) 3.0 Development	$4,420,840
5509	HEDIS Health Outcomes Survey	$4,249,170
5510	ESRD Patient Survey	$500,000
5511	Pittsburgh Research Initiative	$1,499,740
5513	ESRD Public Reporting Initiative	$248,532
5514	Analysis Contract	$449,864
5515	Senior Risk Reduction	$3,291,258
5516	Hospital Satisfaction Survey	$1,700,000
6149	Validation of Managed Care Data for Risk Adjustment	$6,388,706
5081 B	Systematized Nomenclature of Medicine	$350,000
Total		$243,486,514

SOURCE: Personal communication, C. Lazarus, March 17, 2005.

TABLE A.5   Evaluation of Task 1 in 7th SOW

Task	Setting	Domains	Performance Measures
1a	Nursing home	Chronic care (percentage of residents with listed condition)	Pain Infections (pneumonia, urinary tract infections, etc.) Pressure sores Pressure sores (with additional risk adjustment) Loss of ability in some basic daily tasks Physical restraints
		Postacute care (percentage of short-stay residents with listed condition)	Pain Walk as well or better Delirium Delirium (with additional risk adjustment)
		Provider satisfaction	

Task	Setting	CMS Priority	Performance Measures
1b	Home health	Health status improvement	11 OBQI/OASIS measures[c] (getting dressed, bathing, confusion, medication management, ambulation, toileting, transferring, pain when moving, emergency care, acute hospitalization)
		Provider satisfaction	

Statewide Improvement		Identified Participant Improvement	
Target	Scoring Weights[a]	Target	Scoring Weights[a]
8% averaged improvement on three to five publicly reported quality-of-care measures	0.8—identified participant score	8% averaged improvement on three to five publicly reported quality-of-care measures	0.44 × (actual improvement/target improvement)
80% "satisfied" response rate	0.05	80% "satisfied" response rate	0.15

Statewide Improvement		Identified Participant Improvement	
Target	Scoring Weight[b]	Target	Scoring Weight[b]
N/A		30% of HHAs in the state must have statistically significant improvement in at least one OBQI / OASIS measure	0.8
80% "satisfied" response rate	0.05	80% "satisfied" response rate	0.15

continues

TABLE A.5 Continued

Task	Setting	CMS Priority	Performance Measures
1c	Hospital	Clinical measures	Acute myocardial infarction, heart failure, pneumonia, and surgical infection
		Provider satisfaction	

Task	Setting	CMS Priority	Performance Measures
1d	Physician's office	Chronic disease care (diabetes)	Biennial retinal exam, annual hemoglobin A1c testing, biennial testing of lipid profile
		Preventive services (cancer screening)	Biennial screening mammography
		Preventive services (adult immunization)	Influenza immunization, pneumococcal immunization
		Provider satisfaction	

Statewide Improvement		Identified Participant Improvement	
Target	Scoring Weights[d]	Target	Scoring Weights[d]
8% improvement in combined topic average (average score for a condition, based on improvement in the four sets of indicators)	0.75	N/A	
80% "satisfied" response rate	0.25		

Statewide Improvement		Identified Participant Improvement	
Target	Scoring Weights[e]	Target	Scoring Weights[e]
8% improvement in combined topic average[f]	0.8—identified participant score	8% improvement in diabetes and cancer screening measures	0.44 × (actual improvement/target improvement)
		80% "satisfied" response rate	0.2

continues

TABLE A.5 Continued

Task	Setting	CMS Priority	Performance Measures
1e	Rural or underserved population	Primary evaluation	QIO must show reduction in disparity between a nonunderserved reference group and targeted underserved group
		Secondary evaluation	Full description of targeted intervention group demographics and characteristics
			Documentation of rationale for why a specific intervention was chosen for a particular population
			Quantitative demonstration of intervention effectiveness compared with the outcome for a reference group

Task	Setting	CMS Priority	Performance Measures
1f[b]	Medicare+ Choice Organizations	All areas	Will use Medicare+Choice quality review organizations or accreditation organization evaluations of QAPI projects to determine if expected improvement was demonstrated
		Provider satisfaction	

NOTE: If a Quality Improvement Organization (QIO) scores below 0.6 on any quantitative subtask (Tasks 1a to 1e and 2b), its contract will be reevaluated by a Centers for Medicare and Medicaid Services panel. OBQI/OASIS = Outcome-Based Quality Improvement/Outcome and Assessment Information Set; N/A = not applicable; HHA = Home Health Agency; QAPI = Quality Assessment and Performance Improvement.

[a]A passing score is a score ≥ 1.0. The total possible score for Task 1a is 1.0, which is equal to the statewide score + identified participant satisfaction rate + satisfaction rate = (0.8 − identified participant score) + 0.44 × (identified participant actual improvement/target improvement) + (0.2 satisfaction rate).

[b]A passing score is a score ≥ 1.0. The total possible score for Task 1b is 1.0, which is equal to the (statewide score) + (satisfaction rate) = (0.8 statewide score) + (0.2 satisfaction rate).

[c]See Table A.3 for measures.

[d]A passing score is a score of ≥ 1.0. The total possible score for Task 1c is 1.0, which is equal to the (statewide score) + (satisfaction rate) = (0.75 statewide score) + (0.25 satisfaction rate).

Statewide Improvement		Identified Participant Improvement	
Target	Scoring Weights[g]	Target	Scoring Weights[g]
Demonstrated reduction in disparity	1.0	N/A	
	0.2		
	0.2		
	0.2		

Statewide Improvement		Identified Participant Improvement	
Target	Scoring Weights	Target	Scoring Weights
Technical assistance given; QAPI improvement	0.5	N/A	
80% "satisfied" response rate	0.5		

[e]A passing score is a score of ≥ 1.0. The total possible score for Task 1d is 1.0, which is equal to the (statewide score) + (identified participant score) + (satisfaction rate) = (0.8 – identified participant satisfaction rate) + [0.44 × (identified participant actual improvement/target improvement)] + (0.2 satisfaction).

[f]Elements of combined topic average: administrative claims (used to measure diabetes and mammography measure rates for fee-for-service beneficiaries). The weighted average of Health Plan Empoyer Data and Information Set data will be used to derive diabetes and mammography measures of rates for Medicare+Choice organizations(if applicable). The Consumer Assessment of Healthcare Providers and Systems survey will be used to derive immunization rates statewide.

[g]A passing score is a score ≥ 1.0. The total possible score for Task 1e is 1.6, which is equal to (primary evaluation score) + (secondary evaluation score) = (1.0 primary evaluation score) + (0.6 secondary evaluation score).

[h]Task 1f is not a pass-fail task.

TABLE A.6   Evaluation of Task 1a in 8th SOW

Task	Setting	Dimension of Performance	Performance Measures
1a	Nursing home	Clinical performance measure results[b]	Pressure ulcers among high-risk residents
			Physical restraints
			Management of depressive symptoms
			Management of pain in chronic (long-stay) residents

Statewide Improvement		Identified Participant Improvement	
Targets	Scoring Weights (18% of total[a])	Targets	Scoring Weights (82% of total[a])
		Identified Participant Groups 1 and 2	IPG 1: 0.094 8.5% of total score
		Baseline <10.5%: achieve RFR of ≥15%	IPG 2: 0.625 5.7% of total score
		Baseline 10.5%–15%: achieve RFR of ≥25%	
		Baseline >15%: achieve RFR of ≥35%	
		Identified Participant Group 1	IPG 1: 0.094 8.5% of total score
		Baseline <4%: achieve RFR of ≥15%	
		Baseline 4%–10%: achieve RFR of ≥35%	
		Baseline >10%: achieve RFR of ≥60%	
		Identified Participant Group 2 Achieve 10% RFR	IPG 2: 0.625 5.7% of total score
		Baseline <10%: achieve RFR of ≥30%	IPG 1: 0.094 8.5% of total score
		Baseline ≥10%: achieve RFR of ≥40%	
		Baseline <5%: achieve RFR of ≥25%	IPG 1: 0.094 8.5% of total score
		Baseline 5%–8%: achieve RFR of ≥35%	

continues

TABLE A.6 Continued

Task	Setting	Dimension of Performance	Performance Measures
		Process improvement	Extra credit: Process change implementation
		Organization culture change	Target setting[b]

Statewide Improvement		Identified Participant Improvement	
Targets	Scoring Weights (18% of total[a])	Targets	Scoring Weights (82% of total[a])
		Baseline >8%: achieve RFR of ≥50%	
Document at least one of the following processes of care for 50% of new admissions for: • Skin inspection and pressure ulcer risk assessment • Depression screening and treatment • Evaluation of the necessity and alternatives for the use of physical restraints • Pain assessment and treatment	Extra credit: 0.05 for each, totaling 0.2 18% of total score		
At least 25% of nursing homes in the state set targets for high-risk pressure ulcers and physical restraints. QIO sets own statewide target for high-risk pressure ulcers and physical restraints	0.1 9% of total score	All participants in Identified Participant Groups 1 and 2 must set targets for high-risk pressure ulcers and physical restraints	

continues

TABLE A.6 Continued

Task	Setting	Dimension of Performance	Performance Measures
			Data collection on experience of care[b]
		Satisfaction and knowledge/ perception[b]	

Task	Setting	Dimension of Performance	Performance Measures
1b	Home health	Clinical performance measure results[d]	OASIS publicly reported measures[e]
			Acute care hospitalization

Statewide Improvement		Identified Participant Improvement	
Targets	Scoring Weights (18% of total[a])	Targets	Scoring Weights (82% of total[a])
		Identified Participant Groups 1 and 2 must have ≥90% of nursing homes collect and monitor satisfaction experience of care for each of the following: • Residents, annually • Staff, annually • Retention of certified nursing assistants, annually	IPG1: 0.0925 for each survey 8.4% of total for each survey IPG2: 0.0375 for each survey 3.4% of total for each survey
At least 80% score on satisfaction and knowledge/perception surveys	0.1 9% of total score		

Statewide Improvement		Identified Participant Improvement	
Targets	Scoring Weights (53% of Total[c])	Targets	Scoring Weights (47% of total[c])
Meet or exceed target RFR for one QIO-selected measure OASIS publicly reported measure	0.1 (0.13 max) 10% of total score	Average rate of group must meet or exceed identified participant group target RFR for one home health agency–selected measure[b]	0.09 (0.11 max) 9% of total score
Meet or exceed 30% RFR for acute care hospitalization measure[b]	0.19 (0.22 max) 19% of total score	Average rate of group must meet or exceed identified participant group target RFR for acute care hospitalization measure[b]	0.27 (0.32 max) 27% of total score

continues

TABLE A.6 Continued

Task	Setting	Dimension of Performance	Performance Measures
		Systems improvement[b]	Telehealth
		Process improvement	Immunization assessment survey[b]
			Incorporation of immunizations into computer
		Organization culture change	Survey tool to measure organizational culture change

Statewide Improvement		Identified Participant Improvement	
Targets	Scoring Weights (53% of Total[c])	Targets	Scoring Weights (47% of total[c])
		Implementation by identified participant group of telehealth meeting CMS telehealth guidelines	0.05 5% of total score
50% minimum response rate	0.05 5% of total score		
Achieve 50% RFR (or 80% statewide performance) on the percentage of home health agencies that incorporated influenza or pneumococcal immunizations, or into comprehensive patient assessments	0.09 (0.11 max) 9% of total score		
		Implement CMS survey tool	0.02 2% of total score
		Implementation of quality improvement activity and submission of a plan of action based on results of organizational culture change survey	0.04 4% of total score

continues

TABLE A.6   Continued

Task	Setting	Dimension of Performance	Performance Measures
		Organization culture change	Extra credit: Target setting
		Satisfaction and knowledge/perception	

Task	Setting	Dimension of Performance	Performance Measures
1c1	Hospital	Clinical performance measurement results	Appropriate care measure[b,g]
		Clinical performance measurement and reporting	Measures reporting[b]
			Assistance to hospitals to ensure data are timely, valid, and complete[b]
		Process improvement	Surgical Care Improvement Project (SCIP)

Statewide Improvement		Identified Participant Improvement	
Targets	Scoring Weights (53% of Total[c])	Targets	Scoring Weights (47% of total[c])
At least 25% of non-identified participant group home health agencies set targets for acute care hospitalization and other OASIS measures	Extra credit: 0.07	At least 50% of identified participant group home health agencies set targets for acute care hospitalization and other OASIS measures	Extra credit: 0.05
At least 80% score on satisfaction and knowledge/perception surveys	0.1 10% of total score		

Statewide Improvement		Identified Participant Improvement	
Targets	Scoring Weights (27% of total[f])	Targets	Scoring Weights (73% of total[f])
		At least 75% of hospitals must achieve 50% RFR	0.3 (0.4 max)[b] 27% of total score
25% of hospitals must report on the set of 22 HQA measures[g]	0.1 9% of total score		
More than 95% of hospitals submitting data to QIO Data Warehouse	0.1 9% of total score		
		At least 50% identified participant group hospitals achieve an overall RFR ≥25% on SCIP process measures for surgical site infections and venous thromboembolis[b,g]	0.3 27% of total score

continues

TABLE A.6 Continued

Task	Setting	Dimension of Performance	Performance Measures
		Systems improvement	Use of CPOE, bar coding, or telehealth[b]
		Satisfaction and knowledge/perception[b]	

Task	Setting	Dimension of Performance	Performance Measures
1c2	Critical access hospital or rural hospital	Clinical performance measure results	One quality improvement measure selected by each critical access hospital
		Clinical performance measurement and reporting	Reporting of Hospital Quality Alliance measure set[b]

Statewide Improvement		Identified Participant Improvement	
Targets	Scoring Weights (27% of total[f])	Targets	Scoring Weights (73% of total[f])
		Extra credit: Achieve overall RFR ≥25% for other SCIP process measures	Extra Credit[i]: 0.1 max
		Percentage of hospitals completing assessment tool	0.2 18% of total score
		Percentage of hospitals demonstrating improvement at remeasurement	
At least 80% score on satisfaction and knowledge/perception surveys	0.1 9% of total score		

Statewide Improvement		Identified Participant Improvement	
Targets	Scoring Weights (64% of total[j])	Targets	Scoring Weights (36% of total[j])
RFR >10%	Weight = number of critical access hospitals reporting/ total number of critical access hospitals		
Extra credit: RFR >20%			
50% of nonreporting critical access hospitals report on at least one Hospital Quality Alliance measure topic	Score = (weight × 0.5) + {weight × 0.1 × [(actual RFR − 0.1)/ 0.1]} 0.6 max for both clinical		

continues

TABLE A.6 Continued

Task	Setting	Dimension of Performance	Performance Measures
			Extra credit: Reporting on transfer measures for new acute myocardial infarction and/or emergency department
		Systems improvement	Use of CPOE, bar coding, or telehealth
		Organizational change	Hospital safety culture assessment
		Satisfaction and knowledge/perception[b]	

Statewide Improvement		Identified Participant Improvement	
Targets	Scoring Weights (64% of total[j])	Targets	Scoring Weights (36% of total[j])
Extra credit: 100% of nonreporting critical access hospitals report on at least one Hospital Quality Alliance measure topic	performance measure results and reporting Weight = number of critical access hospitals not reporting/total number of critical access hospitals Score = (weight × 0.5) + {weight × 0.1 × [(% newly reporting − 0.5)/0.1]}		
Extra credit: Work with critical access hospitals to promote reporting on these measures and identify a quality improvement project	Extra credit[k]: 0.2 max		
		Extra credit: At least one nonreporting critical access hospital works on CPOE, bar coding, or telehealth and achievement of evaluation criteria	Extra credit: 0.05
		Percentage achieving RFR ≥1% from results of safety culture assessment	0.4[j,k] 36% of total score
At least 80% score on satisfaction and knowledge/ perception surveys	0.1 9% of total score		

continues

TABLE A.6 Continued

Task	Setting	Dimension of Performance	Performance Measures
1d1	Physician practice	Clinical performance measure results	Statewide support for Physician Voluntary Reporting Program[g]
			Statewide quality improvement by working with public health, provider groups, and others to support prevention and disease-based care processes
			Assistance to Medicare Advantage plans
			Assistance to End-Stage Renal Disease Networks
			Medicare Management Demonstration Project
		Clinical performance measurement and reporting[m]	Export data
		Process improvement[m]	Care management process to meet individual's health needs through the practice site systems survey
		Systems improvement[m]	Production and use of information from electronic systems
		Satisfaction and knowledge/perception[b]	

Statewide Improvement		Identified Participant Improvement	
Targets	Scoring Weights (17% of total[l])	Targets	Scoring Weights (83% of total[l])
Improvement, as evaluated by project officer	0.1 8.3% of total score		
		Report on at least one DOQ measure: Preexisting electronic systems (10% of sites did not have them; 20% of sites did)	0.2 0.2
		Adoption of care management process: Electronic clinical information systems (30% of sites did not have them; 75% sites did)	0.2 0.2
		Produce and use electronic clinical information for 75% of sites without preexisting electronic clinical information systems[b]	0.2 17% of total score
At least 80% score on satisfaction and knowledge/ perception surveys	0.1 8.3% of total score		

continues

TABLE A.6 Continued

Task	Setting	Dimension of Performance	Performance Measures
1d2	Underserved populations	Clinical performance measure results	Claims-based clinical measures[g]
		Clinical performance measurement and reporting	Task 1d1 activities
		Systems improvement	Promotion of culturally and linguistically appropriate service (CLAS) standards
		Process improvement	Cultural competency education
		Satisfaction and knowledge/perception[b]	

Statewide Improvement		Identified Participant Improvement	
Targets	Scoring Weights (35% of total[n])	Targets	Scoring Weights (65% of total[n])
≥4% absolute improvement for all underserved populations for diabetes, mammography, and adult immunization measures	0.25 25% of total score		
Promote improvement in rates for applicable underserved populations		Select underserved populations that at least equal the underserved population in the state to complete Task 1d1 activities	
		Use Office of Minority Health Theme 3 tool with 80% completion rate to promote adoption of CLAS standards[b]	0.25 25% of total score
		≥80% primary care physicians complete both Themes 1 and 2 of Office of Minority Health tool[b]	0.4 40% of total score
At least 80% score on satisfaction and knowledge/ perception surveys	0.1 10% of total score		

continues

TABLE A.6 Continued

Task	Setting	Dimension of Performance	Performance Measures
1d3	Part D prescription drug Benefit	Clinical performance measure results	

NOTE: RFR = Reduction in failure rate; IPG = identified participant group; QIO = Quality Improvement Organization; OASIS = Outcome and Assessment Information Set; CMS = Centers for Medicare and Medicaid Services; CPOE = Computerized Provider Order Entry; CAHPS = Consumer Assessment of Healthcare Providers and Systems.

[a]The Task 1a score is equal to (0.5 clinical performance measure scores) + (0.5 organization culture change scores) + (0.1 satisfaction and knowledge/perception score) + (0.2 extra credit); total score = 1.1; total possible score = 1.3.

[b]Core activities. If a QIO does not complete these specific activities, its contract may be subject to reevaluation by a Centers for Medicare and Medicaid Services panel.

[c]The Task 1b score is equal to (0.65 clinical performance measure score) + (0.05 systems improvement score) + (0.14 process improvement score) + (0.06 organization culture change score) + (0.1 satisfaction and knowledge/perception score) + (0.27 extra credit); total score = 1.0; total possible score = 1.27.

[d]The total points for these measures are scaled on the basis of percent improvement above or below the target RFR. Extra credit is available for scoring above the target RFR, indicated here by (max).

[e]Except acute care hospitalization and emergent care; see Table A.3 for measures.

[f]The Task 1c1 score is equal to (0.3 clinical performance measure score) + (0.2 clinical performance measurement and reporting scores) + (0.3 process improvement score) + (0.2 systems improvement score) + (0.1 satisfaction and knowledge/perception score); total score = 1.1; total possible score = 1.3.

Statewide Improvement		Identified Participant Improvement	
Targets	Scoring Weights[o]	Targets	Scoring Weights[o]
	Measures to be developed by consensus review process	Implementation of a quality improvement project	To be determined by Government Task Leader
	CAHPS	For QIOs electing to work on self-management of medication therapy	

[g]See Table A.3 for measures.

[h]Extra credit for the Appropriate Care Measure Identified Participant Group is based on recruitment of hospitals.

[i]Partial credit is also given. QIOs achieving at least 25% RFR on three measures will receive 0.05 point; QIOs achieving at least 25% RFR on four measures will receive the full 0.1 point.

[j]The Task 1c2 score is equal to (0.6 clinical performance measure score and clinical performance measurement and reporting score) + (0.4 organization culture change) + (0.1 satisfaction and knowledge/perception score); total possible score = 1.35.

[k]Extra credit for these activities are scaled on the basis of the percentage of critical access hospitals achieving the target RFR.

[l]The Task 1d1 score is equal to (0.1 clinical performance measure score) + (0.4 clinical performance measurement and reporting score) + (0.4 process improvement score) + (0.2 systems improvement score) + (0.1 satisfaction and knowledge/perception score); total score = 1.2.

[m]The total points for these activities are scaled on the basis of the ability of participants without electronic clinical information systems to produce clinical information.

[n]The Task 1d2 score is equal to (0.25 clinical performance measure score) + (0.25 systems improvement score) + (0.4 process improvement score) + (0.1 satisfaction and knowledge/perception score); total score = 1.0.

[o]"Passing" for Task 1d3 is to be determined by the Task 1d government task leader.

TABLE A.7 Comparison of Deliverables for the 7th and 8th Scopes of Work

7th SOW Deliverables	8th SOW Deliverables
Task 1a: Nursing Homes	
Development and implementation of a quality improvement plan in which 3 to 5 of the 10 nursing home quality-of-care measures were targeted for statewide improvement	Development of alternative Task 1a criteria (applicable to WY, AK, DC, and PR)
Development and implementation of a plan to partner with nursing home stakeholders	Lists of the identified participants for groups 1 and 2
List of the identified participants	Indicate whether QIO will work on process improvement measures and which nursing homes will submit data for these measures
Contact name for each identified participant	Set targets for the measures for high-risk pressure ulcers and measures for physical restraints (management of depressive symptoms and management of pain in patients with chronic pain are optional) with the help of nursing homes at the statewide level
	Submit statewide targets for the measures of high-risk pressure ulcers and for physical restraints; submissions for measures of management of depressive symptoms and management of pain in chronic pain are optional
	Documentation of PARTner activity codes
	Documentation of baseline and annual remeasurement rates for resident satisfaction
	Documentation of baseline and annual remeasurement rates for staff satisfaction
	Documentation of annual certified nursing assistant or nursing aids turnover rate
	Quarterly submission of mandatory process of care data (optional)
Task 1b: Home Health	
QIO training of home health agencies on OBQI	Lists of the clinical performance of identified participant group and their plans of action
List of identified participants	Lists of the systems improvement and organization culture change identified participant group

TABLE A.7   Continued

7th SOW Deliverables	8th SOW Deliverables
List of contact information for each participant	Selected statewide OASIS measure Acute care hospitalization strategic plan Acute care hospitalization strategic plan final report Systems improvement and organization culture change identified participant group survey results Systems improvement and organizational culture change identified participant group plans of action Statewide survey results of statewide immunization practices Documentation of PARTner activity codes
Task 1c1: Hospitals	
List of contact information for every hospital in the state	Update data on Provider Reporting System List of identified participants for acute care measure, surgical care improvement project, and systems improvement and organization culture change identified participant groups Documentation of contact with local American College of Surgeons president Results of baseline readiness/adoption tool for CPOE, bar coding, or telehealth Results of remeasurement readiness/adoption tool for CPOE, bar coding, or telehealth Systems improvement and organizational culture change hospitals' plans for CPOE, barcoding, and telehealth implementation plans
Task 1c2: Critical Access Hospitals	
N/A	Submission of critical access hospital measure set Report of quality improvement activities on at least one critical access hospital measure List of participants for identified participant group Final report of quality improvement activities with all reporting critical access hospitals

continues

TABLE A.7   Continued

7th SOW Deliverables	8th SOW Deliverables
	Submission of the Rural Organizational Safety Culture Change interventions and change models tested/implemented
	Baseline results and methods of safety culture survey
	Report of Rural Organizational Safety Culture Change intervention and change models implemented
	Remeasurement results of safety culture survey

Task 1d1: Physician Practice

7th SOW Deliverables	8th SOW Deliverables
List including each identified participant along with his or her Unique Physician Identification Number via PARTner	Assistance given to Medicare Advantage plans
List of contact information for each participating physician office	Assistance provided to support Physician Voluntary Reporting Program and other statewide work
	Recruitment plan
	Work plan indicating the technical assistance activities offered to identified participant physician practice sites, including those sites in Task 1d2
	List of physician practices sites receiving QIO assistance
	Strategy and assistance for electronic submission of DOQ measures
	Office System Survey assessing status of identified participant group for electronic clinical information production and use
	Updated environmental scan
	List of physician practice sites with applications of interest for QIO assistance
	List of physician practice sites using EHR due to work of QIO
	Information depicting QIO efficiencies
	Office System Survey of identified participant groups

Task 1d2: Physician Practice: Underserved Populations

7th SOW Deliverables	8th SOW Deliverables
N/A	Identify Task 1d1 underserved identified participants
	Identify CLAS identified participants
	Report efforts to reach underserved populations
	Report CLAS results

TABLE A.7   Continued

7th SOW Deliverables	8th SOW Deliverables

Task 1d3: Physician Practice/Pharmacy: Part D Prescription Drug Benefit

N/A	Assessment of environment for electronic prescribing and continuous quality improvement
	QIO staff/training plan
	Baseline levels of performance
	Submission of two concept papers for quality projects to be developed with Medicare Advantage and other prescription drug plans
	Submission of one project proposal for a quality project to be developed with Medicare Advantage and other prescription drug plans
	Plan interventions and develop interventional materials
	Identify annual quality measure targets
	Report required information on providers involved in projects
	Directory of contacts within each prescription drug plan

Task 1e: Underserved and Rural Beneficiaries

Submission of approved 6th SOW plans targeting an underserved population	N/A
Submission of plan if new project was chosen	
Report of final results	

Task 1f: Medicare Advantage

Plan of action to invite Medicare+Choice organizations to participate in Tasks 1a to 1e	N/A
Submit list of contacts for all Medicare+Choice organizations	

NOTE: SOW = scope of work; QIO = Quality Improvement Organization; PARTner = Program Activity Reporting Tool; OBQI = Outcome-Based Quality Improvement; OASIS = Outcomes and Assessment Information Set; CPOE = computerized provider order entry; N/A = not applicable; DOQ = Doctor's Office Quality; EHR = Electronic Health Record; CLAS = culturally and linguistically appropriate service.

B

Private-Sector Organizations Offering Services Related to Quality Improvement

TABLE B.1   Private-Sector Organizations Offering Services Related to
Quality Improvement

Organization Name	Contact Information	Date Founded (Status)	Board Information
Abt Associates Inc.	55 Wheeler Street Cambridge, MA 02135 Phone: (617) 492-7100 http://www.abtassociates.com	1965 (FP)	13 members
American Institutes for Research (AIR)	1000 Thomas Jefferson Street, NW Washington, D.C. 20007 Phone: (202) 403-5000 http://www.air.org	1946 (NFP)	13 members

Office Sites (Number of Employees)	Main Activities Related to Performance Measurement and Quality Improvement	Primary Customers	Revenue
5 offices across the U.S. (1,000+)	Apply health economics, evaluation research, survey research, and other measurement sciences to public health policy, technical assistance, and regulation assessment Assignments have included: • Measuring the impact of public health programs, including projects at the state and federal levels • Improving the health of disparate populations • Assessing the cost-effectiveness of drugs and therapies • Evaluating the benefits of new technology • Determining the outcomes of health plan subscribers • Measuring the health effects of environmental hazards	• Governments • Funding organizations • Foundations • Nonprofit institutions • Business and industry worldwide	N/A
9 offices across the U.S.; international offices in 9 countries (1200+)	Health care research and policy analysis. Collaborate to: • Develop and test concepts for prevention and public health campaigns and initiatives • Monitor and assess subsequent changes in attitudes, behavior patterns, and media coverage • Carry out specific projects to improve quality data on delivery of care and performance measurement for substance-abuse and mental health services • Conduct a new project on assessing quality of life for sickle cell patients	• Federal and state governments • Foundations • Private health care and research organizations • Universities	$182 million for 2004

continues

TABLE B.1   Continued

Organization Name	Contact Information	Date Founded (Status)	Board Information
CareScience, Inc.	3600 Market Street, 7th Floor Philadelphia, PA 19104 Phone: (888) 223-8247 http://www.carescience.com	N/A (FP)	N/A
Center for Health Care Strategies	P.O. Box 3469 Princeton, NJ 08543-3469 Phone: (609) 895-8101 Fax: (609) 895-9648 http://www.chcs.org	1995 (NFP)	8 names, with titles and affiliations

Office Sites (Number of Employees)	Main Activities Related to Performance Measurement and Quality Improvement	Primary Customers	Revenue
Philadelphia, PA (NA)	• Provide care management tools for health care data collection, data mining, quality reporting, public reporting, and clinical process redesign • Advise on performance improvement, redesign of care management infrastructure, improvement of clinical processes and resource utilization, and administrative and physician leadership development • Organize public educational events and training for health care professionals and leaders, such as monthly forums and a national conference • Offer technology to support improvements in performance and clinical outcomes through organizational and cultural change management, monitoring, and continuous quality improvement • Provide training in data analysis and improve data analysis skills • Offer comprehensive hands-on training	Hospitals and health systems; alliances with California Health Care Foundation, Joint Commission on Accreditation of Healthcare Organizations, and others	N/A
Princeton, NJ (30)	Technical assistance and training to help states, health plans, and consumer organizations use managed care effectively to: • Improve quality of services • Improve health services for low-income families and people with severe illnesses and disabilities • Reduce racial and ethnic health disparities • Increase community options for people with disabilities	• State officials • Health plan leaders • Consumer organizations across the country	N/A

continues

TABLE B.1 Continued

Organization Name	Contact Information	Date Founded (Status)	Board Information
Cerner Corporation	2800 Rockcreek Parkway Kansas City, MO 64117 Phone: (866) 221-8877 http://www.cerner.com/public	1979 (FP)	8 names, with titles, affiliations, and photos

Office Sites (Number of Employees)	Main Activities Related to Performance Measurement and Quality Improvement	Primary Customers	Revenue
7 offices across the U.S.; international offices in 9 countries (Associates: worldwide, 6,255; Kansas City, 4,031)	Outcomes Management solutions enable organizations to measure, predict, and improve outcomes at multiple levels: • APACHE—prospective and current information at the point of care • Critical Outcomes—collected knowledge from critical care database • Health Facts—national research database and industry benchmark • Surveillance Insights—use of health department reporting, surveillance, and data mining to decrease nosocomial infections Executable Knowledge for Regulatory Standards provides alerts/rules, order sets, documentation and reports from major regulatory and quality assurance groups IQHealth® creates a web-based location for recording, tracking, and exchanging personal information for common chronic conditions Multum—drug knowledge for integration into a clinical information system or via Internet access Innovations include: • Lighthouse—development of a data-driven, clinical optimization process to enable physician and nursing behavior changes • Genomics Data Model—to store, represent, and manipulate the data representation of personal genomic information	Health organizations, e.g.: • Hospitals • Health systems • Physician practices • Home health organizations	N/A

continues

TABLE B.1   Continued

Organization Name	Contact Information	Date Founded (Status)	Board Information
Eclipsys	1750 Clint Moore Road Boca Raton, FL 33487 Phone: (561) 322-4321 Fax: (561) 322-4320 http://www.eclipsys.com	1995 (FP)	6 names, with titles, and affiliations
Epic Systems Corporation	5301 Tokay Blvd. Madison, WI 53711-1027 Phone: (608) 271-9000 Fax: (608) 271-7237 http://www.epicsystems.com	1979 (FP)	N/A

Office Sites (Number of Employees)	Main Activities Related to Performance Measurement and Quality Improvement	Primary Customers	Revenue
16 offices across the U.S. and 3 in Canada (2000)	Offers services for: • Clinical transformation • Clinical knowledge management • Outsourcing (information technology, information management, revenue cycle management) • Remote hosting • Customer relationship management and support • Software implementation • Product education and training • Integration and streamlining of care delivery with a shared electronic health record, single health data repository, and workflow-enhancing documentation	1500+ health care organizations, including: • 60,000 physicians • 400,000 nurses • 70,000 administrative support staff • 35,000 ancillary staff	Within U.S. totaled $293.1 million in 2004; outside U.S. totaled $16 million in 2004
Madison, WI (2100)	Develop and install large-scale health care software systems that: • Provide shared, complete, longitudinal electronic health records for providers, affiliates, and patients across the care continuum • Promote patient safety and health care quality • Improve disease management by identifying at-risk patients, guiding providers through best-practice care standards, and using integrated web access to engage patients	Large health care organizations	N/A

continues

TABLE B.1   Continued

Organization Name	Contact Information	Date Founded (Status)	Board Information
Health Dialog Services Corporation	60 State Street, Suite 1100 Boston, MA 02109 Phone: (617) 406-5200 http://www.healthdialog.com	1995 (FP)	9 members
HealthGrades	500 Golden Ridge Road Suite 100 Golden, CO 80401 Phone: (303) 716-0041 http://www.healthgrades.com	1999 (FP)	5 names, with titles and affiliations (in biography)

Office Sites (Number of Employees)	Main Activities Related to Performance Measurement and Quality Improvement	Primary Customers	Revenue
Corporate office in Boston, MA, with 5 call centers across the U.S. (900+)	Care management services to help individuals become more engaged in their care and have more effective relationships with their physicians, e.g.: • Predictive modeling to identify individuals for coaching • Health coaching for individuals and families • Physician support • Program measurement and reporting Analytic solutions: • Examination of unwarranted variations in care • Provider measurement services • Patient profiles • Opportunity analyses for each plan	Approximately 16 million individuals with access to services through relationships with more than 30 health plan and employer clients, including: Blue Cross and Blue Shield (BCBS) of Michigan and other states, Health Care Services Corporation, American Standard, Fidelity, Excellus BCBS, Noridian (BCBS of North Dakota), Definity Health, and others	N/A
Golden, CO (105)	Business solutions, including independent, third-party ratings and advisory services, to help providers assess and improve their quality of care: • Identify quality improvement opportunities • Implement evidence-based, best-practice process improvement strategies for hospital patients • Work with the nation's top-performing hospitals to build and maintain a reputation for excellence	• Physicians • Consumers • Hospital executives • Employers • Health plans • Benefit managers • Liability insurers	N/A

continues

TABLE B.1   Continued

Organization Name	Contact Information	Date Founded (Status)	Board Information
HealthShare/ THA	6225 U.S. Highway 290 East Austin TX 78723 Phone: (512) 465-1070 http://www.healthshare-tha.com	1969 (FP)	15 members
IDX	40 IDX Drive Burlington, VT 05402-1070 Phone: (802) 862-1022 Fax: (802) 862-6848 http://www.idx.com	1969 (FP)	10 names, with titles and affiliations
Ingenix	12125 Technology Drive Eden Prairie, MN 55344 Toll-free: (800)-INGENIX Phone: (952) 833-7100 Fax: (952) 833-7201 Email: info@ingenix.com http://www.ingenix.com	N/A (FP)	9 names, with titles and affiliations; UnitedHealth Group board: 12 names
Institute for Clinical Systems Improvement	8009 34th Ave South Suite 1200 Bloomington, MN 55425 Phone: (952) 814-7060 Fax: (952) 858-9675 http://www.icsi.org	1993 (NFP)	16 names, with titles and affiliations

Office Sites (Number of Employees)	Main Activities Related to Performance Measurement and Quality Improvement	Primary Customers	Revenue
4 offices in Texas (13)	Offers services for patient data, group purchasing, and insurance. Provides quality initiatives for: • Clinical quality, operational, and patient satisfaction benchmarking • Continuous performance monitoring • Core measures solutions • Quality improvement analysis and reporting	Subsidiary of the Texas Hospital Association: • Hospitals • Health care organizations	N/A
9 offices across the U.S. and 1 office in London, UK (N/A)	Offers services for specialty work-flow solutions: • Patient management • Support of patient care through a comprehensive lifetime patient record • An encompassing image and information management solution for cardiology and radiology	• Hospitals • Group practices • Academic medical centers • Integrated delivery networks	$521 million in 2004
20 offices in the U.S. in addition to international locations (N/A)	Offers database tools, data management services, and consultation to improve business processes that depend on complete, timely, and accurate provider data: • Data assessment report • Data enhancement • Deceased provider analysis • National health care databases	• 3,000+ hospitals and 250,000 physicians • 2,000 payers and other intermediaries • 100 Fortune 500 companies • 183 pharmaceutical and biotechnology companies	Expected fiscal year 2005 revenues of $800 million
Bloomington, MN (25)	Offers services for: • Evidence-based health care • Support for clinical and service improvement • Patient education resources • Outreach to the health care community and the general community	55 hospitals and medical groups (ranging from 5 to 1,000 physicians), representing 8,300 hospital beds and 7,600 physicians	$3.5 million per year

continues

TABLE B.1   Continued

Organization Name	Contact Information	Date Founded (Status)	Board Information
Institute for Healthcare Improvement	20 University Road, 7th Floor Cambridge, MA 02138 Phone: (617) 301-4800 Toll-Free: (866) 787-0831 Fax: (617) 301-4848 http://www.ihi.org/ihi	1991 (NFP)	16 names, with titles, affiliations, and photos
Learn, Empower, Achieve, Produce—LEAP (Life Services Network)	911 N. Elm Street, Suite 228 Hinsdale, IL 60521 Phone: (630) 325-6170 or 2 Lawrence Square Springfield, IL 62704 Phone: (217) 789-1677 http://www.lsni.org/ LEAPbrochure.pdf	1999 (FP)	N/A

Office Sites (Number of Employees)	Main Activities Related to Performance Measurement and Quality Improvement	Primary Customers	Revenue
Cambridge, MA (70+)	Offers services to: • Provide solutions ready for action • Provide knowledge about quality improvement • Create communities of users with common interests and the opportunity to interact with experts Offers materials such as books, white papers, audio, video, and moderated discussion communities Offers additional programs: • IMPACT Network • 100K Lives Campaign • Conferences and training • Collaborative learning • Pursuing Perfection • Transforming Care at the Bedside	• Health care providers and organizations • Hospitals	N/A
Hinsdale, IL; Springfield, IL (N/A)	A long-term care workforce development and retention program for staff, including train-the-trainer modules and workshops to: • Build positive relationships with residents and families • Foster capable work teams • Develop effective communication techniques • Make participants feel valued and effective • Release "hidden" talents	• NFP long-term care communities and nursing home staff (nurse managers, physicians, nurses, administrators, social workers) • Developed in partnership with Life Services Network of Illinois and Mather Lifeways	N/A

continues

TABLE B.1   Continued

Organization Name	Contact Information	Date Founded (Status)	Board Information
Mathematica Policy Research, Inc.	P.O. Box 2393 Princeton, NJ 08543-2393 Phone: (609) 799-3535 http://www.mathematica-mpr.com	1968 (FP)	13 members

Office Sites (Number of Employees)	Main Activities Related to Performance Measurement and Quality Improvement	Primary Customers	Revenue
Princeton, NJ; Cambridge, MA; Washington, DC (~500)	Collects data through surveys, administrative databases, and other methods; analyzes data; evaluates programs; summarizes policy implications; and identifies solutions: • Evaluated specific demonstrations of pay-for-performance programs • Evaluates Medicare demonstration projects for disease management and care coordination • Developed clinical quality, outcomes, utilization, and program management measures • Evaluated implementation of Hospital Quality Alliance measures and Hospital Compare • Evaluated impact of public reporting of quality measures on hospitals through a national survey of hospital executives • Conducted case studies of hospital transformational change with respect to quality of care • Provides technical assistance and training to the Centers for Medicare and Medicaid Services (CMS) and all states in developing a Medicaid Statistical Information System	• Federal and state agencies • Health care industry • Foundations	Approximately $90 million in 2005

continues

TABLE B.1   Continued

Organization Name	Contact Information	Date Founded (Status)	Board Information
McKesson Corporation	McKesson Corporation Headquarters One Post Street San Francisco, CA 94104-5296 Phone: (415) 983-8300 http:/www.mckesson.com	1833 (FP)	10 names, with titles, affiliations, and photos
Medstat	777 E. Eisenhower Parkway Ann Arbor, MI 48108 Phone: (734) 913-3000 http://www.medstat.com	1981 (FP)	N/A

Office Sites (Number of Employees)	Main Activities Related to Performance Measurement and Quality Improvement	Primary Customers	Revenue
Corporate office in San Francisco, CA; 300+ facilities nationwide (24,000+: 21,000 in the U.S., 3,000 international)	• Integration of pharmacy information management with computerized physician order entry applications and clinical data entry • Disease management services • Performance management and clinical information solutions Process improvement: • Identify opportunities using data collected through current hospital reporting initiatives • Aggregate measures • Include evidence-based guidelines and real-time alerts into clinical work flow • Use daily management tools to measure performance against targets • Measure the impact of care improvement processes on quality Improve financial performance through: • Medical necessity compliance checks • Submission of a "clean claim"	• 200,000 physicians • 25,000 retail pharmacies • 10,000 long-term care sites • 5,000 hospitals • 2,000 medical–surgical manufacturers • 750 home care agencies • 600 health care payors • 450 pharmaceutical manufacturers	$80 billion in 2005
8 offices across the U.S. (650)	Offer services: • Integration and organization of multiple databases • Evaluation of health care patterns, trends, and clinical performance issues • Data mining and modeling capabilities • Strategies resulting from targeted analyses and benchmarking • Credentialed research to study outcomes and economic impact • Creation of clinical and financial comparison data for benchmarking • Training and education • Privacy and security advice on the Health Insurance Portability and Accountability Act (HIPAA)	• Employers • Government health programs • Health plans • Hospitals • Health systems • Pharmaceutical companies • Researchers	Part of the Thomson Corp., which had revenues of $8.10 billion in 2004

continues

TABLE B.1 Continued

Organization Name	Contact Information	Date Founded (Status)	Board Information
My InnerView Inc.	2620 Stewart Avenue Wausau, WI 54401 Phone: (715) 848-2713 http://www.myinnerview.com	N/A (FP)	N/A
New York Association of Homes and Services for the Aging (NYAHSA) Subsidiary: NYAHSA Services, Inc., which manages product development and marketing of EQUIP	150 State Street, Suite 301 Albany, New York 12207-1698 Phone: (518) 449-2707 http://www.equipforquality.com	N/A (NFP) (Subsidiary: FP)	5 members

Office Sites (Number of Employees)	Main Activities Related to Performance Measurement and Quality Improvement	Primary Customers	Revenue
Wausau, WI (N/A)	Offers Learn™, a series of self-directed training modules with the Quality Profile™ and Risk Monitor™ web tracking systems to collect, benchmark, and use quality data and satisfaction surveys; ready-to-use resources such as competencies, presentation visuals, trainer's scripts, staff handouts, and evaluation tools; and a web-based "Culture Change Staging Tool" Provides guidelines and best practices to: • Interpret report findings • Take planned actions • Set performance targets • Monitor risks and performance over time • Address customer service and the resolution of customer concerns	• Managers and leadership teams within long-term care organizations • Partnership with the American Health Care Association	N/A
Albany, NY (N/A)	EQUIP software and client support helps long-term care facilities: • View individual resident, unit, or facilitywide and benchmarking data • Create visual reports and graphs of quality issues • Gain access to current and comprehensive information on long-term care, including new research and updates on clinical practice guidelines • Improve quality of care, manage risk, and control costs	400+ primarily NFP long-term care facilities nationwide	N/A

continues

TABLE B.1 Continued

Organization Name	Contact Information	Date Founded (Status)	Board Information
Pacific Business Group on Health (PBGH)	221 Main Street, Suite 1500 San Francisco, CA 94105 Phone: (415) 281-8660 http://www.cchri.org	Initially convened (1993) and now manages California Cooperative Healthcare Reporting Initiative (CCHRI) (NFP)	Governed by an executive committee consisting equally of purchasers, health plans, and health care providers

Office Sites (Number of Employees)	Main Activities Related to Performance Measurement and Quality Improvement	Primary Customers	Revenue
San Francisco, CA (N/A)	Members of the collaborative work together to: • Collect and report standardized, reliable health plan and provider performance data • Promote the use of accurate and comparable quality measures within health care • Create efficiency in data collection leading to reduced burden and cost to all participants • Maintain a forum for multiple plan–provider and provider–provider collaboration on quality improvement initiatives • Provide a source for expert advice to consumer reporting entities	CCHRI is a collaborative of health care purchasers, plans, and providers: • 10 health plans, representing over 85 percent of the commercial health maintenance organization (HMO) population in California • PBGH participating employers representing nearly 3 million employees, retirees, and relatives • Provider organizations, including 159 medical groups (participants in the 2005 Consumer Assessment Survey) and state associations	N/A

continues

TABLE B.1 Continued

Organization Name	Contact Information	Date Founded (Status)	Board Information
		Breakthroughs in Chronic Care Program (2004) under PBGH corporate umbrella (NFP)	Steering committee of representatives from California health plans and physician groups, public health officials, and medical educators
Permedion	350 Worthington Road, Suite H Westerville, Ohio 43082 Phone: (800) 473-0802 Fax: (614) 895-6784 http://www.permedion.com	1974 (NFP)	5–8 physicians plus 1 Medicare beneficiary
Premier	12225 Camino Real San Diego, CA 92130 Phone: (858) 481-2727 http://www.premierinc.com	1996 (FP)	15 names, with affiliations and photos

Office Sites (Number of Employees)	Main Activities Related to Performance Measurement and Quality Improvement	Primary Customers	Revenue
San Francisco, CA (3 employees within PBGH)	Improves service and care for patients with chronic conditions: • Focuses on ambulatory practice redesign by leveraging the improvement infrastructure of physician groups • Coordinates disease management programs between health plans and physician groups	• 4 health plans • 100 physician groups	$1 million per year
Westerville, OH (55)	• Statistical and clinical expertise • Quality review and improvement services • Health care claims analysis • Utilization management • Quality-of-care case review • Medical record review • Validation of performance measures, performance improvement projects, and data quality • Customized services to meet the needs of individual groups	• Federal and state government agencies • Hospitals and other health care providers • Health plans • Other payers • Licensing boards	$4.2 million
4 offices across the U.S. (N/A)	• Participates in CMS pay-for-performance demonstration project • Offers rapid improvement programs, webinars, meetings, conferences, continuing education credits, and tools • Provides group purchasing, insurance, and advisory services • Provides advocacy on policy issues	An alliance of NFPs: • 1,500 hospitals • Health care–related facilities • Health systems	N/A

continues

TABLE B.1   Continued

Organization Name	Contact Information	Date Founded (Status)	Board Information
The RAND Corporation	1776 Main Street P.O. Box 2138 Santa Monica, CA 90401 Phone: (310) 393-0411 http://www.rand.org http://www.rand.org/health	1948; 1960s: RAND Health (NFP)	Board of trustees: 24 members; RAND Health board of advisors: 30 members

Office Sites (Number of Employees)	Main Activities Related to Performance Measurement and Quality Improvement	Primary Customers	Revenue
Corporate office in Santa Monica, CA, with additional offices in Pittsburgh, PA, and Washington, DC RAND Europe: Berlin, Cambridge, Leiden RAND-Qatar Policy Institute (170+ employees in RAND Health)	Research to measure, assess, and improve the quality of health care and to provide reliable decision-support information on quality to patients, providers, and purchasers, e.g.: • Central data repository for several large surveys • Tools for assessing quality of care for children and adults and facilitating medical record review • Consumer Assessment of Health Plans Study (CAHPS)—tool to survey consumers about their health care experiences • Assessing Care of Vulnerable Elders—including development of paper-based tools for medical record abstraction; interventions to improve care for the elderly with dementia, urinary incontinence, and falls • Partners in Care—an integrated approach to improving care for depression in primary care • Use of large claims datasets for modeling the impact of changes in reimbursement, benefit design, availability of health information technology, and effectiveness of treating various conditions on future Medicare expenditures	Research sponsors— governmental agencies, foundations, private-sector organizations	$251 million for year ending 9/26/2004 (RAND total); $52 million (RAND Health total)

continues

TABLE B.1 Continued

Organization Name	Contact Information	Date Founded (Status)	Board Information
Resolution Health, Inc.	1625 The Alameda, Suite 400 San Jose, CA 95126 Phone: (408) 882-0678 http://www.resolutionhealth.com	October 2003 (FP)	6 members
Solucient, LLC	1007 Church Street, Suite 700 Evanston, IL 60201 Toll-Free: (800) 366-PLAN Phone: (847) 424-4200 http://www.solucient.com http://100tophospitals.com	2001 (FP)	N/A

Office Sites (Number of Employees)	Main Activities Related to Performance Measurement and Quality Improvement	Primary Customers	Revenue
San Jose, CA; Columbia, MD (40)	Health care data analysis and intervention. Provides a variety of services that: • Describe the quality of care provided to a population at a particular time and over time • Identify patient-specific opportunities to improve the quality, safety, and coordination of care • Provide actionable patient-specific information to physicians, other care managers and patients to enable them to improve quality, safety and coordination of care • Profile the quality of care delivered by individual physicians and physician groups • Help individuals make better health care purchasing decisions • Reduce medical costs while maintaining or improving quality of care	• Health plans/ insurers • Large self-insured employers • Unions • Third-party administrators • Disease management companies • Pharmacy benefit management companies • Benefit consultants	N/A
4 offices across the U.S. (500+)	• Provide information products serving the health care industry • Maintain a large health care database • Provide tools and assistance for health care managers to improve the performance of their organizations	3,100+, including: • 2,000 hospitals • 12 state hospital associations • 16 of the 20 largest pharmaceutical manufacturers in the U.S. • 100 major payors, including 15 Blue plans • Biomedical and biotechnology companies • Consultants	N/A

continues

TABLE B.1 Continued

Organization Name	Contact Information	Date Founded (Status)	Board Information
Wellspring Innovative Solutions, Inc.	2149 Velp Avenue, Suite 500 Green Bay, WI 54303 Phone: (920) 434-0123 http://www.wellspringis.org	1994 (NFP)	7 members

NOTE: NFP = not-for-profit organization; FP = for-profit organization; N/A = not available.

Office Sites (Number of Employees)	Main Activities Related to Performance Measurement and Quality Improvement	Primary Customers	Revenue
Green Bay, WI (N/A)	Consulting services on: • Clinical care processes • Embedding continuous quality improvement into daily practice • Recruitment and retention strategies • Data-based decision making • Presurvey planning and preparation • A model in which educational modules, workshops, and follow-up for delivery of improved quality of care are used to create a multidisciplinary approach to resident-centered care • Consulting on culture change and improvement in quality measures to provide educational modules for clinical changes and empowerment of front-line caregivers	• Core charter group comprising 11 independent NFP skilled nursing facilities throughout eastern Wisconsin • Alliances of nursing homes around the U.S. • QIO community, including HealthInsight (Utah and Nevada QIOs)	

C

Approaches to Evaluation Design

The Institute of Medicine committee recommends that the Centers for Medicare and Medicaid Services (CMS) undertake formal evaluations to assess the Quality Improvement Organization (QIO) program as a whole, as well as the effectiveness of the individual interventions occurring within the work of the contract, as discussed in Recommendation 7 in Chapter 5. This recommendation is important for many reasons, including the need to evaluate whether goals have been reached, as well as to learn which types of interventions are most effective.

Many types of study designs exist, and each one has its own strengths and weaknesses. Challenges exist with all design types, including the identification of "cases" and "controls" (sampled from appropriate providers), refined definition of the "disease" (quality improvement), and confounding factors (such as the voluntary nature of the program). One overarching limitation is due to the fact that the QIO program itself is voluntary and thus presents issues of selection bias

The following sections present a brief definition of each design model, some strengths and weaknesses of the design model, and specific suggestions as to how the study design might be applied to the QIO program. Multiple studies will be needed because of the complexity of the QIO program and the multitude of provider settings and intervention targets. CMS will need to consider not only how to use these studies to evaluate individual interventions but also how to assess the program as a whole, which will be much more complicated and which will require multiple approaches.

CASE-CONTROL STUDY DESIGN

A case-control study is a retrospective study that attempts to link an effect to a cause. In the typical clinical study, one might look at the relationship between exposure to a drug and the risk of cancer. In such an example, one assembles "cases" (those who have the disease) and "controls" (those who do not have the disease). Cases and controls are then compared with respect to their "exposures" to relevant agents that might be causally related to the disease. One then obtains the relative risk of being exposed to an agent in those who have the disease.

Given this framework, the case-control design can be used to evaluate the impacts of QIO interventions in the following way: the selected cases would demonstrate improvements in quality (the "disease"), whereas the controls would not demonstrate any improvements. The cases and the controls are both providers. The exposure is QIO intervention activities. A population-based case-control study would examine cases with the disease from a specified geographic area, with the controls also sampled from the same area. A hospital-based case-control study would sample the cases and the controls from the same hospital.

One needs to control for any other provider or environmental characteristics that could confound the results, such as factors that might be independent predictors of improvements in quality, independent of the QIOs themselves. One would thus need to make sure that the cases and the controls match on variables that are related to improvements in quality, such as participation in other quality improvement efforts or willingness to participate. (This might mean that both cases and controls would have to be sampled from a population of providers who volunteered to work with QIOs.) As a result of the case-control study, the relative risk of demonstrating improvements in quality when the case is exposed to the QIO program is calculated.

One challenge is how the "disease" is defined. Several options exist and would best be tailored to the specific goals described in the scope of work (SOW). For example, if one of the goals of the SOW is to improve the rate of use of beta-blockers in hospitalized patients with myocardial infarction, that outcome would be the equivalent of the "disease" under study. For a program as complex as the QIO program, a number of key outcomes need to be evaluated, so more than one study is needed. Therefore, the SOW must clearly define these desired outcomes so that an evaluation can truly represent what the QIOs were charged with accomplishing.

Another challenge in designing the case-control study (as is also the case in many of the study designs described below) will be to identify the cases and the controls. More than one study is necessary to focus on the different settings and groups that are "exposed" to the QIOs. Cases and controls must be sampled from the same provider setting at the state, national, or other level, as appropriate.

Because the QIO program is multidimensional, the "exposure" aspect of the study will have to be carefully developed. For example, an "exposure" might be whether the providers have been engaged in projects with QIOs. The other essential aspect of defining the exposure would be to achieve more granularity, which would include the quality, intensity, and characteristics of the QIO interventions. The more precise the definition of this exposure becomes, the less the risk involved in obtaining confounding variables that bias the results.

Confounding factors have made it difficult to evaluate quality improvement interventions that are multifaceted and that take place in dynamic, complex systems types of environments. Cases and controls must be matched on variables that, independently of the QIO program, might lead to improvements in quality. Examples include public reporting and payment policies. Other variables on which cases and controls may be matched are those that may not necessarily be causally related to quality improvement, such as provider size and provider location.

RANDOMIZED CONTROLLED TRIAL

In a randomized controlled trial, researchers randomly assign patients to an experimental intervention or an alternative treatment (placebo or standard treatment). Randomized treatment allocates controls for potential measured and unmeasured confounding factors, making this experimental design the "gold standard" for the evaluations of treatments if it is properly powered and well performed (Cook et al., 1995).

In the QIO program, a randomized controlled trial could be done on a large scale. Again, the variable of "willingness to participate" must be considered. If the entire population to be randomized includes only those providers who are willing to participate with the QIOs, then providers who want to work on quality improvement but who are assigned to the control group would have to be willing to not receive QIO assistance.

The use of a randomized controlled trial design in the evaluation of quality improvement interventions faces other challenges. First, the unit of intervention is often at the provider, clinic, or hospital level, so the level of randomization must also be at this higher level. Thus, the availability of a study sample that is large enough to adequately test the intervention can be an issue. Second, interventions cannot be blinded to the subject receiving it or to those delivering the assistance. As discussed above, the "treatment" is assistance from the QIO, and the "control" equals no QIO assistance. Thus, care must be taken to control for cross-contamination of the control arm (receipt of assistance from other sources) as well as avoid bias in the evaluation of study end points. Other limitations of confounding factors may be applicable, as may the factor of "readiness for change."

The literature includes a growing number of examples of randomized controlled trials of quality improvement interventions. Kiefe and colleagues performed a successful randomized controlled trial of provider feedback among clinicians in Alabama (Kiefe et al., 2001). Similarly, Ferguson and colleagues performed a successful national randomized controlled trial of bypass surgery quality interventions to promote the adoption of process measures among 359 hospitals (Ferguson et al., 2003).

NONEQUIVALENT CONTROL GROUP STUDY DESIGN

In the nonequivalent control group design, subjects are not randomly assigned to a control or an experimental group. Instead, an intervention group is chosen, and a second group not receiving the intervention is chosen as a control group. The primary risk associated with this design is that the control group may be far from equivalent to the experimental group. The prototypical use of this design has been in the education field, in which one classroom is used as the experimental group and another is used as the control group. In those cases it is assumed that students are randomly assigned to the classrooms, and hence, there is good reason to believe in the strong similarity among groups.

This study design might be applicable to evaluations of intervention assistance in the QIO program, since participation in the "experiment" is voluntary and those not asking for assistance can be used as the control group. Randomization to the provision of provider assistance does not occur, and although the participating and nonparticipating provider groups are similar, they will not have the exact same characteristics. One strategy might be to compare two regions that are very similar (e.g., in socioeconomic status) and randomly select the region that would receive the intervention and use the other region as a nonequivalent control group. Provider settings such as nursing homes are not randomly assigned to a geographic region. Hence, the dissimilarity risk is much higher, and it would be important to carefully choose the regions so that the nursing homes and the patients are as similar as possible.

This can be a powerful design when there is good reason to believe in the similarity of regions and the likelihood exists that external forces would not affect one region differently from the other. However, this assumption may not be able to be made about many QIOs. For example, a QIO might be asked to evaluate the effectiveness of an intervention to reduce pressure sores in nursing home patients. If a state is large enough, the intervention could be initiated with nursing homes in one region of the state that could act as the experimental group and nursing homes in another region that could act as the control group by not participating in the intervention. This might also be applied to the comparison of the results for a region in one state with the results for a region in another state. The intervention must be carefully documented as to what was actually done and, to the extent possible, must be standardized during both time periods. Furthermore, many of the confounding variables (including readiness for change) and difficulty with definitions discussed in the previous examples apply to this type of study design as well.

CROSSOVER STUDY DESIGN

In the crossover study, researchers randomly assign half of the intervention cases to receive a treatment initially and the other half is used as a control. After some period of time, the control group begins to receive the treatment.

In the QIO program, the crossover study could be used for all the providers who request QIO assistance. Specifically, among those providers requesting assistance, QIOs could randomly assign half of the providers to receive the assistance intervention in the first year, and at the end of the year the evaluation could assess the impact of the intervention on those providers compared with the impact of the intervention on providers that did not receive the assistance. Then, in the second year the two groups "cross over," with the second group receiving the intervention assistance with follow-up assessment of its impact.

This design is likely to be particularly useful because at least some, if not all, of the QIOs do not have the resources and staff needed to meet a large demand for the provision of technical assistance all at once. By staggering assistance activities, it becomes possible not only to target the resources so that an intervention can be implemented well but also, at the same time, to create a control group for more rigorous assessment of whether the intervention makes a difference.

In this case, as discussed for the other examples, the successful implementation of such a design requires a sufficient number of providers, half of whom are willing to wait for the intervention assistance. Checks need to be made to be sure that the randomly assigned providers are comparable on important characteristics (as discussed in previous examples). Also, the intervention must be carefully documented as to what was actually done and, to the extent possible, standardized during both time periods. To induce those providers who do not receive the initial intervention assistance to participate in the evaluation, CMS might consider providing some financial assistance to the groups agreeing to participate in the evaluation.

QUALITATIVE RESEARCH AND ANALYSIS

Qualitative research is an approach to data collection and analysis that focuses on understanding the particularities of specific situations and streams of events by using open-ended data collection methods, such as interviews, focus groups, and observations; by generating highly detailed and contextualized descriptions; and by analyzing data, which are typically in the form of text and, sometimes, images, to identify patterns and themes. All of the previously described studies should include qualitative analysis as a part of their design.

Two significant uses of qualitative methods advance understanding of the effectiveness of QIOs in general and the specific interventions used by QIOs. The first is to use qualitative methods, alone or in combination with other data collection methods, to document in detail the implementation of interventions. The second is to use qualitative methods to explore the institutional and community environments in which the QIOs work; the characteristics of these environments can be viewed as "covariates" to their ability to make progress.

The purpose of documentation is twofold: first, to support the replication (or avoidance) of particular interventions, and second, to assess the "fidelity" of the intervention in comparison with the intent of the intervention. For example, if a QIO uses a collaborative to promote quality improvement activities on a specific aspect of performance, it would be useful to document exactly how the collaborative operated, including how the institutions and the participants in the collaboratives were recruited, the content of their interactions with the QIO and with each other, and the experiences that they report as a result of their participation. Designs of collaboratives vary widely; therefore, if a particular collaborative method is effective, the design should be assessed, disseminated, and replicated. Variation in the circumstances of interventions is to be expected. Some variation will be inconsequential, but it is possible that other variations will significantly influence the outcomes. A sophisticated evaluation design involves qualitative documentation of the implementation, such that outcomes could be linked to implementation in a systematic (although not necessarily a quantitative) way.

Qualitative work is often used in situations in which no clear hypotheses about the factors that influence both processes and outcomes exist or when there is no valid or reliable method for the measurement of those factors. A good example of the use of qualitative methods is the work of Bradley and colleagues in their study of the institutional factors that influenced hospitals' successful quality improvement efforts to promote the use of beta-blockers (Bradley et al., 2001). Using these methods, this research team has made a substantial contribution to early knowledge of these factors. It is noteworthy that work like this can in fact be replicated and, after a time, be used as a foundation for more quantitative measurement and analysis.

SUMMARY

As discussed here, CMS and the QIOs may design multiple types of studies, including those discussed above, to evaluate the effectiveness of interventions and the success of the QIOs. Considering the complexity of the QIO program and the environment under which it operates, no one study type is without challenges or weaknesses. In fact, combined approaches might compensate for some of those weaknesses. Unlike studies of clinical disease or environmental exposure, these studies are confounded by the voluntary nature of the program, the differences in provider settings, variations among interventions, and ethical issues of having control groups that are denied assistance for quality improvement. Although studies of individual, specific interventions could be done with relative ease, designing a comprehensive evaluation of the program overall for the 9th SOW and beyond will be most challenging for the reasons mentioned here. Several different types of study design may need to be included to obtain an accurate picture of the overall success of the program. Each type of study design should be considered and should be employed with rigor. Although these evaluations are difficult to design, they provide important, ongoing feedback for the management of the program as well as contribute valuable information to the quality improvement community as a whole.

REFERENCES

Bradley EH, Holmboe ES, Mattera JA, Roumanis SA, Radford MJ, Krumholz HM. 2001. A qualitative study of increasing beta-blocker use after myocardial infarction: Why do some hospitals succeed? *Journal of the American Medical Association* 285(20):2604–2611.

Cook DJ, Sackett DL, Spitzer WO. 1995. Methodologic guidelines for systematic reviews of randomized control trials in health care from the Potsdam consultation on meta-analysis. *Journal of Clinical Epidemiology* 48(1):167–171.

Ferguson TB Jr, Peterson ED, Coombs LC, Eiken MC, Carey ML, Grover FL, DeLong ER. 2003. Use of continuous quality improvement to increase use of process measures in patients undergoing coronary artery bypass graft surgery: A randomized controlled trial. *Journal of the American Medical Association* 290(1):49–56.

Kiefe CI, Allison JJ, Williams OD, Person SD, Weaver MT, Weissman NW. 2001. Improving quality improvement using achievable benchmarks for physician feedback: A randomized controlled trial. *Journal of the American Medical Association* 285(22):2871–2879.

D

Glossary and Acronyms

GLOSSARY

Activities of daily living. Activities of basic daily life usually done without assistance, such as eating, bathing, dressing, and using the bathroom.

Adverse event. An undesirable and usually unanticipated event or injury in a health care setting, including incidents that have no permanent effect, such as a fall or administration of improper medication.

Apportionment. A distribution of funds for programs as required by law (OMB, 2004).

Benchmarking. Comparison of internal processes with best practices or scores of a comparison group to find new ways to achieve continuous improvement.

Case review. Retrospective review of a medical record by experts to ensure the protection of beneficiaries and the integrity of the Medicare Trust Fund; also involves the review of appeals and complaints filed by beneficiaries (see *quality review*, *utilization review*, and *diagnosis-related group validation review*).

Case Review Information System. Application used by Quality Improvement Organizations to track and report data related to case review activities.

Clinical Data Abstraction Center. Independent organization that contracts with the Centers for Medicare and Medicaid Services to abstract data from medical records.

CMS Abstraction and Reporting Tool. Used by providers, Quality Improvement Organizations, and Clinical Abstraction Data Centers to collect and analyze data on hospital-related quality indicators.

Collaborative. An intervention modality designed to bring together stakeholders working toward quality improvement for the same clinical topic. Participants usually follow the same processes to reach goals and interact on a regular basis to share knowledge, experiences, and best practices.

Communities of practice. Informal groups of people involved in quality improvement efforts on the same topic area. Groups support each other via listserves, teleconferences, and other modalities to share knowledge and best practices. In the Quality Improvement Organization program, these are often organized around a specific task by the Quality Improvement Organizations Support Center.

Conditions of Participation. Standards required of providers for their participation in the Medicare and Medicaid programs. The Centers for Medicare and Medicaid Services designs these standards to improve quality and protect the health and safety of beneficiaries (CMS, 2005b).

Dashboard. A part of QIONet on which data are displayed for Quality Improvement Organization activities on contract tasks.

Data abstraction. Process by which specific information and data are gleaned from medical records.

Data validation. Process by which the accuracy of information and the data gleaned from medical records are assessed.

Diagnosis-related group validation review. A type of case review that ensures that the claim codes match information in the medical record according to documentation of diagnosis, procedures, and discharge status.

Electronic health record. A computerized recording of a patient's health information that is maintained by providers (CMS, 2005c).

Fee-for-service. Financing methodology currently used by Medicare in which providers are reimbursed for each individual procedure or patient encounter.

Government Task Leader. A Centers for Medicare and Medicaid Services representative who has direct responsibility for oversight of a specific task or special study of the Quality Improvement Organization contract.

Identified participants. Providers with whom Quality Improvement Organizations work intensively on specific quality improvement projects.

Implicit review.   Subjective decision making during case review activities, based on individual professional judgment.

Knowledge transfer.   A collective exchange of ideas regarding how to best promote or provide high quality.

Medicare Advantage (formerly Medicare+Choice).   Health plan offered by an organization (a public or private risk-bearing entity licensed by the state and certified by the Centers for Medicare and Medicaid Services) to all Medicare beneficiaries in a single service area at the same premium and level of cost sharing (CMS, 2005a).

Medicare Quality Improvement Community (MedQIC).   A public website that serves as an informational resource for quality improvement activities and that is run by a Quality Improvement Organization Support Center.

Patient safety.   Prevention of harm caused by errors of commission and omission.

Payment error rate.   The rate of incorrect amounts of payments, including both overpayments and underpayments as well as both inappropriate denials and inappropriate payments.

PDSA cycle.   A methodology for continuous quality improvement: *p*lan for a change in a process, *d*o a trial of the planned change, *s*tudy the results, and *a*ct to implement the next steps on the basis of the results.

Performance measurement.   "Measurement of data that show the progress toward specific results that are the intended outcome of specific actions, thus providing a way to evaluate the actions" (Top 10 by 2010, 2005).

Physician access.   Designates an organization that has arrangements for local physicians to perform case review activities, including at least one physician for every generally recognized specialty and subspecialty.

Physician sponsored.   Designates an organization that has at least 20 percent of physicians in the state as owners or members or that has 10 percent as owners or members and represents an additional 10 percent through other means.

Program activity reporting tool.   Application used by Quality Improvement Organizations to report on deliverables and by Centers for Medicare and Medicaid Services to monitor deliverables and approve project plans.

Project Officer.   A Centers for Medicare and Medicaid Services representative who directly oversees and monitors a specific individual Quality Improvement Organization contract.

Prospective payment system. Financing methodology currently used by Medicare in which services are reimbursed at a predetermined, fixed amount on the basis of coding for the services provided.

Provider. An individual or group of individuals (or an institution) who provide health care services to beneficiaries. Providers in the Quality Improvement Organization program include hospitals, nursing homes, home health agencies, physicians, and pharmacies/pharmacists.

Public reporting. "Providing the public with information about the performance or quality of health services or systems for the purpose of improving the performance or quality of the services or systems" (Healthcare Infection Control Practices Advisory Committee, 2005).

QIONet. A protected intranet website used by the Quality Improvement Organization community to share and report information.

Quality assurance. "The process of looking at how well a medical service is provided. The process may include formally reviewing health care given to a person, or group of persons, locating the problem, correcting the problem, and then checking to see if what you did worked" (CMS, 2005a).

Quality improvement. A set of techniques for continuous study and improvement of the processes of delivering health care services and products to meet the needs and expectations of the customers of those services and products. It has three basic elements: customer knowledge, a focus on processes of health care delivery, and statistical approaches that aim to reduce variations in those processes (IOM, 1990).

Quality Improvement Organization. Organization under contract with the Centers for Medicare and Medicaid Services to assist Medicare providers with quality improvement and to review quality and cost issues for the protection of Medicare beneficiaries and the Medicare Trust Fund.

Quality Improvement Organization Support Center. A Quality Improvement Organization (QIO) funded under a support contract to act as a central resource on a specific task or area of need for the entire QIO program community.

Quality improvement plan. Devised by providers with Quality Improvement Organization assistance to correct for concerns found during case review activities, such as treatment patterns that do not meet standards of care; also known as a *corrective action plan*, when in conjunction with a sanction.

Quality of care. The degree to which health services for individuals and populations increase the likelihood of desired health outcomes and are consistent with current professional knowledge (IOM, 1990).

Quality review. A type of case review that examines whether the care provided met recognized standards, was medically necessary, was performed in the appropriate setting, and was provided economically with adequate documentation.

Reduction in failure rate. The change in performance from the baseline to follow-up (absolute improvement) divided by the difference between baseline and perfect (100 percent) performance; also known as *relative improvement*.

Root-cause analysis. Process for identifying the fundamental cause(s) of an error or inefficiency in processes or outcomes.

Scientific Officer. A Centers for Medicare and Medicaid Services representative who provides scientific or clinical expertise to all Quality Improvement Organizations.

Scope of work. A section of the statement of work that provides an overall nontechnical description of Quality Improvement Organization program activities.

Six aims. Safe: avoiding injuries during care that is intended to help. Effective: providing services based on scientific knowledge and refraining from providing services to those not likely to benefit (avoiding underuse and overuse, respectively.) Patient-centered: providing care that is respectful of and responsive to individual patient preferences, needs, and values. Timely: reducing delays for those who receive and give care. Efficient: avoiding waste, including waste of equipment, supplies, ideas, and energy. Equitable: providing care that does not vary in quality because of characteristics such as gender, ethnicity, geographic location, and socioeconomic status (IOM, 2001).

Special studies. Performed under Task 4 of the Quality Improvement Organization (QIO) core contract. These studies are on topics not addressed by Tasks 1 to 3 and are performed by QIOs with Centers for Medicare and Medicaid Services (CMS) approval. They are usually solicited by CMS. These studies are often pilot projects that may lead to future work for the QIO program as a whole.

Standard Data Processing System. The information system for the Quality Improvement Organization (QIO) program, it contains many data and reporting tools and was designed and developed in response to the ongoing information requirements of the QIOs and other affiliated partners to fulfill their contractual requirements with the Centers for Medicare and Medicaid Services (CMS). This system interfaces with CMS, 53 QIOs, and Clinical Data Abstraction Centers.

Statement of work. Part of the Quality Improvement Organization core contract that delineates detailed work requirements, a list of deliverables, evaluation criteria, and a budget.

Support contracts.   These activities contribute to the operation of the Quality Improvement Organization (QIO) program as a whole but are not a part of the core contract. Contracts are usually awarded to organizations that do not hold QIO core contracts.

Survey and Certification.   Reviews by State Survey Agencies (or other Centers for Medicare and Medicaid Services agents) to determine compliance of Medicare providers with Conditions of Participation.

Technical assistance.   The process by which Quality Improvement Organizations work with providers, managed care organizations, and other stakeholders to improve patient outcomes. This includes root-cause analysis, assistance with the implementation of interventions and systems changes, facilitating knowledge transfer, assisting with data collection, and coordinating efforts with other stakeholders.

Transformational change.   The Centers for Medicare and Medicaid Services' (CMS's) vision that, through the adoption of certain strategies (measurement and reporting, health information technology adoption, process redesign, and organization culture change), the Quality Improvement Organization program, along with other efforts, can lead to measurable changes in the health care delivery system to align with the Institute of Medicine's six aims and CMS's vision of "the right care for every patient every time" (Pugh, 2005).

Transparency.   "The clarity with which a regulation, policy, or institution can be understood anticipated. Depends on openness, predictability, and comprehensibility" (Deardorff, 2005).

Utilization review.   A type of case review that examines the medical necessity and reasonableness of services or items provided, such as for the necessity of admission and proper coding.

ACRONYMS

AHQA	The American Health Quality Association
BIPA	Benefits Improvement and Protection Act of 2000
CAC	Consumer Advisory Council
CAHPS	Consumer Assessment of Healthcare Providers and Systems
CART	CMS Abstraction and Reporting Tool
CDAC	Clinical Data Abstraction Center
CEO	chief executive officer
CMS	Centers for Medicare and Medicaid Services
CPOE	Computerized Provider Order Entry

CRIS   Case Review Information System

DHHS   U.S. Department of Health and Human Services
DRG   diagnosis-related group

EHR   electronic health record
EMCRO   Experimental Medical Care Review Organization
EMTALA   Emergency Medical Treatment and Labor Act
ESRD   end-stage renal disease

FMIB   Financial Management Investment Board (Centers for
                    Medicare and Medicaid Services)
FY   fiscal year

HCFA   Health Care Financing Administration
HEDIS   Health Plan Employer Data and Information Set
HINN   hospital-issued notice of noncoverage
HPMP   Hospital Payment Monitoring Program

IHI   Institute for Healthcare Improvement
IOM   Institute of Medicine
IPG   identified participant group

MedPAC   Medicare Payment Advisory Commission
MedQIC   Medicare Quality Improvement Community
MMA   Medicare Modernization Act

NODMAR   Notice of discharge and Medicare appeal rights
NQCB   National Quality Coordination Board

OASIS   Outcome and Assessment Information Set
OBQI   Outcome-Based Quality Improvement (system)
OBRA   Omnibus Budget Reconciliation Act

PARTner   Program Activity Reporting Tool
PEPPER   Program for Evaluating Payment Patterns Electronic Re-
                    ports
PRO   Peer Review Organization
PSRO   Professional Standards Review Organization

QAPI   Quality Assessment and Performance Improvement (project)
QIO   Quality Improvement Organization
QIOSC   Quality Improvement Organization Support Center

SDPS   Standard Data Processing System
SOW   scope of work

TOPS   Transmittal of Policy System (a document)

REFERENCES

CMS (Centers for Medicare and Medicaid Services). 2005a. *Glossary.* [Online]. Available: http://www.cms.hhs.gov/glossary [accessed November 15, 2005].

CMS. 2005b. *Conditions of Participation.* [Online]. February 3. Available: http://www. cms.hhs.gov/cop [accessed November 15, 2005].

CMS. 2005c. *8th Statement of Work (SOW), Version #080105-1.* [Online]. Available: http:// www.cms.hhs.gov/qio [accessed November 4, 2005].

Deardorff AV. 2005. *Deardorff's Glossary of International Economics.* [Online]. Available: http://www-personal.umich.edu/~alandear/glossary [accessed November 15, 2005].

Healthcare Infection Control Practices Advisory Committee. 2005. *Guidance on Public Reporting of Healthcare-Associated Infections.* [Online]. February 28. Available: http:// www.consumersunion.org/campaigns/PublicReportingGuide [accessed November 15, 2005].

IOM (Institute of Medicine). 1990. *Medicare: A Strategy for Quality Assurance,* Vol. 1. Washington, DC: National Academy Press.

IOM. 2001. *Crossing the Quality Chasm: A New Health System for the 21st Century.* Washington, DC: National Academy Press.

OMB. 2004. *OMB Circular Number A-11: Preparation, Submission, and Execution of the Budget.* [Online]. Available: http://www.whitehouse.gov/omb/circulars/a11/current_year/a_11_2004.pdf [accessed November 15, 2005].

Pugh MD. 2005. Final report: CMS Quality Group Planning Project QIOSC contract 500-02-WA02 final report (revised). Pueblo, CO: Pugh Ettinger McCarthy Associates, LLC.

Top 10 by 2010. 2005. *Glossary of Sustainable Indicator Terms.* [Online]. Available: http:// www.top10by2010.org/glossary.pdf [accessed November 15, 2005].

E

Committee Biographies

Steven A. Schroeder, M.D., *Chair, Main Committee,** is distinguished professor of health and health care, Division of General Internal Medicine, Department of Medicine, University of California, San Francisco (UCSF), where he also heads the Smoking Cessation Leadership Center. The Center, funded by The Robert Wood Johnson Foundation, works with leaders of American health professional organizations and health care institutions to increase the rate at which patients who smoke are offered help to quit. Between 1990 and 2002 he was president and chief executive officer (CEO) of The Robert Wood Johnson Foundation. During his term of office the foundation made grant expenditures of almost $4 billion in pursuit of its mission of improving the health and health care of the American people. During those 12½ years the foundation developed new programs in substance abuse prevention and treatment, care at the end of life, and health insurance expansion for children, among others. In 1999, it reorganized into health and health care groups, reflecting the twin components of its mission. Dr. Schroeder graduated from Stanford University and Harvard Medical School, and trained in internal medicine at the Harvard Medical Service of Boston City Hospital and in epidemiology as an Epidemic Intelligence Service Officer of the Centers for Disease Control and Prevention (CDC). He held faculty appointments at Harvard, George Washington, and UCSF. At both George Washington and UCSF he was founding medical

---

*Member of the Main Committee on Redesigning Health Insurance Performance Measures, Payment, and Performance Improvement Programs.

director of a university-sponsored health maintenance organization (HMO), and at UCSF he founded the company's division of general internal medicine. Dr. Schroeder has produced more than 260 publications in the fields of clinical medicine, health care financing and organization, prevention, public health, and the workforce. He recently completed his term as chairman of the American Legacy Foundation and chair of the International Review Committee of the Ben Gurion School of Medicine. He is a member of the editorial board of the *New England Journal of Medicine* and the Harvard Overseers, and a director of the James Irvine Foundation, the Save Ellis Island Foundation, and the Charles R. Drew University of Medicine and Science. He holds six honorary doctoral degrees and has received numerous awards.

Stephen M. Shortell, Ph.D., M.P.H., *Chair, QIO Subcommittee,**† is a prominent researcher in health policy and organization behavior at the University of California (UC), Berkeley and is dean of the School of Public Health. Dr. Shortell is known as a leading academic voice advocating reform of the nation's health system. His research has helped establish determinants of health outcomes and quality of care for health care organizations. As Blue Cross of California distinguished professor of health policy and management, Dr. Shortell holds a joint appointment at UC Berkeley's School of Public Health and the Haas School of Business. He also is affiliated with UC Berkeley's Department of Sociology and UC San Francisco's Institute for Health Policy Studies. Dr. Shortell is an elected member of the Institute of Medicine (IOM) of the National Academies. He has received the Baxter-Allegiance Prize, considered the highest honor worldwide in the field of health services research. He also has received the Distinguished Investigator Award from the Association for Health Services Research and the Gold Medal award from the American College of Healthcare Executives for his contributions to the field. He serves on the boards of the Health Research and Educational Trust and the National Center for Healthcare Leadership. Dr. Shortell received his bachelor's degree from the University of Notre Dame; his master's degree in public health from the University of California, Los Angeles; and his Ph.D. in behavioral science from the University of Chicago. Before coming to UC Berkeley in 1998, he held teaching and research positions at Northwestern University, the University of Washington, and the University of Chicago.

---

*Member of the Main Committee on Redesigning Health Insurance Performance Measures, Payment, and Performance Improvement Programs.

†Member of the Quality Improvement Organization Subcommittee.

Anne-Marie J. Audet, M.D.,[†] is vice president at The Commonwealth Fund, where she directs the Quality Improvement and Efficiency Program. She joined the Fund in November 2000 to launch this new program. Dr. Audet has worked in the field of quality improvement for more than 15 years and brings a deep understanding of its science, as well as an appreciation of the barriers and enablers that come into play when knowledge must be translated into real-world situations. At the national level, Dr. Audet previously worked in the development of evidenced-based clinical guidelines and policy analysis at the American College of Physicians. At the state level, in 1994 she joined the Massachusetts Peer Review Organization and helped lead the implementation of the state's new Medicare Health Care Quality Improvement Program contract. Before joining the Fund, Dr. Audet served as director of the Office for Clinical Effectiveness/Process Improvement at Beth Israel Deaconess Medical Center in Boston, where she was responsible for the development of quality measurement systems, physician profiles of quality and efficiency, educational programs, and institutionwide medication safety initiatives. She also participated in a number of quality improvement programs within Caregroup, an integrated network of care. While at the Beth Israel Medical Center, she was coeditor of "Clinical Crossroads," a series published monthly in the *Journal of the American Medical Association*. She has published on such topics as quality improvement, practice guidelines, physicians and quality of care, use of information technologies, and public health. She sits on the Board of the Massachusetts Medical Society and Alliance Charitable Foundation. In addition to her M.D., Dr. Audet holds a bachelor of science degree in cell and molecular biology, a master of science in epidemiology and statistics from McGill University, and a masters of science in health policy and management from Harvard University.

Bobbie Berkowitz, Ph.D., R.N., F.A.A.N.,[*] is alumni endowed professor of nursing at the University of Washington (UW) School of Nursing and adjunct professor in the School of Public Health and Community Medicine. She directs the Turning Point initiative funded by The Robert Wood Johnson Foundation and the Center for the Advancement of Health Disparities Research funded by the National Institute of Nursing Research. She serves on the board of directors as vice-chair of Qualis Health, the Quality Improvement Organization (QIO) of Washington State. Before joining UW, Dr. Berkowitz was deputy secretary of health for the Washington State Department of Health. She is a member of the board of trustees for Group Health

---

[*]Member of the Main Committee on Redesigning Health Insurance Performance Measures, Payment, and Performance Improvement Programs.
[†]Member of the Quality Improvement Organization Subcommittee.

Cooperative, a fellow in the American Academy of Nursing, and a member of the Institute of Medicine (IOM). She served as cochair of the IOM Committee on Using Performance Monitoring to Improve Community Health and as vice-chair of the IOM/Transportation Research Board Committee on Physical Activity, Health, Transportation, and Land Use. She holds a Ph.D. in nursing science from Case Western Reserve University.

Donald M. Berwick, M.D., M.P.P.,* is president and CEO of the Institute for Healthcare Improvement (IHI), a not-for-profit organization helping to accelerate the improvement of health care throughout the world. He is clinical professor of pediatrics and health care policy at the Harvard Medical School and professor of health policy and management at the Harvard School of Public Health. He is also a pediatrician, an associate in pediatrics at Boston's Children's Hospital, and a consultant in pediatrics at Massachusetts General Hospital. Dr. Berwick has published over 110 scientific articles in numerous professional journals on subjects relating to health care policy, decision analysis, technology assessment, and health care quality management. He serves on the IOM's Governing Council, and the IOM's Board on Global Health. He is also a member of several editorial boards, including that of the *Journal of the American Medical Association*. A summa cum laude graduate of Harvard College, Dr. Berwick holds a master of public policy degree from the John F. Kennedy School of Government and an M.D. cum laude from the Harvard Medical School.

Bruce E. Bradley, M.B.A.,* is Director of Health Care Strategy and Public Policy, Health Care Initiatives, for General Motors Corporation in Pontiac, Michigan. He is responsible for health care–related strategy and public policy with a focus on quality measurement and improvement, consumer engagement, and cost-effectiveness. General Motors provides health care coverage for over 1.1 million employees, retirees, and their dependents, with an annual expenditure of $5.2 billion. Mr. Bradley joined General Motors in June 1996 after 5 years as corporate manager of Managed Care for GTE Corporation. In addition to his health care management experience at GTE, he spent nearly 20 years in health plan and HMO management. From 1972 to 1980 he was executive director of the Matthew Thornton Health Plan, Nashua, New Hampshire. From 1980 to 1990 he was president and CEO of the Rhode Island Group Health Association in Providence, Rhode Island, a staff model HMO. He was cofounder of the HMO Group (now the Alliance of Community Health Plans), a national

---

*Member of the Main Committee on Redesigning Health Insurance Performance Measures, Payment, and Performance Improvement Programs.

corporation of 15 nonprofit, independent group practice HMOs, and the HMO Group Insurance Co., Ltd. Mr. Bradley has gained recognition for his work in achieving health plan quality improvement and for his efforts in developing the Health Plan Employer Data and Information Set (HEDIS) measures and processes. He is a board member of the National Quality Forum, past member of the board of the Foundation for Accountability, board member of the American Board of Internal Medicine Foundation, past board member of the Academy for Health Services Research and Policy, and founding member and past chair of the Leapfrog Group board. A native of Pelham, New York, Mr. Bradley holds a bachelor's degree in psychology from Yale University (1967) and a master's degree in business and health care administration from the Wharton School at the University of Pennsylvania (1972).

Janet M. Corrigan, Ph.D.,* is president and CEO of the National Committee for Quality Health Care (NCQHC), a nonprofit, nonpartisan education and research institute. Prior to joining NCQHC in June 2005, she was senior board director at the IOM, where she was responsible for the Board on Health Care Services' portfolio of initiatives on quality and safety, health services organization and financing, and health insurance issues. She provided leadership for the IOM's Quality Chasm series, which includes 10 reports produced during her tenure, among them *To Err Is Human: Building a Safer Health System* and *Crossing the Quality Chasm: A New Health System for the 21st Century*. Prior to joining the IOM in 1998, Dr. Corrigan was executive director of the President's Advisory Commission on Consumer Protection and Quality in the Health Care Industry. She serves on the boards of the Baldrige Board of Overseers and the National Center for Healthcare Leadership. She received her doctorate in health services research and a master of industrial engineering degree from the University of Michigan, and master's degrees in business administration and community health from the University of Rochester.

Jack L. Cox, M.D., M.M.M.,† is a physician executive consultant in health care quality improvement. Former group vice president, Product Planning, and chief medical officer for Premier, Inc., a national health care alliance of over 1,500 not-for-profit hospitals, Dr. Cox led the clinical product and technology evaluation team for Group Purchasing Services. He was responsible for providing clinical support/leadership to Group Purchasing Services,

---

*Member of the Main Committee on Redesigning Health Insurance Performance Measures, Payment, and Performance Improvement Programs.

†Member of the Quality Improvement Organization Subcommittee.

Supply Chain Consulting, Informatics/Performance Services, and the Safety Institute. Dr. Cox's broad background includes over 20 years of clinical experience, 13 years in teaching and research with faculty appointments to five medical schools, and over 18 years as a health care executive. He is a board-certified family physician, a fellow of the American Board of Family Practice, and a fellow of the American College of Physician Executives, and holds a master's degree in medical management from Tulane University. Prior to joining Premier, Dr. Cox was regional medical director for Intermountain Healthcare in Utah and served on its corporate board of trustees. He has published and spoken nationally and internationally on various aspects of health care, including preventive care, quality improvement, health care management, and safety.

Karen Davis, Ph.D.,* is president of The Commonwealth Fund, a national philanthropy engaged in independent research on health and social issues. A nationally recognized economist, she has had a distinguished career in public policy and research. She served as deputy assistant secretary for health policy in the U.S. Department of Health and Human Services from 1977 to 1980 and holds the distinction of being the first woman to head a U.S. Public Health Service agency. Prior to her government career, Dr. Davis was a senior fellow at the Brookings Institution in Washington, D.C., a visiting scholar at Harvard University, and an assistant professor of economics at Rice University. She was chair of health policy and management at the Johns Hopkins Bloomberg School of Public Health from 1981 to 1992. She also serves on the board of Geisinger Health System. She is the recipient of the 2000 Baxter-Allegiance Foundation Prize for Health Services Research, and the 2006 Academy Health Distinguished Investigator Award. She is a former president of Academy Health. Dr. Davis received her doctorate in economics from Rice University and was awarded an honorary doctorate in humane letters from The Johns Hopkins University in 2001.

Nancy-Ann Min DeParle, J.D.,* is a senior advisor to JPMorgan Partners, LLC, and adjunct professor of health care systems at the Wharton School of the University of Pennsylvania. From 1997 to 2000, she served as administrator of the Health Care Financing Administration (HCFA), now the Centers for Medicare and Medicaid Services (CMS). Before joining HCFA, Ms. DeParle was associate director for health and personnel at the White House Office of Management and Budget. From 1987 to 1989 she served as the

---

*Member of the Main Committee on Redesigning Health Insurance Performance Measures, Payment, and Performance Improvement Programs.

Tennessee commissioner of human services. She has also worked as a lawyer in private practice in Nashville, Tennessee, and Washington, D.C. She is a member of the Medicare Payment Advisory Committee; a trustee of The Robert Wood Johnson Foundation; and a board member of Cerner Corporation, DaVita Guidant Corporation, Triad Hospitals, and the National Quality Forum. Ms. DeParle received a bachelor's degree from the University of Tennessee; bachelor's and master's degrees from Oxford University, where she was a Rhodes Scholar; and a J.D. degree from Harvard Law School.

Elliott S. Fisher, M.D., M.P.H.,* is Professor of Medicine and Community and Family Medicine, where he is director of the Institute for the Evaluation of Medical Practice at the Center for the Evaluative Clinical Sciences, Dartmouth Medical School, Hanover, New Hampshire, and senior associate of the VA Outcomes Group, Veterans Administration Medical Center, White River Junction, Vermont. He is a general internist and former Robert Wood Johnson clinical scholar with broad expertise in the use of administrative databases and survey research methods in health systems evaluation. His research has focused on exploring the causes and consequences of variations in clinical practice and health care spending across U.S. regions and among health care providers.

Richard G. Frank, Ph.D.,* is Margaret T. Morris professor of health economics in the Department of Health Care Policy at Harvard Medical School. He is also a research associate with the National Bureau of Economic Research. Dr. Frank is a member of the IOM. He advises several state mental health and substance abuse agencies on issues related to managed care and financing of care. He also serves as coeditor for the *Journal of Health Economics*. Dr. Frank was awarded the Georgescu-Roegen prize from the Southern Economic Association for his collaborative work on drug pricing, the Carl A. Taube Award from the American Public Health Association for outstanding contributions to mental health services and economics research, and the Emily Mumford Medal from Columbia University's Department of Psychiatry. In 2002 Dr. Frank received the John Eisenberg Mentorship Award from National Research Service Awards.

Robert S. Galvin, M.D.,* is director of global health care for General Electric (GE). He is in charge of the design and performance of GE's health programs, totaling over $3 billion annually, and oversees the 1 million pa-

---

*Member of the Main Committee on Redesigning Health Insurance Performance Measures, Payment, and Performance Improvement Programs.

tient encounters that take place in GE's 220 medical clinics in more than 20 countries. Drawing on his clinical expertise and training in Six Sigma, Dr. Galvin has been an advocate and leader in extending the benefits of this methodology to health care. He has focused on issues of market-based health policy and financing, with a special interest in promoting transparency and reforming the payment system. He is a past member of the Strategic Framework Board of the National Quality Forum and is currently on the board of the National Committee for Quality Assurance. He is a co-founder of the Leapfrog Group, the founder of Bridges to Excellence, and a member of the Advisory Group of the Council on Health Care Economics and Policy. Dr. Galvin is widely published on issues affecting the purchaser side of health care. He is professor adjunct of medicine at Yale, where he directs the seminar series on the private sector for the Robert Wood Johnson Clinical Scholars fellowship. He is a fellow of the American College of Physicians.

David H. Gustafson, Ph.D.,[*†] is a research professor at the University of Wisconsin, Madison, where he directs the Center of Excellence in Cancer Communications (designated by the National Cancer Institute) and the Network for the Improvement of Addiction Treatment (supported by The Robert Wood Johnson Foundation and the federal government's Center for Substance Abuse Treatment). His research focuses on the use of systems engineering methods and models in individual and organizational change. Much of his research centers on the development and evaluation of health systems to support people facing serious health problems such as cancer. His randomized controlled trials and field tests have helped in understanding the acceptance, use, and impact of e-health on quality of life, behavior change, and health service utilization. His research has also contributed to organizational improvement, with particular attention to models that predict and explain organizational change. Dr. Gustafson is a fellow of the Association for Health Services Research and of the American Medical Informatics Association and a fellow and past vice-chair of the board of IHI. He also chaired the recent Federal Science Panel on Interactive Communications in Health and is chair of the eHealth Institute. He is a member of the University of Wisconsin Athletic Board.

---

[*]Member of the Main Committee on Redesigning Health Insurance Performance Measures, Payment, and Performance Improvement Programs.
[†]Member of the Quality Improvement Organization Subcommittee.

Jeff Kang, M.D., M.P.H.,[†] is chief medical officer for CIGNA HealthCare and is responsible for the company's medical strategy and policy. This includes evidence-based coverage decisions, benefit design, consumer decision support, disease management, case management, utilization management, quality measurement and improvement, and pharmacy. Before joining CIGNA HealthCare, Dr. Kang was chief clinical officer for CMS and director of its Office of Clinical Standards and Quality. There he was responsible for Medicare technology assessment and coverage policy. His responsibilities also encompassed setting quality standards for Medicare participating hospitals and facilities; leading CMS's quality measurement, improvement, and patient safety activities; managing Medicare's Peer Review Program; and leading CMS's overall clinical direction and purchasing initiatives. His experience in Washington, D.C., began in 1994, when he joined the national health care reform debate as a White House fellow. Currently, Dr. Kang is cochair of the National Quality Forum's Steering Committee for Standardizing Ambulatory Care (physician) Performance Measurement and a member of the cHealth Initiative Leadership Council. He is board certified in internal medicine and geriatrics and was on the Clinical Faculty at Harvard Medical School. He received an M.D. degree from the University of California, San Francisco, and an M.P.H from the University iof California, Berkeley.

Mary Anne Koda-Kimble, Pharm.D.,[*] is dean of the School of Pharmacy at the University of California, San Francisco (UCSF), where she teaches and has cared for patients at the UCSF Diabetes Center. She holds the Thomas J. Long Endowed Professorship and previously served as chair of the Department of Clinical Pharmacy. Dr. Koda-Kimble received her Pharm.D. from UCSF and joined its faculty in 1970, where she was involved in developing an innovative clinical pharmacy curriculum. She is a member of the United States Pharmacopoeia board of trustees and was vice-chair of the Accreditation Council of Pharmaceutical Education Board of Directors. She is past president of the American Association of Colleges of Pharmacy and has served on the California State Board of Pharmacy, the Food and Drug Administration's (FDA) Nonprescription Drugs Advisory Committee, and many other boards and task forces of national professional associations. Dr. Koda-Kimble is frequently invited to address national and international groups and has produced many publications, the best known of which is *Applied Therapeutics*, a text widely used by health professional students and practitioners throughout the world.

---

[*]Member of the Main Committee on Redesigning Health Insurance Performance Measures, Payment, and Performance Improvement Programs.
[†]Member of the Quality Improvement Organization Subcommittee.

Alan R. Nelson, M.D.,*† is an internist–endocrinologist who was in private practice in Salt Lake City, Utah, until becoming CEO of the American Society of Internal Medicine (ASIM) in 1992. Following the merger of ASIM with the American College of Physicians (ACP) in 1998, Dr. Nelson headed the Washington Office of ACP–ASIM until his semiretirement in January 2000; he currently serves as special advisor to the executive vice president/ CEO of the College. He was president of the American Medical Association and currently serves as a member of the Medicare Payment Advisory Commission, which advises Congress on Medicare issues. A member of the IOM, he was chair of the IOM Committee on Ethnic and Racial Disparities in Health Care and is a coeditor of the study report, *Unequal Treatment: Confronting Racial and Ethnic Disparities in Health Care*. Dr. Nelson attended Utah State University and received his M.D. from Northwestern University in 1958.

Gregg Pane, M.D., M.P.A.,† was recently appointed by Mayor Anthony Williams as the District of Columbia Acting Director of Health. In this role, he will direct a $1.5 billion, 1,400-employee agency responsible for Medicaid, health safety net issues, public health, and hospital bioterrorism preparedness. He previously served as vice president for clinical quality and medical director of the Office of Public Policy Initiatives of the Henry Ford Health System, serving as the System's chief quality officer and leading initiatives in the quality and public financing of health care. He has also been chief policy and planning officer for the Veterans Health Administration in Washington, D.C. He was among the key senior executives who reengineered the Veterans Administration's infrastructure and helped set the standard for national quality initiatives in health care.

Barbara R. Paul, M.D.,† is senior vice president and chief medical officer of BEI, a leading provider of elder care headquartered in Fort Smith, Arkansas. She was previously director of CMS's Quality Measurement and Health Assessment Group. While at CMS, she led the launch of U.S. Department of Health and Human Services Secretary Tommy G. Thompson's Nursing Home Quality Initiative and Home Health Quality Initiative and played a key role in the agency's overall quality measurement and public reporting work. She represented the agency on the boards of the National Quality Forum and the Leapfrog Group. Dr. Paul is an internist who was in full-time practice in Napa, California, from 1987 to 1999 in a small group

---

*Member of the Main Committee on Redesigning Health Insurance Performance Measures, Payment, and Performance Improvement Programs.
†Member of the Quality Improvement Organization Subcommittee.

practice affiliated with Queen of the Valley Hospital and with Kaiser Permanente. She served as director of women's health services and chair of the Department of Medicine at Queen of the Valley Hospital and was active with the California Medical Association, where she chaired its Council on Ethical Affairs and served on its board of trustees. Dr. Paul earned a bachelor of science degree in biochemistry from the University of Wisconsin, Madison, and an M.D. from the Stanford University School of Medicine.

Norman C. Payson, M.D.,* having completed his turnaround assignment, retired as chairman and CEO of Oxford Health Plans, Inc. in November 2002. Oxford Health Plans is a prominent greater New York health plan with 1.5 million members. Dr. Payson was recruited to the CEO position in 1998 after Oxford experienced severe operational and financial challenges and then led its successful turnaround. Prior to joining Oxford, he was cofounder and CEO of Healthsource, Inc., from its inception in 1985 until its sale to CIGNA Corporation in 1997. During his tenure, Healthsource grew to 3 million members in 15 states. Dr. Payson is a graduate of the Massachusetts Institute of Technology and received his M.D. at Dartmouth Medical School.

William A. Peck, M.D.,*† became Alan A. and Edith L. Wolf distinguished professor of medicine and director of the Washington University Center for Health Policy in 2003. From 1989 to 2003 he served as dean of Washington University School of Medicine and vice chancellor for medical affairs (executive vice chancellor from 1993 to 2003), and president of the Washington University Medical Center. Dr. Peck was awarded an honorary doctor of science degree from the University of Rochester in 2000. His academic activities include original investigations in bone and mineral metabolism and extensive clinical teaching, as well as patient care experience. His major scientific contributions include the first method for studying directly the structure, function, and growth of bone cells; demonstration of mechanisms whereby hormones regulate bone cell function; and examination of the causes of osteoporosis. Dr. Peck was founding president of the National Osteoporosis Foundation. He serves on the boards of Allied Health Care Products, Angelica Corporation, TIAA-CREF Trust Company, and Research!America (vice-chair), and is a trustee of the University of Rochester. Dr. Peck is past chairman of the American Association of Medical Colleges.

---

*Member of the Main Committee on Redesigning Health Insurance Performance Measures, Payment, and Performance Improvement Programs.

†Member of the Quality Improvement Organization Subcommittee.

He has served on many editorial boards and was a consultant for major pharmaceutical companies.

Eric D. Peterson, M.D., M.P.H.,[†] is an associate professor of medicine and associate vice-chair for quality at Duke University Medical Center. He is also codirector of Cardiovascular Research, as well as the director of CV Outcomes Research and Quality at the Duke Clinical Research Institute. His formal research training includes an M.P.H. from Harvard University, with special emphasis in biostatistics. Dr. Peterson received a Paul Beeson Faculty Scholar Research Award in geriatric cardiology. He has a strong record of funding from the National Institutes of Health (NIH) and currently oversees two active NIH R01 awards. He has authored more than 150 peer-reviewed publications, multiple book chapters, and invited editorials. He is principal investigator for the Data Coordinating Centers for the Society of Thoracic Surgeons' National Cardiac Surgery Database, the American College of Cardiology's National Cardiac Database, the American Heart Association's Get with the Guidelines Database, and the CRUSADE National Quality Improvement Initiative. He sits on multiple national committees for the American Heart Association, the American College of Cardiology, and the Veterans Health Administration and cochaired the Working Group on Outcomes Research of the National Heart, Lung, and Blood Institute.

Neil R. Powe, M.D., M.P.H., M.B.A.,[*] is professor of medicine, professor of health policy and management, and professor of epidemiology at the Johns Hopkins University School of Medicine and the Johns Hopkins Bloomberg School of Public Health. He also is director of the Welch Center for Prevention, Epidemiology and Clinical Research, an interdisciplinary research and training center at the Johns Hopkins Medical Institutions focused on population-based and health services research. Dr. Powe's research has involved clinical epidemiology, technology assessment, patient outcomes research, and health services research in many areas of medicine. He has also studied physician decision making and other determinants of the use of medical practices, including payers' decisions about insurance coverage for new medical technologies; the effect of financial incentives on the use of technology; efficiency and outcomes in for-profit versus nonprofit health care institutions; and the relationships among hospital volume, technology, and outcomes. He has extensive experience in developing and measuring

---

[*]Member of the Main Committee on Redesigning Health Insurance Performance Measures, Payment, and Performance Improvement Programs.
[†]Member of the Quality Improvement Organization Subcommittee.

outcomes and quality of care for chronic kidney disease and is author of more than 250 articles. Dr. Powe received his M.D. from Harvard Medical School, M.P.H. from Harvard School of Public Health, and M.B.A. from the University of Pennsylvania. He completed his residency at the Hospital of the University of Pennsylvania, where he was also a Robert Wood Johnson Clinical Scholar and fellow in the Division of General Internal Medicine. Dr. Powe is a member of the American Society of Clinical Investigation, the Association of American Physicians, and the American Society of Epidemiology.

Christopher Queram, M.A.,* has been president/CEO of the Wisconsin Collaborative for Healthcare Quality (WCHQ) since November 2005. The Collaborative is a nonprofit, 501c3, voluntary consortium of organizations learning and working together to improve the quality and cost-effectiveness of health care for the people of Wisconsin. The Collaborative develops and reports comparative measures of healthcare performance; designs and promotes quality improvement initiatives; and advocates for enlightened policy to support its work. Prior to joining WCHQ, Mr. Queram served as CEO of the Employer Health Care Alliance Cooperative (the Alliance) of Madison, Wisconsin, a health care purchasing cooperative owned by more than 160 member companies in south central Wisconsin. In addition to his responsibilities at WCHQ, Mr. Queram is a board member of the Joint Commission on Accreditation of Healthcare Organizations and Delta Dental of Wisconsin, a member of the "Principals" for the Hospital Quality Alliance (HQA), and a member of the steering committee for the Wisconsin Hospital Association's CheckPoint quality reporting initiative. Previously, he served as board member of the Leapfrog Group and the National Quality Forum, as well as a member of the IOM's Committee on the Consequences of Uninsurance and President Clinton's Advisory Commission on Consumer Protection and Quality in the Health Care Industry. Mr. Queram holds a master of arts degree in health services administration from the University of Wisconsin, Madison, and is a fellow in the American College of Healthcare Executives.

Robert D. Reischauer, Ph.D.,* is president of the Urban Institute, a nonprofit, nonpartisan policy research and education organization that examines the social, economic, and governance problems facing the nation. He served as director of the Congressional Budget Office (CBO) between 1989 and 1995 and was CBO's assistant director for human resources and deputy

---

*Member of the Main Committee on Redesigning Health Insurance Performance Measures, Payment, and Performance Improvement Programs.

director during 1977 to 1981. Dr. Reischauer has been a senior fellow in the Economic Studies Program of the Brookings Institution (1986–1989 and 1995–2000) and senior vice president of the Urban Institute (1981–1986). He is an economist with an undergraduate degree from Harvard and a Ph.D. in economics and a master's in international affairs from Columbia University. Dr. Reischauer is a member of the Harvard Corporation and serves on the boards of several educational and nonprofit organizations. He is vice-chair of the Medicare Payment Advisory Commission and served as chair of the National Academy of Social Insurance's project "Restructuring Medicare for the Long Term" from 1995 through 2004.

William C. Richardson, Ph.D.,* is president and CEO emeritus of the W. K. Kellogg Foundation of Battle Creek, Michigan. Before joining the foundation in August 1995, Dr. Richardson was president of The Johns Hopkins University, a position he had held since 1990. He was also professor of health policy and management at the university. Dr. Richardson is a member of the IOM, a fellow of the American Academy of Arts and Sciences, and a member of the American Public Health Association. He has served on the boards of the Council of Michigan Foundations and the Council on Foundations (trustee and chair). He also serves on the board of directors of the Kellogg Company, CSX Corporation, the Bank of New York, and Exelon Corporation. Dr. Richardson is a graduate of Trinity College and the University of Chicago.

Cheryl M. Scott, M.H.A.,* is currently president emerita for Group Health Cooperative (GHC), one of the the nation's largest consumer-governed, nonprofit health care systems. From 1997 to 2004, she was GHC's president and CEO. Prior to assuming her position in 1997, she served as GHC's executive vice president/chief operating officer. Ms. Scott is a clinical professor in the Department of Health Services at the University of Washington. At the national level, she served on the board of the Alliance of Community Plans (trustee and chair) and the board of America's Health Insurance Plans. She currently serves as board chair for the Health Technology Center and is a trustee for the Washington State Life Sciences Discovery Fund. Ms. Scott received a bachelor's degree in communications and a master's degree in health administration from the University of Washington.

Shoshanna Sofaer, D.P.H.,† is Robert P. Luciano professor of health care policy at the School of Public Affairs, Baruch College, New York City. She

---

*Member of the Main Committee on Redesigning Health Insurance Performance Measures, Payment, and Performance Improvement Programs.
†Member of the Quality Improvement Organization Subcommittee.

received master's and doctoral degrees in public health from the University of California, Berkeley. She has served on the faculties of the University of California, Los Angeles, School of Public Health and the George Washington University Medical Center. Her primary research interests include providing information to consumers and patients on the performance of the health care system; assessing the impact of quality, cost, and other comparative information on consumers, patients, providers, and systems; developing consumer-relevant performance measures; and assessing the effectiveness of multistakeholder efforts such as coalitions, partnerships, and collaboratives in improving health and health care. She is an expert in evaluation research, with particular emphasis on appropriate designs for formative and summative assessments of both the implementation and outcomes of innovative programs. She specializes in the use of qualitative and mixed methods in health services and policy research. Dr. Sofaer served as a member of the IOM Committee on the Consequences of Uninsurance; she chaired the subcommittee that produced the committee's sixth and final report, which addressed principles and recommendations.

Samuel O. Thier, M.D.,* is professor of medicine and professor of health care policy at Harvard Medical School. He was president and CEO of Partners HealthCare System from 1996 to 2002. From 1994 to 1997 he was president of the Massachusetts General Hospital; he was Brandeis University's president during the previous 3 years. He served 6 years as president of the IOM and 11 years as chair of the Department of Internal Medicine at Yale University School of Medicine, where he was Sterling professor. Dr. Thier is an authority on internal medicine and kidney disease and is also known for his expertise in national health policy, medical education, and biomedical research. Born in New York, he attended Cornell University and received his medical degree from the State University of New York at Syracuse in 1960. He served on the medical staff of Massachusetts General Hospital as an intern, resident, chief resident in medicine, and chief of the renal unit, and held a faculty appointment at Harvard. Prior to joining the faculty of Yale in 1975, he was professor and vice-chair of the Department of Medicine at the University of Pennsylvania. He has received several honorary degrees and the UC Medal of the University of California, San Francisco. He has served as president of the American Federation of Clinical Research and chair of the American Board of Internal Medicine and is a master of the American College of Physicians, a fellow of the American Academy of Arts and Sciences, and a member of the American Philosophical Society. Dr. Thier is a director of Charles River Laboratories, Inc., The

---

*Member of the Main Committee on Redesigning Health Insurance Performance Measures, Payment, and Performance Improvement Programs.

Commonwealth Fund (chair), the Federal Reserve Bank of Boston, and Merck & Co., Inc., and a member of the Board of Overseers of TIAA-CREF and the Board of Overseers of Cornell University Medical College.

Gail R. Wilensky, Ph.D.,* is a senior fellow at Project HOPE, an international health education foundation, where she analyzes and develops policies relating to health reform and to ongoing changes in the medical marketplace. Dr. Wilensky testifies frequently before congressional committees; acts as an advisor to members of Congress and other elected officials; and speaks nationally and internationally before professional, business, and consumer groups. From 2001 to 2003, she cochaired the President's Task Force to Improve Health Care Delivery for Our Nation's Veterans, which addressed health care for both veterans and military retirees. From 1997 to 2001 she chaired the Medicare Payment Advisory Commission, which advises Congress on payment and other issues relating to Medicare, and from 1995 to 1997 she chaired the Physician Payment Review Commission. Previously, she served as deputy assistant to President G. H. W. Bush for policy development, advising him on health and welfare issues. Prior to that, she was administrator of HCFA, overseeing the Medicare and Medicaid programs. Dr. Wilensky is an elected member of the IOM and its Governing Council, serves as a trustee of the Combined Benefits Fund of the United Mineworkers of America and the American Heart Association, and is on the Advisory Board of the National Institute of Health Care Management. She is an advisor to The Robert Wood Johnson Foundation and The Commonwealth Fund, immediate past chair of the Board of Directors of Academy Health, and a director on several corporate boards. Dr. Wilensky received a bachelor's degree in psychology and a Ph.D. in economics at the University of Michigan.

INSTITUTE OF MEDICINE STAFF BIOGRAPHIES

Rosemary A. Chalk is director of the Board on Children, Youth and Families (BCYF) and also serves as director of the Redesigning Health Insurance Performance Measures, Payment, and Performance Improvement Programs (PPPI) project at the IOM. She has been a senior staff member of the IOM and the Division on Behavioral and Social Sciences and Education of the National Academies for almost 19 years, directing studies on vaccines and immunization finance, educational finance, family violence, child abuse and neglect, and research ethics. She took on the role of BCYF director in Sep-

---

*Member of the Main Committee on Redesigning Health Insurance Performance Measures, Payment, and Performance Improvement Programs.

tember 2003 and began directing the PPPI project in April 2005. For 3 years (2000 to 2003), Ms. Chalk was a half-time study director at the IOM and also directed the child abuse/family violence research area at Child Trends, a nonprofit research center in Washington, D.C., where she conducted studies on the development of child well-being indicators for the child welfare system. Over the past decade, Ms. Chalk has directed a range of projects sponsored by the William T. Grant Foundation, the Doris Duke Charitable Foundation, the Carnegie Corporation of New York, The David and Lucile Packard Foundation, and various agencies within the U.S. Department of Health and Human Services. Earlier in her career, Ms. Chalk was a consultant and writer for a broad array of science and society research projects. She has authored publications on issues related to child and family policy, science and social responsibility, research ethics, and child abuse and neglect. She was the first program head of the Committee on Scientific Freedom and Responsibility of the American Association for the Advancement of Science from 1976 to 1986 and is a former section officer for that organization. She served as a science policy analyst for the Congressional Research Service at the Library of Congress from 1972 to 1975. She has a bachelor's degree in foreign affairs from the University of Cincinnati.

Karen Adams, Ph.D., M.T. (A.S.C.P.), is senior program officer at the IOM. She is currently lead staff member on the Performance Measurement and Pay for Performance Subcommittees of the IOM's congressionally mandated study Redesigning Health Insurance Performance Measures, Payment, and Performance Improvement Programs. Her prior work at the IOM includes serving as study director of the Committee on Priority Areas for National Action: Transforming Health Care Quality and co-study director of the 1st Annual Crossing the Quality Chasm Summit: A Focus on Communities. Before joining the IOM, she held the rank of assistant professor in the Department of Medical and Research Technology, University of Maryland School of Medicine, and was also academic coordinator of the undergraduate medical technology program. Dr. Adams received an undergraduate degree in medical technology from Loyola College, a master's degree in management from the College of Notre Dame, and a doctorate in health policy from the University of Maryland. During her doctoral studies she was awarded an internship at the Agency for Healthcare Research and Quality, during which she researched more than 30 years of innovations in medical informatics. She is also certified as a medical technologist by the American Society of Clinical Pathologists.

Samantha M. Chao, M.P.H., is senior health policy associate for the IOM's Board on Health Care Services. She completed a master's degree in health policy at the University of Michigan School of Public Health. As part of her studies, she interned with both the Michigan Department of Community Health and the American Heart Association to promote the study of chronic disease and disease prevention.

Contessa Fincher, Ph.D., M.P.H., joined the IOM's Board on Health Care Services in 2004 as a program officer. She is a recent graduate of the University of Alabama at Birmingham, where she studied administration–health services, with a focus on outcomes research. She has an M.P.H. from the University of Texas School of Public Health at Houston, with a concentration in health services research. Her postdoctoral work was completed at Wyeth Research in the Department of Global Health Outcomes and Pharmacoeconmic Assessment, where she designed cost-effectiveness models as part of her work in cardiovascular disease. Before joining the IOM, she worked briefly as a pharmacoeconomist at the Food and Drug Administration and Abt Associates, a government and pharmaceutical consulting company. Dr. Fincher has published articles in such journals as the *New England Journal of Medicine*, the *American Journal of Cardiology*, and *Ethnicity and Disease*.

Tracy A. Harris, D.P.M., M.P.H., joined the IOM's Board on Health Care Services in 2004 as a program officer. Her work background includes clinical experience and health policy work. Previously, she was trained in podiatric medicine and surgery and spent several years in private practice. In 1999, Dr. Harris was awarded a Congressional Fellowship with the American Association for the Advancement of Science. She spent 1 year working in the U.S. Senate on many issues, including elder fraud, telemedicine, a national practitioners data bank, health professional shortage areas, stem cell research, and malpractice caps. While earning a master's degree, she worked on various projects, including Medicaid disease management and the uninsured. She has a doctor of podiatric medicine degree from the Temple University School of Podiatric Medicine and a master of public health degree with a concentration in health policy from The George Washington University.

Dianne Miller Wolman, M.G.A., is currently lead staff on a Congressionally mandated evaluation of the Quality Improvement Organization Program of Medicare, part of the IOM's Redesigning Health Insurance Project. Prior to this she co-directed a 3-year study of the Consequences of Uninsurance, which produced a series of six reports: Insuring Health. Prior to that she directed the study that resulted in the IOM report, *Medicare Laboratory Payment Policy: Now and in the Future*, released in 2000. She joined the Health Care Services Division of the Institute of Medicine in 1999 as a senior program officer. Her previous work experience in the health field has been varied and focused on finance and payment in insurance programs. She came from the General Accounting Office, where she was a senior evaluator on studies of the Health Care Financing Administration and its management capacity. Previously, she was a policy specialist at a national association representing nonprofit providers of long-term care services. Her earlier positions included policy analysis and management with: the office of the secretary, DHHS; a peer review organization; a governor's task force on access to health care; and a third-party administrator for very large health plans. In addition, she was policy director for a state Medicaid rate setting commission. She has a master's degree in government administration from Wharton Graduate School, University of Pennsylvania.

Index

T